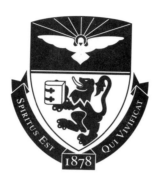

access to
Clinical
education

Leg Ulcers

Christine Moffatt is an internationally known expert in the field of leg ulceration. Having run the Riverside leg ulcer project in London, she is now Director of the Centre for Research and Implementation of Clinical Practice based at Thames Valley University. The Centre, as part of its remit, continues to undertake clinical and organisational research in Tissue Viability and Service development. Christine is widely published and retains her clinical expertise through nurse consultancy at UCL Hospitals and St George's Hospital, London, as well as teaching the English National Board N18 Leg Ulcer Management course at Thames Valley University.

Peter Harper is module leader for the English National Board Course N18 Professional Development in Leg Ulcer Management. He has considerable experience in the post-registration education of nurses and provides educational support to the Centre for Research and Implementation of Clinical Practice which has close links with the Wolfson Institute of Health Sciences at Thames Valley University. He is actively involved in clinical practice as a specialist nurse at the University College Hospital London Leg Ulcer Clinic.

For Churchill Livingstone:

Commissioning Editor: Ellen Green
Project Manager: Valerie Burgess
Project Development Editor: Mairi McCubbin
Designer: Judith Wright
Illustrator: Robert Britton
Copy-editor: Sue Beasley
Page Layout: Kate Walshaw
Indexer: Liza Weinkove
Sales Promotion Executive: Hilary Brown

access to Clinical education

Leg Ulcers

Christine Moffatt
MA RGN NDN
Director of Education and Clinical Practice,
The Centre for Research and Implementation of Clinical Practice,
Wolfson Institute of Health Sciences, Thames Valley University,
London, UK

Peter Harper
BSc(Hons) RGN RNT
Senior Lecturer, Wolfson Institute of Health Sciences,
Thames Valley University, London, UK

Educational Consultant, Access to Clinical Education series
Diane Marks-Maran
BSc RGN DipN(Lond) RNT
Associate Director, Wolfson Institute of Health Sciences, and
Head of the Centre for Teaching and Learning in Health Sciences,
Thames Valley University, London, UK

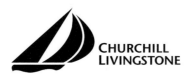
CHURCHILL
LIVINGSTONE

NEW YORK EDINBURGH LONDON MELBOURNE SAN FRANCISCO AND TOKYO 1997

CHURCHILL LIVINGSTONE

Medical Division of Pearson Professional Limited
Distributed in the United States of America by Churchill Livingstone Inc.,
650 Avenue of the Americas, New York, N.Y. 10011, and by associated
companies, branches and representatives throughout the world.

© Pearson Professional Limited 1997

First edition 1997

ISBN 0 443 05533 5

British Library of Cataloguing in Publication Data
A catalogue record for this book is available from the British Library.

Library of Congress Cataloging in Publication Data
A catalogue record for this book is available from the Library of Congress

The
publisher's
policy is to use
**paper manufactured
from sustainable forests**

Produced by Longman Singapore Publishers Pte Ltd
Printed in Singapore

Contents

The plate section is between pages 102 and 103.

Preface

The management of leg ulceration has changed dramatically during the last 10 years. This is perhaps largely due to the increased use of effective compression therapy in the treatment of venous ulcers which are the predominant type. The realisation that, at last, something can be done for what has been considered for many years to be a chronic intractable condition, has also affected practitioners caring for those with leg ulcers. The shift from treating the symptoms to treating the cause has inspired many practitioners to adopt a more systematic, research-based approach to care. As a result, much has been written about the subject and as practitioners and providers of health care have become aware of the improvement in care there has also been a demand for educational programmes. Programmes now available range from single study days to longer courses such as the English National Board course N18.

This book represents a slightly different approach. Whilst the intended learning outcomes and content are essentially based on ENB N18, the book enables practitioners to study when and where they choose. It is primarily aimed at nurses but could equally be of use to any health care professional as a reference, because we have gone to great lengths to ensure that our review of the literature is both current and comprehensive.

The activities, scenarios and case studies are intended as means through which to explore and improve your own clinical practice, as well as provide some variety in the learning process. We hope you find the process of working through this book a fulfilling experience, both in terms of consolidating what you already know about the management of leg ulceration and in providing you with new knowledge.

Finally, we would like to thank our families, friends and colleagues for their support during the production of this book.

London, 1997

C. M.
P. H.

Acknowledgements

The publishers would like to thank Moya Morison, Perth, for acting as a Critical Reader for this book; and the Community and District Nursing Association for their assistance in field testing the books in the ACE series.

We are also grateful to the following for permission to reproduce the following articles in the Reader:

Bailliere Tindall for Reader 2—Torrance C 1986 The physiology of wound healing. (Nursing 5) Nursing UK 3(5): 162–168

BMJ Publishing Group for Reader 1—Callam M J, Ruckley C V, Harper D R, Dale J J 1985 Chronic ulceration of the leg: extent of the problem and provision of care. British Medical Journal 290: 1855–1856

Journal of Tissue Viability for Reader 15—Cameron J 1995 The importance of contact dermatitis in the management of leg ulcers. Journal of Tissue Viability 5(2): 52–55

Macmillan Magazines Ltd for: Reader 3—Silver I A 1994 The physiology of wound healing. Journal of Wound Care 3(2): 106–109; Reader 5—Moffatt C J, Franks P J 1994 A prerequisite underlining the treatment programme: risk factors associated with venous disease. Professional Nurse June 1994, 637–642; Reader 6—Pinchcofsky-Devin G 1994 Nutrition and wound healing. Journal of Wound Care 3(5): 231–234; Reader 7—Plassman P 1995 Measuring wounds. Journal of Wound Care 4(6): 269–272; Reader 8—Vowden K R, Vowden P 1996 Hand-held Doppler assessment for peripheral arterial disease. Journal of Wound Care 5(3): 125–128; Reader 9—Moffatt C, O'Hare L 1995 Ankle pulses are not sufficient to detect impaired arterial circulation in patients with leg ulcers. Journal of Wound Care 4(3): 134–138; Reader 10 —Williams I M, Picton A J, McCollum C N 1993 The use of Doppler ultrasound 1: arterial disease. Wound Management 4(1): 9–12; Reader 11—Picton A J, Williams I M, McCollum C N 1993 The use of Doppler ultrasound 2: venous disease. Wound Management 4(1): 13–15; Reader 12—Morison M J 1989 Wound cleansing —which solution? Professional Nurse, February 1989, 220–225; Reader 13—Moffatt C 1995 Graduated compression hosiery for venous ulceration. Journal of Wound Care 4(10): 459–462;

New England Journal of Medicine for Reader 14 —Caputo G M, Cavanagh P R, Ulbrecht J S, Gibbons G W, Karchmer A W 1994 Assessment and management of foot disease in patients with diabetes. New England Journal of Medicine Sept 29 1994, 854–860.

About the series   *Diane Marks-Maran*

This book has been designed to enable nurses to improve their specialist knowledge and understanding of an important area of clinical practice. To help you to make the most of this learning package, we have designed this introductory section as a guideline for those of you who are new to open and distance learning.

Who is this book for?

This book is for nurses in either hospital or community settings, or in the private sector, who provide wound care to a variety of patients or clients and who want to take the opportunity, through this learning package, to ensure that their knowledge and skills are up to date and that their practice is evidence based.

What is the best way for me to use this learning package?

This depends upon what you want to gain from completing the package. At one level, this book is an excellent way to update your clinical knowledge and skill through open learning. Open learning means that you complete the package in your own time and at your own pace, taking as long as you like, reading selectively from the text and focusing on those aspects that are important to you. You complete no assessment and merely complete the activities within the package for your own interest.

At another level, in addition to updating clinical knowledge and skill, you may wish to complete this book as part of fulfilling your PREP requirements. In this case, you will need to show evidence in your professional portfolio of how this package has improved your clinical practice.

At a third level, as well as updating your clinical knowledge and skill, you may be planning to undertake further study at your local university to gain, for example, a post-registration qualification and a further academic award. In this case, completing this package and successfully passing the written assessment at the end of the book may be used to gain academic credits towards your planned academic award if the university of your choice has approved this programme of study.

What do the learning outcomes mean?

More and more, colleges and universities are aware of the need to make explicit the exact requirements for completing a module or programme successfully. Learning outcomes are one way of doing this.

Learning outcomes indicate the specific knowledge, skills and understandings you will be exposed to in the learning package. They also tell you what your assessment will entail. Additionally, if you are planning to use this book towards achieving your PREP professional requirements, you may find the learning outcomes a useful basis for submitting evidence of learning within your personal professional profile.

What do I need to do to complete this book for my PREP requirements?

Completing this book can be used towards fulfilment of your PREP requirements to show evidence of your continued learning. The UKCC has sent you a package of information entitled 'PREP and You' which explains how to complete a personal professional profile to show evidence of learning and improvement in practice. If you have not received this information, the UKCC will be happy to send you the package. In addition, issue 17 of the UKCC magazine *Register* (Summer 1996) gives a comprehensive guide to writing your personal professional profile. Completing the written assessment at the end of this book provides one piece of evidence you can include in your profile even if you do not submit it for marking to gain academic credits; recording your reflection on learning as a result of completing this package is another form of evidence to include in your profile.

What do I need to do if I want to gain academic credits for completing this book?

Some universities have accredited this learning package at both diploma level (level 2) and degree level (level 3). Accreditation has been awarded on the basis of the expected learning outcomes for the package and for the written assessment at the end of the package. You can only receive academic credits for completing the written assessment and achieving a pass grade for that assessment. You can receive academic credits at level 2 if you successfully pass the associated assessment and achieve the level 2 learning outcomes; you will receive level 3 credits if you successfully pass the level 3 assessment at the end of the package and achieve the associated learning outcomes. This means that you can use this package towards your future study to gain a Diploma in Higher Education in Nursing or a BSc in nursing.

Prior to undertaking the assessment, you should find out from the university of your choice whether they will accredit this learning pack. If they have done so, you will be able, for a registration fee, to submit your assessment for marking. If you successfully pass the assessment, you will get the credits that your university has chosen to award this learning package. Thames Valley University (TVU) has already accredited this package and would be willing to undertake this service for you. Other universities will follow shortly. The university of your choice may, however, accept the credits awarded you by institutions such as TVU through their APL/APEL process. A visual illustration of how to use this learning package is given in Figure 1.

What exactly does level 2 study mean?

When we talk about a package or course being at level 2 or level 3 it means that the work expected of you is assessed at a certain level. Level 2 normally equates to the second year of a full-time degree programme, at the end of which students would achieve a Diploma in Higher Education. However, modern education allows students to take various routes, including part-time and distance learning modes.

At level 2 you are expected to:

- demonstrate good understanding of relevant concepts and issues
- make appropriate use and application of relevant research
- demonstrate the ability to solve problems
- analyse a range of information and apply this knowledge to practice
- demonstrate the ability to construct arguments and evaluate the relevance of issues to your professional practice.

Level 2 means that you are expected to demonstrate the ability to collect information and apply that information to solve a simple but unpredictable problem or a complex but predictable problem in your practice. Level 2 also means that you are

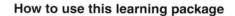

How to use this learning package

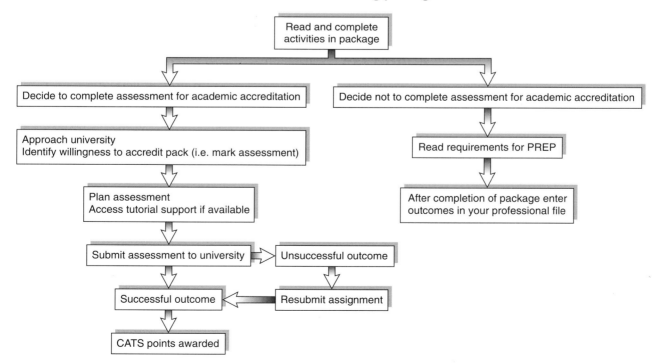

Fig. 1 How to use this learning package.

expected to manage care within broad guidelines for defined activities and to demonstrate knowledge and understanding of the subject and the variety of ideas and frameworks which may be applied to this subject. A level 2 student is one who also demonstrates the ability to analyse a variety of types of information with minimum guidance, can apply major theories of discipline and can compare alternative methods or techniques for gathering data. Within a level 2 learning package you will show that you can use a range of ideas and information towards a given purpose, such as solving a particular patient problem or situation, and can select appropriate techniques of evaluation, demonstrating that you are able to evaluate the relevance and significance of information you have collected.

In addition, when given a complex task to undertake, a level 2 student should demonstrate that she or he can choose an appropriate set of actions in sequence to complete the task, and can evaluate individual performance in terms of strengths and weaknesses. Level 2 students can challenge received opinion, adopt flexible approaches to study, identify their own learning needs and undertake activities to improve their own performance. At level 2 you are expected to demonstrate that you can study autonomously in completing straightforward study tasks. In tackling problems you should demonstrate that you can identify the key elements of a problem and choose appropriate methods for resolving problems.

What does level 3 study mean?

Level 3 study refers to a range of more advanced academic skills and equates to the third year of a full-time degree course. In addition to level 2 skills you are expected to:

- demonstrate a comprehensive and detailed knowledge of a major subject area
- critically analyse new or abstract information and relate this to your professional practice
- design creative solutions to problems
- critically evaluate evidence which supports conclusions or recommendations
- demonstrate the ability to sustain analytical argument whilst being aware of controversies and critical standpoints
- demonstrate the ability to develop a constructive, independent and original line of thought.

At level 3, you are expected to be able to demonstrate that you can work with complex and unpredictable situations, apply a wide range of innovative and standard techniques and demonstrate autonomy in planning and managing resources within broad guidelines. Your written assessments at level 3 should show that you can incorporate awareness of personal responsibility and a critical ethical dimension into your written work. A level 3 student demonstrates a comprehensive and detailed knowledge of a major subject area with the ability to demonstrate specialisation and yet realise that knowledge within a specialism is always growing and changing. A level 3 student can analyse new and/or abstract data without guidance and can transform abstracted data and concepts towards a given purpose with minimum guidance. In addition, a level 3 student can also design novel solutions to problems and can critically evaluate evidence which supports conclusions or recommendations. The students can select appropriate responses to a situation from a repertoire of actions and can evaluate their own performance and the performance of others.

In addition, people who are working at level 3 can manage their own learning using a wide range of resources, can seek and make use of feedback and can apply their own criteria for judging their performance. Problem solving at level 3 involves demonstrating confidence and flexibility in identifying and defining complex problems and applying appropriate knowledge and evidence to their solutions.

I have never studied using an independent method before. How can I get help in developing the study skills I need to work in this way?

Studying independently through open and distance learning is very different from taking a course at a college or university. It affords nurses the opportunity to study at their own pace, in their own environment and in their own time. Distance learning is especially beneficial for nurses who do not have access to a university-based course, owing to geographical, work or domestic constraints or situations. However, studying through open or distance learning does require good study skills and time-management skills to make the most of the learning package. We would recommend that you read one of the many guides to study skills which are available for students. This will give you practical advice on how to get the most out of learning packages such as this one. We particularly recommend the following two books:

- Goodall C 1995 *A Survivor's Guide to Study Skills and Student Assessments*. Churchill Livingstone, Edinburgh
- Parnell J, Kendrick K 1994 *Study Skills for Nurses*. Churchill Livingstone, Edinburgh.

In addition, study skills packs may be available from the university accrediting the package; tutorial support may also be offered. Thames Valley University is able to provide learning support in the form of feedback, tutorial support and advice to nurses undertaking this book. Details of the tutorial support available from TVU, as well as the amount and cost, are obtainable from:

Jean Clayton
APL Manager
Wolfson School of Health Sciences
Thames Valley University
32–38 Uxbridge Road
London W5 2BS
Tel: 0181 280 5230
Fax: 0181 280 5125
e-mail: jean.clayton@tvu.ac.uk

What types of learning activities will I be undertaking in this book?

In order to make this book interesting and varied, the authors have included a wide range of activities for you to complete. One type is reading activities. These are interesting and informative parts of the package which are designed to give you important information and knowledge about the subject. Sometimes a reading activity will request that you read an article from a journal on a particular subject or aspect of care. This article can be found in the Reader at the back of the book. Reading activities are often followed by self-assessment questions (SAQs). SAQs are designed to enable you to test your understanding of what you have read and draw together some of the important points in the reading you have just completed. Sometimes SAQs are included to assess your prior learning (e.g. one SAQ might ask you to write your own definition of a wound) or are in the form of short true/false questions.

Another type of activity in the package is that which asks you to describe something that currently happens in your own practice. You may be asked to reflect on some previous experience or patient. This may be followed by a feedback section where the author enables you to analyse your practice or previous experience against the literature, research and evidence. Another activity may ask you to look at a photograph and make certain observations. This will be followed by some kind of feedback to check your observations with those of the author. Other activities may include completing a chart or diagram, followed by feedback from the author of the package.

As you can see, undertaking a learning package is not the same thing as reading a book! It involves you in a wide variety of activities to find information, use information, analyse information and make clinical judgements. You will always be given some sort of feedback from the activities within the package.

You mentioned a Reader at the end of this package. What is it?

The Reader is a selection of articles from various professional journals about the subject you are studying in the learning package. We recognise that some nurses are undertaking distance learning study because they do not have easy access to a college or university in their geographical area and therefore may not have access to some of the journals which specialise in the subject of this learning package. For this reason, we are including a Reader within the book. Some of the learning activities within the package ask you to read certain articles from the Reader and answer questions about those articles. Other articles are just related to the subject and are useful for you to have as reference material and to help you complete your written assessment.

There seem to be a lot of terms used in this book. How can I be sure that I am understanding these terms in the way I am supposed to?

To help you understand the terminology in this book the following glossary will be helpful.

Critically analyse. To critically analyse something means to look at a wide range of information about a subject or issue, to identify the strengths and weaknesses of the arguments for or against something, draw conclusions based on the diverse information available to you and defend your conclusions with reference to the widest possible sources of information. At level 2, students should be able to analyse a range of information with minimum guidance, apply major theories of a discipline and compare alternative methods or techniques for obtaining data (SEEC 1996). Level 3 critical analysis means that students can analyse new and/or abstract data and situations without guidance using a wide range of techniques appropriate to the subject being studied (SEEC 1996).

Define. When you are asked to define something in a learning activity, what you are being asked to do is to write the meaning of something, e.g. a wound is ....

Demonstrate knowledge. Demonstrating knowledge involves showing that you know relevant facts, principles and concepts and that you can select these appropriately to make a clinical decision and justify that decision. Knowledge is demonstrated by defining, naming, listing or identifying parts of a whole as well as interpreting information through explaining and describing facts and applying facts to solve a problem or to give an example of a situation.

Describe. When you are asked to describe something, you are being asked to interpret information. This means that you must first show that you have the information and then give your interpretation of it.

Evaluate. Evaluating involves assessing or re-assessing a situation, criticising it, identifying strengths and weaknesses, discriminating or judging something. In nursing, evaluation often involves making a judgement of care given as compared to evidence or research.

Reflect. Reflection is thinking in a structured way in order to learn something from your experiences as a nurse and to make a decision or take an action as a result of your thinking. There are a number of frameworks for reflection, each of which offers structured questions to think through a situation and learn from it. At the end of structured reflection is some sort of learning which points you in new directions for the way you practise as a nurse.

When I complete the activities in this book and write my assessment, how should I reference my essay?

It is important to cite references appropriately. There are a number of ways of referencing and, so long as you select a recognised method and are consistent in your approach, it does not matter which one you use. You should seek guidance from the university who will be marking your assessment about their preferred referencing system. Details of some approaches to referencing can be found in the two study skills books which were identified earlier.

REFERENCE

SEEC 1996 Guidelines on levels and generic levels descriptors. South East England Consortium/Wales HE CATS

Introduction

The pack is organised into six separate sections, falling into two main parts. The first, Sections 1–5, describes the origins of leg ulceration, patient assessment and professional intervention. The second, Section 6, uses a series of case studies to explore the reality of care.

We would suggest that those of you who are relatively new to the field of leg ulceration begin with Section 1 and work through the pack sequentially. Those of you who have perhaps more experience could start with the case studies in Section 6 and use Sections 1–5 for reference/revision as necessary. For example, you might read through Case Study 1 which discusses a patient with venous ulceration and then read about the origin of venous disease in Section 3.

Section 1 sets the scene for you by looking at the extent to which leg ulceration is present in the population, as well as identifying some of the main political, economic and social factors which relate to the management of leg ulcers.

Section 2 provides you with the main anatomical and physiological factors you need to know to help you understand the aetiology of leg ulceration and how treatments work.

Section 3 discusses the causes and effects of leg ulceration in relation to the altered anatomy and physiology. These range from venous ulceration, the most common origin, through the complexities of mixed aetiologies to far less common origins such as malignancy.

Section 4 addresses the complex business of assessment which for the purposes of discussion is broken into seven stages. A fictitious scenario is used to illustrate the points made.

Section 5 describes the range of professional interventions available and their appropriate delivery based on comprehensive assessment. Intervention is discussed in the context of a multidisciplinary approach to care.

Section 6 contains the case studies which are based on the experience of real patients and deal with the many different types of ulceration you will come across. They also illustrate the uniqueness of every patient's experience and provide a vehicle through which new content can be discussed which is specific to the care of the person in question. You will be asked to imagine yourself in a particular role within the scenarios, which may be different from your own. This will hopefully give you insight into a variety of different professional roles.

Learning outcomes

LEVEL 2 LEARNING OUTCOMES

At the end of this package nurses will demonstrate that they can:

1. explain and discuss the scope and nature of the problem of leg ulcers, including their origins and related anatomy and physiology
2. critically analyse the assessment and professional intervention given to patients with leg ulcers, taking into account relevant research evidence.

LEVEL 3 LEARNING OUTCOMES

At the end of this package nurses will demonstrate that they can:

1. critically evaluate leg ulcer management practices in their place of work and the extent to which these practices reflect local and national guidelines, technological advances and research evidence
2. examine critically the multidisciplinary approach to leg ulcer management with particular reference to the contribution to quality care which can be made by a leg ulcer specialist nurse.

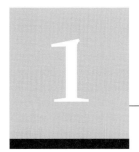

Leg ulceration: setting the scene

Introduction

If you talk to friends, relatives, colleagues or neighbours it is highly likely some of them will know someone who has a leg ulcer. We know it is a big problem and a huge drain on resources but to find out just how large a problem it is, we have to look at epidemiological research. This section explores some of the work in this area as well as the social, economic and political factors which influence the situation.

LEARNING OUTCOMES

When you have completed this section you should be able to:

- summarise major epidemiological trends in leg ulceration
- distinguish the social and environmental factors which influence leg ulceration
- discuss some of the political and financial implications of leg ulcer management in relation to nursing practice.

1.1 EPIDEMIOLOGY

Epidemiology is the study of disease in relation to a particular group of people (or 'population') (Barker & Rose 1984). Before we look at the epidemiology of leg ulceration, it is important to clarify some of the terminology used.

Some of the most common terms you will come across relate to measuring the levels of leg ulceration in the population. The first activity looks at three of them.

Activity   5 MINUTES

Write down in your own words what you think the following terms mean:

1. prevalence
2. incidence
3. risk factors.

FEEDBACK

1. Prevalence—refers to the total number of cases identified at a given point in time.
2. Incidence—refers to the number of new cases that develop over a given time span.

It is important not to confuse the terms prevalence and incidence. If for instance you were looking at the spread of HIV and AIDS in a particular population, prevalence would tell you how many people have the disease and incidence would show you how quickly the disease was spreading. An examination of epidemiological studies in relation to leg ulceration gives quite considerable insight into prevalence but little information on incidence.

3. Risk factors—refer to factors which predispose an individual to a higher risk of developing a disease and also to factors implicated in the progression, severity and outcome of the disease process.

Activity   5 MINUTES

Why do we need to know the prevalence and incidence of leg ulceration? Suggest four ways in which this information might be used.

FEEDBACK

If you know the extent of the problem and the rate at which it is developing, you can:

1. plan the efficient use of your current resources
2. estimate resource requirements in the future
3. identify risk factors to aid preventive measures and target particularly vulnerable groups
4. identify changes in the pattern of the disease.

The measurement of incidence and prevalence is, however, problematic. Fletcher (1995) states

> the optimum method is to estimate the prevalence (of leg ulcers) from a random or total sample of the at risk population, using a standardised clinical examination. The disadvantages of this approach are that very large surveys are needed for conditions with a relatively low prevalence.

She suggests three other approaches (research designs):

1. A survey approach using postal questionnaires, but warns that results are dependent on response rates and the validity of the questionnaire used.
2. A case study approach which involves a known population such as an individual case load, the total number of patients visiting a particular hospital outpatient clinic or health care trust. Findings from such an approach cannot be generalised beyond the members of the group in question.
3. Opportunistic surveys which also use a known population, but these are not considered as reliable as approaches based on randomisation.

Large-scale epidemiological studies suggest that between 1 and 2% of the population will suffer from a leg ulcer at some point in their lives (Callam et al 1985, Cornwall et al 1986, Nelzen et al 1991, Lindholm 1993). Although the highest prevalence of leg ulceration is found in the elderly, Callam et al (1985) found that over a third of those who developed a leg ulcer did so before the age of 50 and two-thirds before the age of 65.

These studies indicate that ulceration is more common in women than in men. The reasons for this gender difference are unclear, although it is suggested that they relate to high risk of deep vein thrombosis and varicose veins during pregnancy plus increased longevity. The epidemiological studies that have been undertaken have concentrated on measuring the prevalence of the condition. Approximately 80 000 to 100 000 people are suffering with a current leg ulcer and for every current ulcer there are four people with a healed ulcer that may recur. Very little is known of the true incidence of leg ulceration; however, the recurrence rates are known to be high. Two-thirds of patients will experience two or more episodes of ulceration, and 21% of patients will have more than six episodes (Callam et al 1985). Recent work suggests that even with effective prevention strategies, 25% of venous ulcers will recur within 1 year (Moffatt & Dorman 1995). Many ulcers remain unhealed for more than 10 years; the Riverside Study (Moffatt et al 1992) identified a patient who had an unhealed ulcer for 63 years.

Demographic changes suggest a dramatic increase in the very elderly (Rose 1993). This is particularly relevant when considering the increased prevalence of ulceration within this group and the obvious health economic implications that result from it. Cornwall et al (1986) identified a 50% increased risk of concurrent arterial disease in this group which may complicate treatment.

While the epidemiological studies provide invaluable evidence of the size of the problem, they may in fact understate it. The major studies rely on the reporting of cases known to professionals; recent evidence suggests that there may be a number of patients who choose to treat their own ulcer (Moffatt et al 1992).

Activity   40 MINUTES

Read Article 1 in the Reader (p. 118) and answer the following questions.

1. The survey identified 1477 people with chronic leg ulcers. What process did the researchers use to identify these patients?
2. Was ulceration more common in men or women?
3. What percentage of ulcers were open at any one time?
4. Do you think the results of this study could be extrapolated (generalised) to the UK as a whole? Give your reasons.
5. What does the study show about who provides the care to people with leg ulcers?
6. According to the study, what age group, in women, had the highest prevalence of chronic leg ulcers?

· ·

FEEDBACK

1. A postal survey was targeted at general practitioners, district nurses, occupational health services, old peoples' homes, physiotherapy departments, hospital outpatient departments and hospital inpatient departments.
2. Women outnumbered men by a ratio of 2.8 to 1.
3. 20–25% of ulcers are thought to be open at any one time.
4. The results could be generalised to other similar communities but great care should be taken to ensure that 'like' is being compared with 'like'. The results of a similar postal survey in an inner city community might be very different.
5. The study shows that most patients are managed by the primary care team.
6. Women aged 75–84 years had the highest prevalence of chronic leg ulcers.

· ·

1.2 THE SOCIAL CONTEXT

Social class

It is vital to have a good understanding of the social background of your patients as this could have direct influence on the success of your proposed intervention.

Activity | **120 MINUTES**

Carry out a comprehensive assessment of the social background of the next five patients you encounter with leg ulcers. Your assessment should include consideration of the following:

- social role
- economic status
- lifestyle
- home environment
- relationships and family and social support.

Then, for each patient, consider whether there is any evidence that social class has played a part in the development and healing of his or her leg ulcer. Note down the reasons for your answers.

FEEDBACK

A number of authors (Callam et al 1988, Moffatt & Franks 1994, Franks et al 1995) have tried to explore this difficult and complex issue. They refer to the anecdotal perception that leg ulceration is more common in members of the lower socioeconomic groups. Little empirical evidence is available to support this view but there is some agreement that there is a relationship between healing rates and social class, i.e. once people in the lower class groups have an ulcer it takes longer to heal. The factors underlying this phenomenon have not been clearly identified. However, it is reasonable to surmise that factors such as the patient's home environment may be relevant. Franks et al (1995) for instance, found significant evidence to support the proposition that patients with central heating had improved healing rates. There is, however, a danger in treating these variables too simplistically. The study referred to by Franks drew subjects from an inner city area where the quality of heating in private accommodation was poor in relation to that found in council housing.

However, there is some recent evidence involving the use of a case control study which does provide some indication of a connection between social class

and leg ulceration. A case control study endeavours to match one individual patient with the disease to another person of similar age and sex who does not have the disease. The study by Fowkes & Callam (1994) found that the case control group collectively contained more subjects in the higher social class groups I and II than the group of patients with ulcers (who were predominantly in the lower social classes). Phillips et al (1994) found a significant correlation between social class and effects on finance, including time lost from work and job loss. There is obvious scope for further work in this area.

Establishing conclusive evidence with regard to social context factors involves reference to many subtle variables. These include:

- role responsibilities
- availability of practical support, e.g. the need to buy provisions
- geographic location, e.g. rural or urban
- family structure
- distribution of health service resources, etc.

Quality of life

A related area which presents similar measurement problems is that of assessing quality of life (which we will return to later on). Researchers in this field often deliberately choose to ignore complex variables because of the difficulty in quantifying them. Fitzpatrick at al (1992) make the following statement in the first of a series of three articles on the assessment of quality of life:

> The term quality of life misleadingly suggests an abstract and philosophical approach, but most approaches used in medical contexts do not attempt to include more general notions such as life satisfaction or living standards.

The study of quality of life offers great scope for more naturalistic research approaches such as the phenomenological study by Charles (1995).

1.3 THE ECONOMIC CONTEXT

The financial implications of leg ulceration have now been recognised in the UK Health Service. An annual estimated cost of £400 million to the tax payer has been identified. A high proportion of this cost is taken up in the provision of district nurses who spend a considerable amount of time on wound care in general and leg ulcer management in particular (Morison & Moffatt 1994). Whilst many patients with leg ulcers are retired, two-thirds will develop their ulcer before the age of 65. Although little is known about the impact of leg ulceration on personal income Callam et al (1988) found that leg ulceration affected the earning capacity of 40% of those who were still working. 21% had moderate to severe limitations of work owing to long periods of sickness. In 5% of cases this led to loss of employment. There are also direct personal financial implications in prescribing certain treatments. For instance, the application of multilayer compression bandages may mean that the patient requires larger footwear and prescription costs may prove very high.

During the past decade the profile of leg ulceration has changed from a situation which was characterised by a sense of hopelessness for both patients and professionals to one in which many patients can expect their ulcers to heal within a few months. A number of factors have contributed to this. They include the development of effective research-based treatment; the shift of emphasis from acute to community care; and awareness of the high drain on resources of largely ineffective care.

As the size of the elderly population increases in a political climate which seeks to put the patient at the centre of health care and stresses the need for high quality cost-effective services, patients may be less willing to tolerate chronic intractable diseases, such as leg ulceration, which are shown to be amenable to effective treatment.

Leg ulceration has been recognised by the Department of Health as a target area for improvement. A consensus conference involving key professionals in the field, in conjunction with the Department of Health, has developed guidelines which will be made available to assist health authorities and practitioners in providing 'best practice'.

SUMMARY

In this section you have learned the following things.

- It is important to distinguish between incidence and prevalence in epidemiological studies.

- Epidemiological data are used for a variety of purposes and can be collected in different ways.

- Measuring incidence and prevalence can be problematic.

- Leg ulceration is a huge problem affecting 1–2% of the population.

- Social factors can influence the effectiveness of intervention.

- A significant proportion of the health service budget is spent on leg ulceration.

- There can be personal financial consequences of leg ulceration for individual patients.

REFERENCES

Barker D J P, Rose G 1984 Epidemiology in medical practice, 3rd edn. Churchill Livingstone, Edinburgh
Callam M J, Ruckley C V, Harper D R, Dale J J 1985 Chronic ulceration of the leg: extent of the problem and provision of care. British Medical Journal 290: 1855–1856
Callam M J, Harper D R, Dale J J, Ruckley C V 1988 Chronic leg ulceration: socio-economic aspects. Scottish Medical Journal 33: 358–360
Charles H C 1995 The impact of leg ulcers on patients' quality of life. Professional Nurse 10(9): 571–574
Cornwall J, Dore C J, Lewis J D 1986 Leg ulcers: epidemiology and aetiology. British Journal of Surgery 73: 693–696
Fitzpatrick R, Fletcher A, Gore S, Jones D, Spiegelhalter D, Cox D 1992 Quality of life measures in health care: application and issues in assessment, British Medical Journal 305: 1074–1077
Fletcher A 1995 The epidemiology of leg ulcers. In: Cullum N, Roe B (eds) Leg ulcers: nursing management: a research based guide. Scutari, London
Fowkes F G R, Callam M J 1994 Is arterial disease a risk factor for chronic leg ulceration? Phlebology 9: 87–90
Franks P J, Bosanquet N, Oldroyd M I, Moffatt C J, Greenhalgh R M, McCollum C N 1995 Venous ulcer healing: effect of socioeconomic factors in London. Journal of Epidemiology and Community Health 49: 385–388

Lindholm C 1993 Leg ulcer patients clinical studies, from prevalence to prevention in a nurse's perspective. Departments of Dermatology and Surgery, Malmö General Hospital, University of Lund, Malmö, Sweden
Moffatt C J, Dorman M C 1995 Recurrence of leg ulcers within a community ulcer service. Journal of Wound Care 4(2): 57–61
Moffatt C J, Franks P J 1994 A prerequisite underlining the treatment programme: risk factors associated with venous disease. Professional Nurse (June): 637–642
Moffatt C J, Franks P J, Oldroyd M, Bosanquet N, Brown P, Greenhalgh R M, McCollum C N 1992 Community clinics for leg ulcers and impact on healing. British Medical Journal 305: 1389–92
Morison M J, Moffatt C J 1994 A colour guide to the assessment and management of leg ulcers, 2nd edn. Mosby, London
Nelzen O, Berqvist D, Lindehagen A, Hallbrook T 1991 Chronic leg ulcers: an underestimated problem in primary health care among elderly patients. Journal of Epidemiology and Community Health 45: 184–187
Phillips T, Stanton B, Provan A, Law R 1994 A study of the impact on quality of life: financial, social and physiological implications. Journal of the American Academy of Dermatology 31(1): 49–53
Rose P (ed) 1993 Social trends 23. Central Statistical Office, HMSO, London

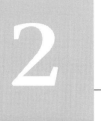

Leg ulcers: related anatomy and physiology

Introduction

Many of the complexities of the management of leg ulceration can be more easily understood if you have a good understanding of the anatomy and physiology of the vascular system of the leg.

LEARNING OUTCOME

When you have completed this section you should be able to describe the anatomical and physiological factors relating to leg ulceration.

2.1 THE VASCULAR SYSTEM

The role of the vascular system is to circulate blood around the body in order to carry substances to and from body tissue cells. According to Hinchliff & Montague (1988), for the vascular system to fulfil its role it must:

- ensure delivery of blood to all tissues
- be flexible and adaptable so that blood flow can be varied according to the metabolic requirement of individual tissue and the body as a whole
- convert a pulsating blood flow in the arteries into a steady flow in the capillaries to facilitate optimal transfer of substances to and from the cells
- return blood to the heart.

The main arteries involved in transporting blood to the legs are shown in Figure 2.1A. It is returned to the heart via the main veins shown in Figure 2.2A. Arteries and veins are similar in structure; both have three layers in cross-section:

- tunica intima—the inner layer made up of single layers of epithelial cells known as the endothelium and some elastic and connective tissue
- tunica media—the middle layer made mostly of smooth muscle and elastic tissues
- tunica adventitia—the outer layer of fibrous connective tissue, fibroblasts and collagen.

These three layers vary in thickness in different parts of the vascular system according to the specific functions of vessels, e.g. the heart is mostly tunica media whereas the smallest vessels, the capillaries, are made of endothelial tissue alone.

2.2 THE ARTERIAL SYSTEM

The function of arteries is to distribute blood to the body tissue. Arteries have strong muscular walls which can relax or constrict as required to regulate what is predominantly rapid blood flow. Small subdivisions of arteries are called arterioles. In addition to the main arteries, Figure 2.1 shows two important aspects of the arterial system in relation to the management of leg ulcers:

1. the process of plaque formation in the lumen of the arteries due to atherosclerosis (Fig. 2.1B; see Sect. 3)
2. the site of the pedal pulses which are used in the assessment of patients with leg ulcers (Fig. 2.1C; see Sect. 4).

The commonest sites for arterial occlusion which may lead to ulceration are:

- lower superficial femoral artery
- aortoiliac vessels
- multiple sites (7% of cases).

2.3 THE VENOUS SYSTEM

The function of the vein is to act as a collection system which returns blood to the heart. The walls of veins are thinner than arteries and are less muscular. They have the ability to dilate and according to Dale (1995) can accommodate approximately 80% of an individual's total blood volume if required. Small subdivisions of veins are called venules.

Figure 2.2 shows, in addition to the main veins, three important aspects of the venous system in relation to the management of leg ulcers.

1. Veins, unlike arteries, have valves which normally allow blood in one direction only (Fig. 2.2B).
2. Venous return of blood is assisted by the action of the calf muscle which acts as a 'pump' (Fig. 2.2C).
3. Varicose veins which become dilated and tortuous cause damage to the valves which in turn causes backflow of blood, resulting in raised pressure in the superficial veins (Fig. 2.2D).

Blood pressure in the venous system of the leg is also affected by gravity and posture. In the upright position it is approximately 90 mmHg. When supine, pressure can fall to approximately 10 mmHg (Dale 1995).

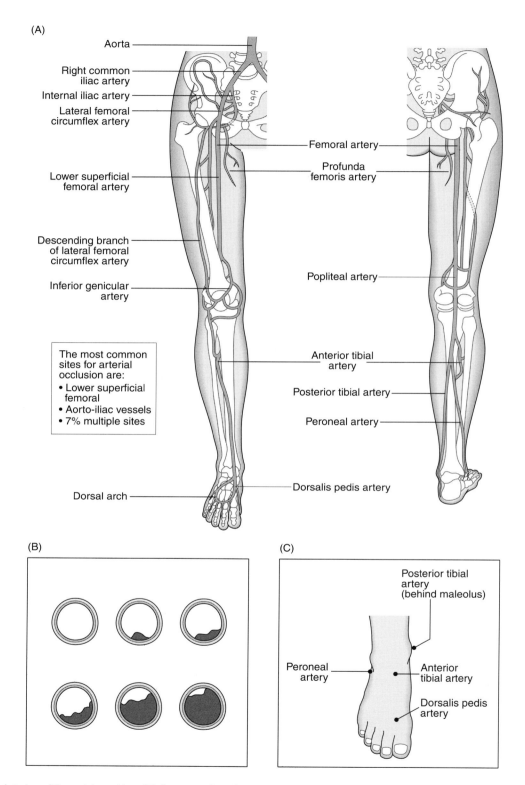

(A)

Aorta

Right common iliac artery

Internal iliac artery

Lateral femoral circumflex artery

Femoral artery

Profunda femoris artery

Lower superficial femoral artery

Descending branch of lateral femoral circumflex artery

Inferior genicular artery

Popliteal artery

The most common sites for arterial occlusion are:
• Lower superficial femoral
• Aorto-iliac vessels
• 7% multiple sites

Anterior tibial artery

Posterior tibial artery

Peroneal artery

Dorsalis pedis artery

Dorsal arch

(B)

(C)

Posterior tibial artery (behind maleolus)

Peroneal artery

Anterior tibial artery

Dorsalis pedis artery

Fig. 2.1 (A) Arteries of the pelvis and leg. (B) Cross-section of artery showing gradual build-up of plaque leading to occlusion of the vessel. (C) Sites of pedal pulses used in the calculation of a resting pressure index.

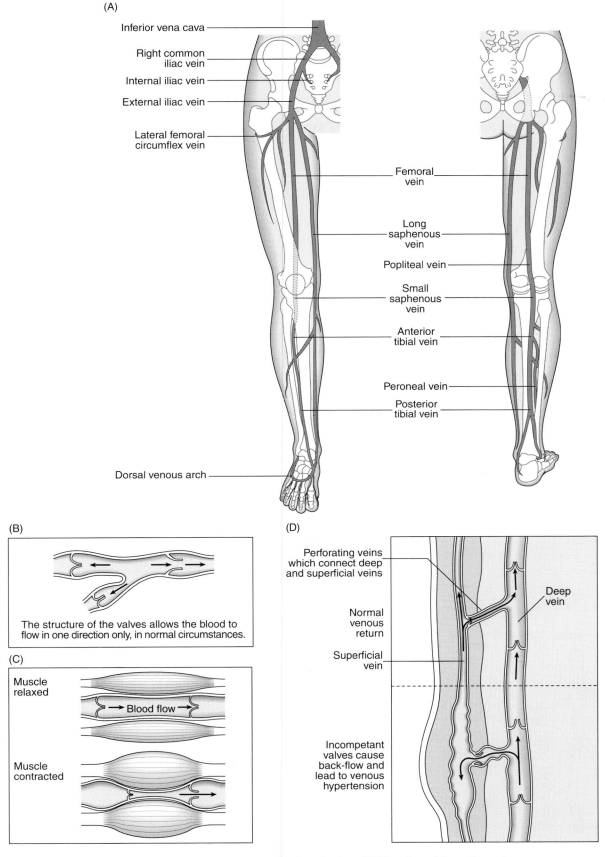

Fig. 2.2 (A) Veins of the pelvis and leg. (B) The structure and function of valves. (C) The effect of the calf muscle pump. (D) Incompetent valves allow backflow of blood from a deep vein into a superficial vein.

2.4 THE MICROCIRCULATION

Figure 2.3 shows a diagrammatic representation of the microcirculation. The physiology of the microcirculation is very complex but it is at this level that theoretical explanations of the origin of ulceration occurs. At the centre of the microcirculation are the capillaries where exchange of fluids, gases, nutrients and waste products takes place. The blood flow in capillaries is steady and slow. The density of capillary networks varies in different tissue and even though they consist of endothelium, the gaps between the cells in the single layer have been observed to vary in different parts of the circulation. Three types of capillary wall have been identified: continuous, fenestrated and discontinuous. Arteriovenous shunts occur in the microcirculation. These short vessels allow rapid transfer of blood from arteries to veins, effectively bypassing the capillaries. Diffusion of fluids and solutes occurs in both directions through the capillary walls from the capillary lumen to the interstitial fluids and vice versa. Despite a high rate of diffusion in both directions, the volume of fluid passing out of the capillaries is very nearly the same as that which passes in. This phenomenon was identified by Starling who proposed that three factors governed the rate of transfer between plasma in the capillaries and fluid in the interstitial spaces (Hinchliff & Montague 1988):

1. the hydrostatic pressure on each side of the capillary wall
2. the osmotic pressure of protein in the plasma and in the tissue fluid
3. the properties of the capillary wall.

Hydrostatic pressure refers to the pressure any fluid exerts, when in a confined space, on the walls of the container.

Osmosis is defined by Tortora & Anagnostakos (1987) as 'the net movement of water molecules through a selectively permeable membrane from an area of high water concentration' to an area of low water concentration. Oedema, often seen in leg ulceration of various origins, is the result of an imbalance in these mechanisms which increases the level of interstitial fluid. The lymphatic system of vessels acts as an 'overflow' for excess fluid.

Self-assessment   10 MINUTES

1. What process causes plaque formation in the arteries?
2. What are the names of the three vessels most commonly used in the palpation of the pedal pulses?
3. Name three common sites for arterial occlusion.
4. What structures facilitate the flow of blood in one direction only through the vein?
5. What 'pump' assists the venous return of blood to the heart?
6. What is the consequence of dilated tortuous veins in which the valves have become damaged and incompetent?
7. What three factors govern the rate of transfer between plasma in the capillary and fluid in the interstitial spaces which can ultimately lead to oedema if the system becomes imbalanced?

FEEDBACK

Your answers should have been as follows.

1. The process of plaque formation in the lumen of the arteries is caused by atherosclerosis.
2. The three vessels most commonly used in the palpation of the pedal pulses are the dorsalis pedis, peroneal and posterior tibial.
3. Three common sites for arterial occlusion are the lower superficial femoral artery, aortoiliac vessels and multiple sites in 7% of cases.
4. The structures which facilitate the flow of blood in one direction through the vein are valves.
5. The pump which assists the venous return of blood to the heart is the 'calf muscle' pump (you may also have identified the 'foot pump' which also facilitates venous return on walking).
6. The consequence of dilated tortuous veins in which the valves have become damaged or incompetent is raised pressure in the superficial veins (venous hypertension).

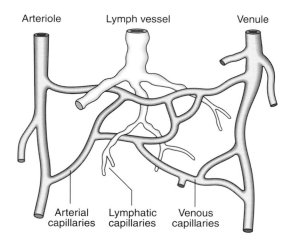

Arteriole   Lymph vessel   Venule

Arterial capillaries   Lymphatic capillaries   Venous capillaries

Fig. 2.3 The microcirculation.

7. The three factors which govern the rate of transfer between plasma in the capillary and fluid in the interstitial spaces are hydrostatic pressure, osmotic pressure and the properties of the capillary wall.

- it synthesises vitamin D
- it signals emotions via the autonomic nervous system
- it acts as an outpost to the immune system
- it provides a frictional surface to facilitate grip.

Ulceration involves a break in the continuity of the skin and damage to underlying tissues resulting in the formation of a wound. The following activity explores the process of wound healing.

2.5 SKIN AND WOUND HEALING

Figure 2.4 is a diagrammatic representation of the skin, which forms the outer protective layer of the body and which is subject to continuous regeneration. The skin has a number of functions:

- it protects you from injury and infection and discourages microbial growth
- it enables you to experience the world and protect yourself through sensation
- it stores fat and water
- it absorbs ultraviolet radiation and excretes carbon dioxide
- it regulates heat, maintaining a constant temperature regardless of the external environment

Activity   60 MINUTES

Read the article in the Reader by Torrance (Article 2, p. 120).

1. Choose one of your own patients and make a list of factors which are influencing the healing of their wound. Use Figure 2.5 to guide your assessment.
2. Suggest which is the most important factor in your list and how you might deal with it.

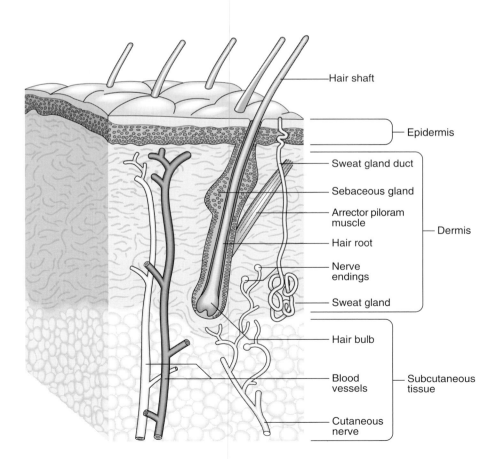

Fig. 2.4 The skin.

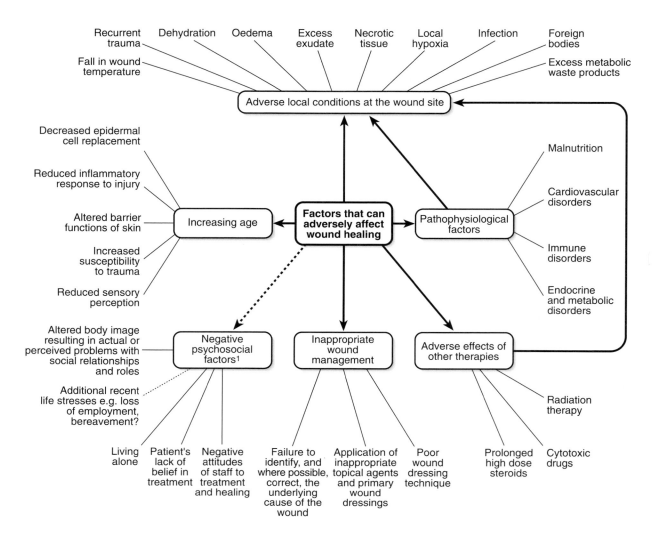

Fig. 2.5 Factors that can adversely affect wound healing (reproduced from Morison & Moffatt 1994 (based on Morison 1992) by kind permission). Note: [1] The direct link between delayed healing and negative psychosocial factors has yet to be unequivocally demonstrated.

FEEDBACK

1. If you identified any factors other than those suggested by Torrance in Article 2 or by Morison & Moffatt in Figure 2.5, make a note of them.
2. The priorities in treating a wound will be different for each patient. In some instances, a poor blood supply might be the dominant factor which is delaying healing, and nursing care alone is unlikely to improve the situation; it may be that reconstructive surgery is required. Sometimes wound healing is delayed by poor dressing technique and inappropriate use of topical agents. In this case the nurse is in a position to rectify the problem once it has been identified. More often than not there are more complex intrinsic and extrinsic factors which combine to delay wound healing. The nurse is better equipped to address these if there is an understanding of the physiological events taking place.

You will have noted the complexity of the wound healing process in the article by Torrance. Since it was written in 1986 researchers have continued to explore this process even further (Silver 1994).

Activity   45 MINUTES

In order to bring you up to date with some of the current issues in wound healing, read the article in the Reader by Silver (Article 3, p. 125).

Two factors involved in the healing process mentioned briefly in the article are oxygen radicals and growth factors. Summarise in your own words what Silver has to say about these factors and then answer the following questions.

1. What are oxygen radicals a side effect of?
2. What do phagocytes use oxygen radicals for?
3. When is the greatest risk of oxygen radical damage?
4. Which phagocytes release growth factors?
5. What does Silver consider to be the most important growth factors?

FEEDBACK

Your answers should have been as follows.

1. Oxygen radicals are a side effect of oxidative phosphorylation—the main system for producing energy.
2. Phagocytes use oxygen radicals for the destruction of bacteria or parasites.
3. The greatest damage from oxygen radicals is likely when blood starts to flow following a hypoxic or ischaemic event.
4. Macrophages release growth factors.
5. Silver identifies the most important growth factors as angiogenic factors, fibroblast growth factors, macrophage colony factor and platelet factor.

SUMMARY

In this section you have learned the following.

- Arteries and veins differ in structure.
- Disease or damage to the structure of veins and arteries contributes to the development of leg ulceration.
- The pedal pulses can be detected in a variety of positions on the foot.
- The diffusion of fluid and solution in the microcirculation is kept in a state of balance by a number of complex factors.
- Wound healing involves a complex cascade of events which can be affected by extrinsic and intrinsic factors.

REFERENCES

Dale J 1995 The anatomy and physiology of the circulation of the leg. In: Cullum N, Roe B (eds) Leg ulcers: nursing management: a research based guide. Scutari, London

Hinchliff S M, Montague S E 1988 Physiology for nursing practice. Baillière Tindall, London

Morison M J 1992 A colour guide to the nursing management of wounds. Wolfe, London

Morison M J, Moffatt C J 1994 A colour guide to the assessment and management of leg ulcers, 2nd edn. Mosby, London

Silver L A 1994 The physiology of wound healing. Journal of Wound Care 3(2): 106–109

Torrance C 1986 The physiology of wound healing. Nursing (UK) 3(5): 162–168

Tortora G J, Anagnostakos N P 1987 Principles of anatomy and physiology, 5th edn. Harper & Row, New York

FURTHER READING

Cohen I K, Diegelmann R F, Lindblad W J 1992 Wound healing: biochemical and clinical aspects. W B Saunders, Philadelphia

Kloth L C, McCullock J M, Feedar J A 1990 Wound healing: alternatives in management, contemporary perspective in rehabilitation. F A Davis, Philadelphia

3 Origins

Introduction

Understanding the origin of your patient's ulcer is one of your primary goals. It is the basis upon which you will build your subsequent plans for intervention. This section explores a wide range of causes and effects, from venous ulceration which is the most common origin to less common origins such as malignancy. Between the two are the mixed aetiologies which are complex and make decision making very difficult for you when deciding how to proceed.

LEARNING OUTCOMES

When you have completed this section you should be able to:

- distinguish the factors contributing to the development of:

  —venous ulceration
  —arterial ulceration
  —diabetic ulceration
  —ulcers related to lymphatic disease
  —vasculitic ulceration occurring in the patient with rheumatoid arthritis

- briefly discuss less common causes of ulceration such as:

  —malignancy
  —haematological disorders
  —infection
  —hypertension
  —trauma
  —iatrogenic
  —factitious.

In the preceding section we have referred to leg ulceration without offering any explanation or definition of the word. We have assumed that someone embarking on this pack would have some understanding of the concept; it is not, however, appropriate to proceed much further without agreeing a definition.

3.1 DEFINING LEG ULCERATION

Activity 15 MINUTES

Try to create your own definition of leg ulceration. Your description should have both descriptive and causative elements.

FEEDBACK

A number of authors have attempted to describe an ulcer. There are some examples in Box 3.1; compare them to your own.

Box 3.1 Definitions of an ulcer

Tissue breakdown on the leg or foot due to any cause.

Cullum (1994)

A leg ulcer is a loss of skin below the knee on the leg or foot which takes more than 6 weeks to heal.

Dale (1995)

An ulcer is a local defect, or excavation, of the surface of an organ or tissue, which is produced by the sloughing of inflammatory necrotic tissue.

Robbins (1967)

A discontinuity of an epithelial surface.

Harding Rains & Mann (1988)

We feel that none of the four examples is comprehensive enough given the complexity of the phenomenon and have combined some of the elements in each in order to create the following working definition for this pack.

A leg ulcer is a breakdown of epidermal and dermal tissue, below the knee on the leg or foot, due to any cause, which fails to heal.

Having now established a working definition, we can proceed to build on what you have already learnt by exploring the different origins of leg ulcers. An understanding of the cause and effect of leg ulceration is essential in making an accurate and comprehensive assessment of your patients and planning treatment for them. We will begin with the leg ulcer you are likely to see most frequently.

3.2 VENOUS ORIGINS

Callam et al (1985) estimated that 70% of leg ulcers are predominantly the result of venous disease.

Activity   10 MINUTES

Read Article 4 in the Reader (p. 129), then make a note of the name of the person who was the first to observe a link between varicose veins and leg ulceration.

• •

FEEDBACK

Despite the lack of knowledge about the anatomy and physiology of venous disease, detailed observation by Hippocrates revealed that he had an understanding of the link between leg ulcers and varicose veins.

• •

If you look again at the chronology in Article 4, you will notice that it was not until much later that a number of writers identified a causative relationship between varicose veins and leg ulceration. In the mid 19th century Gay and Spender recognised that other venous diseases such as deep vein thrombosis could also cause ulceration and from that time used the generic term 'venous ulceration' in preference to varicose. While varicose veins are a common problem affecting approximately 20% of the adult population of the UK, only about 3% will develop a leg ulcer.

Venous hypertension

Venous ulcers are the result of chronic venous hypertension. The factors which contribute to venous hypertension are:

• damage to the valves in the vein with resultant venous reflux (blood flowing backwards down the vein)
• the reflux results in high pressure in the dermal capillary bed and damage to the microcirculation predisposing to ulceration.

Changes in the microcirculation

Patients with venous ulceration have a change in their capillary network. Owing to the high pressure, the capillaries become elongated and it looks as if there is an increase in the number of capillaries, but in fact there are fewer. It has been suggested that this change in the capillaries is due to the development of very small thrombi.

There is much debate over what actually happens at the microvascular level. Researchers are divided into groups of thought. One group believes that lack of oxygen causes venous ulceration at a cellular level, while the other believes that cytotoxic substances cause local tissue breakdown.

Theoretical perspectives

Fibrin cuff theory (Browse & Burnand 1982)

When venous hypertension occurs the single cell wall of the capillary is stretched, enlarging the capillary pores and allowing the passage of large molecules such as red blood cells and protein into the interstitial spaces. One of these proteins is fibrinogen which changes to fibrin at this point and forms bands or cuffs around the outer wall of the capillary. For a number of years it was thought that these cuffs acted as a barrier to the diffusion of oxygen and nutrients, resulting in ulceration of the epidermis. Recent work, however (Herrick et al 1992), suggests that the cuffs are the result rather than the cause of ulceration and that oxygen can diffuse through them. Patients predisposed to ulceration have poor ability to remove (lyse) the fibrin which accumulates. It was noted that the cuffs slowly disappeared during treatment with compression bandaging as the wound healed.

Mechanical theory (Chant 1990)

This theory suggests that ulceration is the result of mechanical stress on the patient's skin. The high pressure in the capillary bed leads to oedema which in turn raises tissue pressure resulting in stretching of the skin. Ulceration is thought to result from tissue ischaemia.

Struckmann (1995) states: 'there is no unequivocal evidence that tissue oxygenation is indeed insufficient in patients with CVI (chronic venous insufficiency)' and that neither the fibrin cuff nor the pericapillary micro-oedema, which certainly exists, has 'been shown to be a significant diffusion barrier to molecules the size of oxygen'.

Because of the criticism of these two previous theories researchers have looked for other explanations.

White cell entrapment theory
(Coleridge Smith et al 1988)

Increased venous pressure causes entrapment of white blood cells in the capillaries. Whilst some researchers think that this may cause a barrier to perfusion, current preference is for the proposition that the cells become activated and release cytotoxic substances resulting in local damage to tissue and ulceration.

The growth factor 'trap' theory
(Higley et al 1995)

Growth factors need to reach the epidermal cells in order to help them to proliferate. Leakage of fibrinogen and protein occurs and these are bound to growth factors which trap them and so prevent normal tissue repair and maintenance of tissue integrity.

You can see that these theories are very complex and a number of authors suggest that the factors may be working in combination, and the theories perhaps describing different aspects of the same phenomenon (Herrick et al 1992, Struckmann 1995).

Skin changes

Chronic venous ulceration results in a number of typical changes to the skin of the lower leg with which you need to be familiar.

Self-assessment 10 MINUTES

1. To what are fibrin cuffs thought to act as a barrier?
2. In mechanical theory, ulceration is thought to result from what condition?
3. What factor is thought to cause white cell entrapment in the capillaries?
4. Leakage of which substances prevents growth factors from reaching epidermal cells?

FEEDBACK

You should have said the following.

1. Fibrin cuffs are thought to act as a barrier to the diffusion of oxygen and nutrients.
2. In mechanical theory, ulceration is thought to result from ischaemia.
3. Increased venous pressure is thought to cause white cell entrapment in the capillaries.
4. Leakage of fibrinogen and protein prevents growth factors from reaching epidermal cells.

Activity 10–15 MINUTES

Look at Plate 8 (between pp. 102 and 103) which shows a typical venous ulcer. Describe in your own words what you can see in terms of site, size, the wound, and surrounding skin.

FEEDBACK

You should have noticed the following points.

The site of the ulcer

The ulcer is on the lateral aspect of the lower leg. This is a very typical position for a venous ulcer. Venous leg ulcers occur in the gaiter region which involves the lower third of the leg and extends to below the malleoli. Many venous ulcers occur on the medial side of the leg but as you see from this picture, they also occur on the lateral aspect. Position is quite an important indication of venous ulceration. It would be unusual to find a venous ulcer occurring on the foot or toes, though not impossible. Sometimes a venous ulcer will extend over the foot owing to maceration from excessive exudate or pressure from tight-fitting shoes.

The size of the ulcer

This is quite a large venous ulcer but they vary considerably in size. Factors influencing size include the underlying venous pathology, the length of time the patient has had the ulcer, the effectiveness of treatment, infection and oedema.

The wound condition

Just by looking at the wound we can tell it is chronic. There is very little evidence of healing. The wound base is yellow due to the presence of slough. It is also likely, owing to the shiny appearance, to have a fibrinous base. Chronic ulcers that do not heal have a collection of fibrinous material which prevents the formation of granulation tissue. You can see areas of red granulation around the edges and dotted throughout the wound, suggesting that the wound will heal given the right environment. Now look at the edges of the wound. These are thickened and there is no pale pink line around the perimeter which would indicate that the wound is healing by epithelialisation. Venous ulcers are not usually very deep and, although they can in severe cases extend into the fascia, they rarely involve bone.

The surrounding skin

The skin looks dry, scaly and discoloured. These skin changes result from leakage of substances from the microcirculation into the surrounding tissue. The brown discoloration is caused by the leakage of red cells which deposit their haem content. The degree of staining varies between patients but to some degree predicts the severity of the underlying disease. Patients who sit in direct contact with fires or radiators may present with pigmentation on the lateral aspect of the leg. This condition is known as erythema ab igne and is frequently confused with the staining seen in venous ulcer patients.

Patients with venous ulceration suffer from a number of dermatological conditions. The commonest presenting skin problem is varicose eczema. The terms 'eczema' and 'dermatitis' tend to be used synonymously. Dermatitis is a non-infective inflammatory disorder of the skin triggered by external or internal factors and sometimes both. Patients complain of intense irritation and weeping. The skin is erythematous and oedematous. Papules and vesicles may develop and the skin eventually forms a crust of scales which fissure. Eczema affects the epidermis and the superficial dermis in the early acute stages; oedema collects in the lower epidermis and causes the keratinocytes to separate. This process is known as spongiosis. As the cells become pulled apart, intra-epidermal vesicles develop. The presenting erythema is due to vascular dilatation in the upper dermis and the accumulation of inflammatory cells. Later, following the acute stage, the epidermis thickens, a process called acanthosis which, in combination with the spongiosis, leads to hyperkeratosis where there is a thick collection of altered keratinocytes causing the scaly appearance seen in these patients. Patients with venous disease may also suffer with contact dermatitis which develops in response to topical agents used in practice.

The development and treatment of contact dermatitis is dealt with in greater depth in Case Study 1 (p. 89).

Patients with venous ulceration may present with other skin conditions such as psoriasis, which may be wrongly diagnosed as varicose eczema because of the underlying venous pathology. Fixed psoriatic-like plaques occurring in isolation may be due to Bowen's disease which is an intraepidermal carcinoma.

Sometimes areas of white tissue are visible rather than areas of pigmentation. This is called *atrophe blanche*. These areas are avascular areas of scar tissue and are very susceptible to tissue breakdown. Debate exists as to why these areas develop and whether they are areas of vasculitis. *Atrophe blanche* is seen in a number of other dermatological conditions including polyarteritis nodosa.

If you were able to feel the leg shown in Plate 8, it would feel hard like wood. This is due to the laying down (induration) of fibrous tissue in the gaiter region. The term lipodermatosclerosis is used to describe this phenomenon (Browse & Burnand 1982). The progressive development of fibrotic tissue can result in a limb that has the appearance of an inverted champagne bottle with gross narrowing at the ankle and a wide oedematous calf. The dry skin condition you see is varicose eczema; the flaky appearance is due to the accumulation of the outer epidermal layer which is forming rapidly and haphazardly. Varicose eczema can be complicated by the use of topical agents which cause an allergic reaction and by pathogenic bacteria causing infected eczema. It is also possible to note an accumulation of oedema around the ankle. Some patients develop a condition known as ankle flare where very small dilated vessels are seen on the medial aspect of the foot. This is particularly common in patients with perforator valve incompetence.

Contributory factors

Section 2 discussed the contribution which the calf muscle pump makes to enhancing venous return. If for some reason the effectiveness of the calf muscle pump is compromised, the effect is to reverse the normal direction of venous flow. Instead of blood being pumped back to the heart, incompetence of the valves in the perforating vein results in the blood being forced into the superficial venous system, thus causing further damage to other valves and ultimately increasing the pressure in the microcirculation.

Activity   5 MINUTES

What factors do you think might inhibit the effectiveness of the calf muscle pump? Try to suggest five of them.

FEEDBACK

The function of the calf muscle pump will be impaired by anything which causes immobility, e.g.:

- paralysis
- arthritis
- joint disease
- obesity
- long periods of inactivity, e.g. sitting with legs down.

Immobility in turn will result in reduction in the contribution which ankle movement makes to venous return (see Sect. 2).

The pattern of the development of venous insufficiency will not be the same in all your patients. Some will have insufficiency of the superficial veins, the perforating veins or the deep veins. In many patients all three will be affected to varying extents. The greater the insufficiency the more likely it is that the patient will develop venous ulcers. Patients with the lowest risk of developing an ulcer have insufficiency in their superficial veins alone, seen as varicose veins. The risk is increased if the perforating and deep veins are also involved. It is yet greater in patients who have had previous deep vein thrombosis, particularly if this has been extensive. The deep vein thrombosis in most cases causes destruction of the valves in the affected area. As the blood attempts to make a new channel through the blockage damage to the valve cusps occurs. This process is known as recanalisation (Negus 1991). In a small proportion of patients, the vein stays permanently blocked. This is known as deep venous obstruction.

Assessment of venous ulceration

Self-assessment   10 MINUTES

What factors, discussed in this section, would you consider important to incorporate into a structured assessment? You should be able to think of seven of them.

FEEDBACK

You could have mentioned the following.

- The presence of varicose veins
- A history of previous varicose vein treatment, e.g. surgery or sclerotherapy
- Immobility—reduced calf muscle pump function
- History of deep vein thrombosis

- Skin changes and condition
- The wound, e.g. position
- Lower limb trauma.

Case Studies 1 and 2 (pp. 89 and 92) explore the assessment and management of venous ulceration.

3.3 ARTERIAL ORIGINS

Atherosclerosis and peripheral vascular disease

As we get older fatty material is deposited on the walls of our arteries and plaques are formed. This process, which begins in early life and leads to narrowing of the lumen of the artery, is called atherosclerosis. Atherosclerosis is the most common cause of arterial ulceration owing to the ischaemia and necrosis caused by the reduced blood supply. Cornwall et al (1986) and Callam et al (1985) suggest that approximately 20% of patients with leg ulcers have arterial insufficiency. Atherosclerosis can affect any artery in the body but it is found more frequently in some vessels than others, e.g. of the brain, the heart, carotid arteries. Approximately 50% of deaths in the UK are due to cardiovascular disease (Rose 1991). Arterial disease also causes peripheral vascular disease. In the leg, common sites are the lower superficial femoral and aortoiliac vessels, and in 7% of patients multiple sites are involved.

Ross (1986) proposes the theory that atherosclerosis develops as shown in Box 3.2.

The severity of the disease varies between patients. The symptoms and degree of ulceration depend on the degree of blockage and the site of occlusion. It is surprising to find that an artery can be 70% blocked and not cause symptoms when the patient is resting. However, these patients often experience intermittent claudication (pain in the calf, thigh or buttocks during exercise) because the diseased vessels cannot dilate sufficiently to cope with the demand for more oxygen.

Box 3.2 The development of atherosclerosis (Ross 1986)

- Monocytes adhere to the internal lining (intima) of the artery.
- This adherence activates the monocyte which becomes macrophagic.
- Macrophages release growth factors.
- Growth factor stimulates the migration and proliferation of vascular smooth muscle cells.
- The altered lining attracts platelets which adhere.
- Lipids, fibrin and other cellular debris accumulate forming plaque.

Other factors relating to this process include:

- the development of calcification of the medial lining of the vessel causing it to become more rigid
- the plaque, relatively harmless in itself, increasingly causes fissures and haemorrhages leading to the development of thrombi and emboli with resultant ischaemia.

With regard to the origin of the disease, Bryant (1992) states: 'although the exact initiating mechanism of atherosclerosis is unknown, the ageing process, lifestyle habits and disease can combine to affect both large and small arteries'.

Ischaemia

Activity   10 MINUTES

Factors which cause ischaemia can be chronic or acute. Think about patients you have nursed. Can you identify any of the causes of ischaemia?

FEEDBACK

You could have mentioned the following.

Acute causes

These include:

- arterial embolism—caused by an embolus blocking a vessel. When it occurs in a major vessel, the patient presents with an acutely ischaemic leg and may not report any known history of arterial disease
- trauma—any major trauma to the lower limb can cause damage to the artery or the venous circulation and may, in rare cases, lead to a fat embolism.

Chronic causes

These include:

- Buerger's disease—a rare peripheral vascular condition causing progressive arterial disease. An alternative term is thromboangiitis obliterans. It is found particularly in young men and is associated with heavy regular smoking. It affects small and medium-size vessels of the extremities, beginning peripherally
- vasospastic disease, e.g. Raynaud's disease
- cold—for example, frostbite causes peripheral ischaemia
- atherosclerosis.

When an artery becomes 90% occluded, many patients will experience rest pain. This is a very important factor suggesting a severely compromised circulation with a significant risk of gangrene which might result in amputation. Patients presenting with more

acute episodes of arterial occlusion are disadvantaged. Many of these patients with chronic disease have learnt to live with their disease and to increase their walking distance despite the development of intermittent claudication. It is believed that many patients gain symptomatic relief by developing new collateral circulation. This involves the enlargement of smaller vessels around the site of the occlusion which compensates for the lost capacity of the main vessel. Whilst many patients have been advised to continue exercising, more recent research has suggested that when patients do so whilst experiencing intermittent claudication metabolites are produced that can lead to heart damage (Edwards et al 1994). Following an acute arterial occlusion due to embolism, the body has not had time to develop a collateral circulation.

Assessment of arterial ulcers

The following activity gives you the opportunity to develop your visual assessment skills.

Activity   15 MINUTES

Look at Plate 2 (between pp. 102 and 103) which shows an arterial ulcer resulting from critical ischaemia (acute). Describe in your own words what you see in terms of the site, size, the wound and the surrounding skin.

FEEDBACK

You should have noticed the following points.

The site of the ulcer

The ulcer in the picture is on the dorsum of the foot. This is a very common site for an arterial ulcer. However, unlike the venous ulcer, an arterial ulceration can occur anywhere on the limb and this is dependent on the site of the arterial occlusion. There are nevertheless certain sites which are more common than others. These include the lateral aspect of the leg and medial malleolus. We have already seen that this was also a common site for venous ulcers.

The size of the ulcer

Whilst arterial ulcers vary in size, this picture shows features which are typical of an arterial ulcer. It is irregular, deep and has a characteristic 'punched-out appearance'. The size relates to the extent of underlying arterial disease and can dramatically increase as the disease progresses or in the presence of infection or uncontrolled oedema.

The condition of the wound

There are a number of features which suggest the wound is 'not healing. The base of the ulcer is covered with an adherent slough and little evidence of granulation tissue. The edges of the wound are rolled. Elevated rolled edges can also be a sign of malignancy.

The surrounding skin

The area around the ulcer looks red and shiny. The reason for this is that the blood vessels in the skin are maximally dilated in an attempt to compensate for the ischaemia. This is a condition known as reactive hyperaemia. The surrounding erythema may have caused you to think that the wound is chronically infected. The shiny appearance of the skin, including the toes, is caused by oedema. You should also notice trophic changes (thickening) in the nails and the absence of any hair.

• •

When patients with this type of ulceration put their legs up, the leg turns pale (blanches) and pain increases. With the legs hanging down (dependent), the foot and toes turn a reddish/blue colour. If you were able to touch the leg it would feel cold. The leg would also be dry due to an absence of sweat glands. You would be able to note how poor the perfusion in the tissue was by applying your thumb to the toenail bed and counting the number of seconds required for the colour to return. This takes longer than 3 seconds to recover in a patient with arterial disease. Pedal pulses would also be difficult to palpate. We will explore the issue of risk factors further in Section 4.

Self-assessment   **15 MINUTES**

The grid in Figure 3.1 contains hidden words which relate to arterial ulceration. Using the clues given, see if you can identify the words in the grid. Words can run in any direction, i.e. backwards, horizontally, vertically, diagonally.

W	U	5	8	9	1	M	U	L	L	A	C
A	1	F	B	L	A	N	C	H	E	L	P
H	P	J	C	F	E	M	O	R	A	L	U
F	L	K	I	C	D	M	L	U	J	D	L
N	A	G	H	E	R	N	D	O	Q	O	S
O	Q	C	P	M	S	I	L	O	B	M	E
K	U	L	O	Q	C	A	W	H	P	T	S
E	E	C	R	A	R	T	E	R	I	A	L
L	B	V	T	T	B	M	G	T	E	A	P
E	T	I	B	T	S	O	R	F	I	B	K
W	O	U	V	E	N	E	R	G	N	A	G
N	H	I	S	R	M	N	S	T	J	L	F

Pain on exercise which is relieved by rest (12 letters)
20% of ulcers are (8)
A cause of acute arterial ulceration (8)
A common artery affected by arterial disease (7)
The foot feels (4)
These are reduced or absent (6)
The nails become (7)
The French word for pale (6)
Death of tissue (8)
A large scale epidemiology study (6-4)
Forms as part of atherosclerosis (6)
Low temperature is needed to cause this one (5-4)

Fig. 3.1 Wordsearch.

• •

FEEDBACK

The words to be found in the grid are:

- claudication
- arterial
- embolism
- femoral
- cold
- pulses
- trophic
- blanche
- gangrene
- Callam 1985
- plaque
- frostbite.

• •

Case Studies 4 and 5 (pp. 97 and 99) explore the assessment and management of arterial ulceration. Case Study 3 (p. 95) explores the more complex situation where a patient has both venous and arterial disease.

3.4 DIABETIC ORIGINS

In this subsection we will consider the development of foot ulceration in patients with diabetes mellitus. It is important to remember that just because someone has diabetes it does not prevent him or her from having the more common types of ulceration, e.g. venous. Foot ulceration in patients with diabetes is due to a very different pathology.

Diabetic risk factors

Foot complications are now the commonest reason for hospital admission in patients with diabetes. Of the 750 000 patients with diabetes in the UK, 4% have undergone amputation and 45 000 have foot ulcers. Of the patients who require an amputation, 42% go on to have a second amputation within 1–3 years and 56% within 3–5 years (Stewart et al 1992). The distressing issue here is that it is claimed that between 50 and 75% of these amputations are preventable with effective management. Recent studies suggest that foot ulceration is more common in those with a previous history of foot ulceration and in patients from lower social class groups (Boulton et al 1994).

We shall now consider the main factors that lead to foot ulceration in the patient with diabetes. These are:

- neuropathy
- ischaemia
- infection.

Peripheral neuropathy

Peripheral neuropathy is probably the single most important cause of foot ulceration and is reported in over 80% of diabetics with this condition (Boulton et al 1986). Fernando et al (1991) demonstrated that patients with other diabetic complications such as nephropathy had an increased risk of developing neuropathic foot ulceration.

Self-assessment   5 MINUTES

Using your current medical knowledge, name the three types of nerves that form the nervous system and which can be affected in the diabetic foot.

FEEDBACK

The three types of nerves are:

- sensory nerves
- motor nerves
- autonomic nerves.

Sensory neuropathy

The sensory nerves supplying the feet and lower legs are damaged leading to progressive loss of sensation and the ability to feel painful stimuli.

In the early stages, patients may be unaware of the condition, while some may complain of severe burning pain, particularly at night. They may also have increased sensitivity to hot and cold.

In the advanced stage, the patients' feet are numb and this numbness may extend to just below the knee. Patients may state that it feels as though they are walking on cushions. This loss of protective sensation results in patients being unable to feel when trauma to their feet is occurring. Common injuries are often the result of foreign bodies, tight shoes or thermal injuries (Young & Boulton 1991). The patient is unaware of the injury and continues to walk on the foot, causing further deterioration.

Motor neuropathy

Motor neuropathy leads to the characteristic foot deformities seen in the patient with diabetes. The neuropathy causes atrophy of the small intrinsic muscles of the foot which are needed to help keep the foot in correct alignment.

The changes associated with motor neuropathy lead to a change in the patient's gait causing a redistribution of pressure during walking. The repetitive stress leads to the formation of calluses on the soles of the feet and the development of perforating ulcers due to tissue breakdown. Figure 3.2 shows the deformities that can occur.

Fluid collects beneath the calluses and can be seen on examination as tiny dark spots in the centre of the callus. This is known as a subkeratotic haematoma. The cavity beneath enlarges and eventually ruptures to the skin surface. There is then significant risk of deep infection leading to osteomyelitis.

Patients with hyperglycaemia produce excessive calluses which cause the tissue to become rigid and inflexible. Patients with diabetes frequently have limited joint mobility leading to foot ulceration (Delbridge et al 1983). Recent work has confirmed that this is a result of increased pressure in conjunction with sensory neuropathy. Areas prone to callus formation are shown in Figure 3.3.

Another common deformity is Charcot's deformity in which there is bony dislocation and collapse of the arch of the foot. This is often described as a 'rocker bottom' deformity.

Autonomic neuropathy

The autonomic nerves control sweating and blood flow. Damage to the autonomic nerves leads to lack of

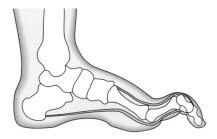

(A) Hammertoes: these develop because of a flexion deformity of the proximal interphalangeal joint. Hammertoe deformities lead to the metatarsal heads being more prominent and bearing more weight. This results in calluses and loss of the protective pad. Claw toe deformity is similar in appearance but is due to the hyperextension of the metatarsal–phalangeal joints.

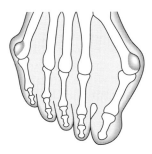

(B) Bunions and bunionettes: these are frequently seen in diabetic patients.

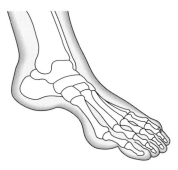

(C) Pes cavus: an excessively high foot arch develops. This is often associated with claw toes and/or callus formation on the dorsal area of the toes and plantar surface of the foot.

Fig. 3.2 Foot deformities in motor neuropathy. (A) Hammertoes: these develop because of a flexion deformity of the proximal interphalangeal joint. Hammertoe deformities lead to the metatarsal heads being more prominent and bearing more weight. This results in calluses and loss of the protective pad. Claw toe deformity is similar in appearance but is due to the hyperextension of the metatarsal–phalangeal joints. (B) Bunions and bunionettes: these are frequently seen in diabetic patients. (C) Pes cavus: an excessively high foot arch develops. This is often associated with claw toes and/or callus formation on the dorsal area of the toes and plantar surface of the foot.

sweating, causing the skin to become dry and cracked. This provides an excellent portal for infection.

Autonomic nerve damage causes the blood vessels to become permanently dilated resulting in poor nutrient exchange. This rush of blood causes a rise in

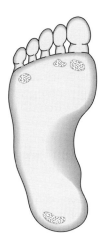

Fig. 3.3 Areas of the foot prone to callus formation.

the venous pressure causing oedema to form. There are small communicating channels called arterio-venous shunts in the foot which normally are kept shut. The dilatation of the vessels allows blood to bypass the capillaries to some extent resulting in nutrient exchange.

Blood flow is increased and pressure in the veins and capillaries is raised leading to oedema which predisposes to ulceration. The patient with autonomic neuropathy has a warm, dry, often numb foot in which the pulses are easily palpated. The foot often appears red.

Peripheral vascular disease in the patient with diabetes

Approximately one-fifth of foot ulcers in patients with diabetes are due to peripheral vascular disease alone (Abbott et al 1990).

Patients with diabetes with peripheral arterial disease tend to have more extensive disease affecting several arteries and affecting both limbs. The more distal arteries such as the peroneal and tibial are often affected.

Boulton et al (1994) state that peripheral vascular disease does not cause ulceration in isolation but that it occurs in combination with other risk factors such as minor trauma and infection which affect the microcirculation.

These patients have the same signs and symptoms as other people with peripheral disease. The ischaemic foot is cold, extremely painful and lacking in pulses as a result of reduced blood flow. It is possible that you may encounter some patients who have both peripheral vascular disease and sensory neuropathy. This makes assessment of these patients very difficult because the sensory neuropathy masks the symptoms of severe peripheral vascular disease in that they have little pain despite the severity of the disease and possibly gangrene.

Microvessel disease

In addition to disease affecting the large blood vessels, people with diabetes have microvascular disease. The tiny capillaries and arterioles become occluded owing to thickening of the blood vessel wall and the collection of debris, thus reducing local blood flow. It is not yet known how much microvessel disease causes foot ulceration but it is thought that it may cause patches of isolated gangrene on the toes. A common site is the big toe, which turns dusky blue and finally black. Later it becomes dry and shrunken. This is termed 'mummified' gangrene. Toes may fall off as a result of autodebridement.

Infection of the diabetic foot

Infection is the most important complication in the patient with diabetic foot ulceration. A number of studies have shown that the patient with diabetes is less able to deal with infection. Japp & Tooke (1994) suggest that the polymorphonuclear leukocytes lose their phagocytic and bactericidal power thus increasing the risk of infection. It is well known that patients with diabetes who develop an acute infection become hyperglycaemic. It is less clear whether hyperglycaemia itself leads to an increased risk of infection (Rayfield et al 1982).

Whereas in many other types of ulcer infection occurs because of a single pathogen, the diabetic is likely to develop an infection due to a number of organisms (polymicrobial). Box 3.3 indicates the organisms frequently found in the infected diabetic foot ulcer. Typically this involves three to six organisms.

Box 3.3 Organisms frequently found in the infected diabetic foot ulcer

Gram-positive cocci
Staphylococcus aureus
Coagulase-negative staphylococci,
  (e.g. S. epidermis)
Streptococci
Enterococci

Gram-negative bacilli
Enterobacteriaceae,
  e.g. Escherichia coli, Proteus spp., Klebsiella, Enterobacter, Pseudomonas aeruginosa

Anaerobes
Bacteroides spp.
Peptostreptococci

Osteomyelitis is a frequent complication of diabetic foot ulceration. In some cases the normal signs of erythema and warmth accompanying cellulitis are absent.

Self-assessment   10 MINUTES

Suggest three changes occurring in the neuropathic foot which may lead to infection.

FEEDBACK

You could have said that:

- the skin is excessively dry and cracked (this allows microorganisms to penetrate)
- there is a lack of sweating (no bactericidal or enzyme activity to reduce infective organisms on the skin)
- there is loss of pain sensation (including the inability to feel the signs of sepsis which therefore may go unrecognised).

Bacteriology

The bacteria affecting the diabetic foot can be divided into two groups: aerobic and anaerobic organisms.

Self-assessment   2 MINUTES

Using your existing nursing knowledge complete the following statements.

Aerobic organisms require   to survive.

Anaerobic organisms require   to survive.

FEEDBACK

You should have said that aerobic bacteria require oxygen to survive, whereas anaerobic organisms can survive in situations where oxygen is limited.

The most common bacterium causing infection in the diabetic foot ulcer is Staphylococcus aureus. The patient with diabetes has an impaired ability to respond to this organism. Streptococci are often found in the diabetic causing rapidly spreading sepsis. The streptococci release hyaluronidase which causes the already damaged capillaries to become more permeable causing oedema. The toxins produced from the streptococci cause tiny thrombi to form in the small blood vessels which are destroyed. This causes local tissue destruction and patches of gangrene.

Anaerobic organisms do not require oxygen to survive. They flourish in the deep tissues of the foot. Organisms such as *Bacteroides* are frequently isolated —as are more harmful bacteria such as *Clostridium perfringens* which in an environment without oxygen can lead to the development of gas gangrene. Aerobic and anaerobic organisms can quickly spread, causing life-threatening septicaemia.

. . . .

Synergistic infection

Occasionally both streptococci and staphylococci cause a rampant cellulitis which spreads rapidly throughout the foot. If this remains untreated it can lead to gangrene and amputation within a few hours.

The following activity helps you to think through ways of differentiating between ulcers due to neuropathy and those related to ischaemia. It also helps you to appreciate how infection complicates the diagnosis and changes the presenting features.

Activity   **20 MINUTES**

Complete Table 3.1 by filling in as many of the signs and symptoms as you can. We have completed those related to temperature to get you started.

. . . .

FEEDBACK

Table 3.2 is the completed table.

. . . .

Table 3.1			
	Neuropathic signs and symptoms	*Ischaemic signs and symptoms*	*Signs and symptoms of infection*
Temperature	Warm	Cold	Warm/hot
Pain			
Pulses			
Pressure index			
Skin			
Sweating			
Callus formation			
Ulcer formation			
Foot deformity			

Table 3.2

	Neuropathic signs and symptoms	Ischaemic signs and symptoms	Signs and symptoms of infection
Temperature	Warm	Cold	Warm/hot
Pain	Numb—neuritic pain	Pain at rest	Throbbing
Pulses	Bounding	Absent or reduced	Dependent on arterial status
Resting pressure index	Elevated/normal	Reduced	Dependent on arterial status
Skin	Dry, cracked, inelastic and fissured	Cold, red or blue on dependency White on elevation	Erythematous and tense
Sweating	Absent	Normal	Normal
Callus formation	Increased during episodes of hyperglycaemia	None	Often occurs beneath calluses
Ulcer formation	Beneath calluses	At any site—often on the medial surface of the forefoot and lateral surface of the 5th metatarsal head	At any site
Foot deformity	Hammer toes, prominent metatarsal heads, Charcot joint, dropped arch	None	Dependent on whether underlying aetiology is neuropathy or ischaemia

Case Study 6 (p. 102) explores the assessment and management of a patient with neuropathic ulceration. Case Study 7 (p. 105) explores the assessment and management of a patient with neuroischaemic ulceration.

A patient with diabetes may present with a number of rarer skin conditions. These include:

- necrobiosis lipoidica diabeticorum in which there are multiple bilateral plaques on the pretibial region which frequently ulcerate and become infected
- granuloma annulare in which lesions occur on the hands and feet.

3.5 LYMPHATIC ORIGINS

Mortimer (1995) states that 'all oedemas, whatever the underlying cause, are due to an imbalance between capillary filtration and lymph drainage'.

Oedema is due to an increase in extracellular fluid in the tissues which results in swelling. Lymphoedema is defined as oedema resulting from lymphatic failure. When the lymphatics fail, large protein molecules accumulate within the tissues. The retention of fluid is largely due to the osmotic force in this trapped protein. Lymph predominantly relies on local changes in the tissue pressure to ensure flow which is achieved by muscular movement and changes in the patient's position. The exception to this is the large lymphatic vessels, containing smooth muscle that contracts, which act as collecting chambers. Mortimer described the lymphatic system using the following analogy: 'It can be compared to the overflow system of a swimming pool which serves to recycle and filter water back to the pool (tissues) which maintain a consistent fluid level (extracellular volume)'.

Lymphoedema occurs more commonly in the limb than the trunk because there are fewer options in the limbs for the development of collateral drainage. Development of lymphoedema has a detrimental effect on the skin and subcutaneous tissue and gives rise to changes which are characteristic of this condition.

The lymphatic system may fail in two ways:

- primary failure—no extrinsic causes can be found, e.g. congenital absence of lymphatic vessels
- secondary failure—this is due to identifiable extrinsic factors, e.g. infections such as filariasis, bacterial lymphangitis, cellulitis, surgical removal, tumour and radiation therapy.

The physiological mechanisms underlying lymphatic failure are:

- obstruction
- obliteration
- reduction in number
- functional failure.

Lymphoedema is commonly seen in patients with chronic venous ulceration (Plate 3, between pp. 102 and 103). There are two functions involved in this process:

- increase in cellular filtration as a result of venous hypertension
- failure of lymph drainage.

Repeated bouts of cellulitis cause progressive destruction of local lymphatics (Bull et al 1993).

On assessment you will notice characteristic skin changes.

- The skin is thickened. This is confirmed by the inability to pinch a fold of skin at the base of the second toe (Stemmer's sign).
- There are pronounced skin creases or folds.
- There is an abnormal build-up of the outer epidermal layer of the skin (hyperkeratosis).
- Frog-spawn-like residues appear which weep lymph following minor trauma. These are dermal lymphatics (lymphangiomas).
- Increasing hyperkeratosis and trapping of lymph leads to papillomatosis.
- The recurrent bouts of cellulitis lead to increasing swelling and deterioration. Although cellulitis is often caused by bacteria, other organisms such as fungi may be implicated.

Occasionally you will see a patient with an intact lymphatic system who has these skin changes as a result of sitting day and night with the legs in a dependent position. This condition is called elephantiasis nostras or the 'armchair syndrome' (Sneddon & Church 1983).

Self-assessment   10 MINUTES

List the four underlying mechanisms in lymphatic failure.

. . . .

FEEDBACK

The four mechanisms are:

- obstruction of the lymphatic vessels
- obliteration of the lymphatic vessels
- reduction in number of the lymphatic vessels
- functional failure of the lymphatic vessels.

. . . .

3.6 VASCULITIC AND OTHER ORIGINS

Many patients with rheumatoid arthritis suffer with leg ulceration. Pun et al (1990) stated that 10% of patients with this condition developed a leg ulcer at some point. However, the patient with rheumatoid arthritis may have a number of factors that lead to ulceration and cause delayed wound healing. It can be very difficult to decide the true ulcer aetiology in these patients (Cawley 1987).

The aetiologies associated with rheumatoid arthritis are:

- vasculitis
- venous disease

- trauma
- arterial insufficiency.

Vasculitis

Vasculitis is an inflammation of the blood vessel wall. It may affect any artery but most frequently affects the vessels in the legs and feet and can be associated with many different diseases.

Many people assume that all patients with ulceration and rheumatoid disease have vasculitic ulcers but in fact Pun et al (1990) found that vasculitis was only present in 18% of such cases.

Vasculitis is also associated with other conditions such as polyarteritis nodosa and systemic lupus erythematosus. Rare diseases such as pyoderma gangrenosum (du Vivier 1993), which involves rapidly spreading ulceration of the limb, are also thought to be due to vasculitis. Considerable debate exists over whether this is true.

A diagnosis of vasculitis is made by taking a biopsy. However, these findings may be unreliable, particularly if the patient has a long-standing ulcer and the rheumatoid disease is in a quiescent stage. The specific investigations required in the assessment of these patients are discussed in Section 4 on assessment.

Activity   5 MINUTES

Plate 4 (between pp. 102 and 103) shows a vasculitic ulcer due to rheumatoid arthritis. Look closely at the picture and note down any unusual signs around the wound edge that suggest this is a vasculitic ulcer.

. . . .

FEEDBACK

You should have been able to see a deep purple edge around the ulcer. This is frequently seen in patients with acute vasculitis. It indicates that the ulcer is extending and the edge is gangrenous and necrotic. Patients with this condition suffer severe pain especially during dressing changes. Because rheumatoid ulcers occur in the gaiter region you can see that they could easily be thought to be due to venous disease.

. . . .

Venous disease

Pun et al (1990) found that 45.5% of patients had venous disease contributing to their ulceration.

Many rheumatoid patients are very immobile and unable to elevate their legs which exacerbates the situation.

Trauma

Pun also found that 45.5% of patients developed their ulceration following trauma (Pun et al 1990). Patients with rheumatoid arthritis are often taking long-term steroid therapy which causes progressive thinning of the skin. Even a mild trauma to their legs can result in an ulcer that does not heal.

Arterial insufficiency

Both Pun et al (1990) and Negus (1991) warn that patients with rheumatoid arthritis are at greater risk of developing arterial disease, with the disease affecting multiple blood vessels and involving the more distal arteries in the calf and foot. Pun et al (1990) found arterial disease was present in 36.4% of patients. Treatment of these patients is often very difficult, with prolonged hospitalisation and poor results following skin grafting.

Self-assessment   10 MINUTES

Answer the following questions.

1. What percentage of patients with rheumatoid arthritis develop a leg ulcer?
2. Complete the following definition. Vasculitis is

3. What percentage of ulcers were found in Pun's study to be due to vasculitis?
4. Name three conditions other than rheumatoid disease which are associated with vasculitic ulceration.
5. How is vasculitis diagnosed?

FEEDBACK

Your answers should have been as follows.

1. 10% of rheumatoid patients develop a leg ulcer.
2. Vasculitis is an inflammation of the blood vessel wall.
3. In Pun's study 18% of ulcers were due to vasculitis.
4. Three other conditions associated with vasculitic ulceration are polyarteritis nodosa, pyoderma gangrenosum and systemic lupus erythematosus.
5. Vasculitis is diagnosed by biopsy.

The rest of this section briefly considers some of the rarer causes of leg ulceration. However, it is not possible to do true justice to the many complex conditions that may lead to ulceration, which are beyond the scope of this pack.

3.7 MALIGNANCY

Malignancy in leg ulceration is very rare. However, occasionally an ulcer may go through a malignant change.

Plate 5 (between pp. 102 and 103) shows a patient with a chronic venous ulcer that has undergone malignant change. If you look at the picture you can see the raised wound edges and the atypical appearance of the wound bed. This was a typical venous ulcer and has developed into a squamous cell carcinoma called a Marjolin's ulcer after the doctor who first described the development of carcinomas in the scars of burns patients many years after the event. Squamous cell carcinomas may also present as primary cancers. They rarely occur below the age of 45 and are commoner in men. They may spread rapidly into the surrounding tissues and metastasise through the lymphatic system.

Now look at Plate 6 (between pp. 102 and 103). This is another example of a skin cancer, in this case a basal cell carcinoma. Basal cell carcinomas are slow-growing, locally invasive tumours usually presenting in middle or old age. They generally occur on the face, although as this picture shows, they may occur on the leg. The lesions generally grow slowly as a nodule or papule, eventually ulcerating. The lesion heals spontaneously becoming a scab which when removed bleeds but never completely heals. Basal cell carcinomas if left will eventually invade deeper structures.

Other types of skin cancer are sometimes found, and malignant melanomas in particular are reported to be on the increase.

A melanoma is a malignant tumour arising from melanocytes. It may arise from a pre-existing mole or naevus or from normal epidermis. Patients at greatest risks are:

- those with frequent solar exposure
- those with a large number of moles
- those with a family history of melanoma
- those with a previous trauma.

Melanomas usually occur late in life but a third occur in the third and fourth decade. In the UK slightly more females suffer than men, and in women the leg is the commonest site while in men it is the trunk.

Melanomas are classified into four types (see Table 3.3).

Table 3.3 Classification of melanomas	
Type	*Features*
Superficial spreading melanoma	Commonest type. Spreads rapidly, eventually becomes nodular as vertical spread develops
Nodular malignant melanoma	The most dangerous. Rapid spread, by vertical invasion. Varied pigment and ulceration
Acral lentiginous malignant melanoma	Arises on palm or sole
Lentigo malignant melanoma	Arises in an area of lentigo. Papule, nodule or plaque appearance

The prognosis of patients presenting with a melanoma is closely linked to the thickness of the lesion and whether metastases have developed. For patients with deep lesions, only about 30% will still be alive at 5 years, whilst of those with very superficial lesions of less than 1 mm depth, 99% will survive. Patients who have had a melanoma are at significant risk of developing a second tumour.

3.8 HAEMATOLOGICAL ORIGINS

A number of haematological disorders are associated with leg ulceration. These include sickle cell disease, polycythemia and thalassaemia. The mechanisms leading to ulceration are complex and are the subject of debate. In many of these conditions tiny thrombi develop in the microcirculation, leading to tissue ischaemia and the development of punched-out, painful ulcers. Patients with sickle cell disease and thalassaemia tend to be younger, whereas polycythemia is found in older patients.

3.9 INFECTION

Infection is often a result rather than a cause of leg ulceration. However, in tropical climates ulceration may develop following infection causing tropical ulcers. One example of this is yaws (tropical granulomatous spirochaetal disease). Ulceration may develop in childhood and fail to heal. Treatment involves high-dose penicillin. Patients with acquired immune deficiency syndrome often present with severe, infective skin lesions. Drug addicts who inject drugs into their veins often develop intractable leg ulceration as a result of phlebitis and infection from dirty needles. These patients are also at increased risk of developing AIDS. AIDS patients may present with Kaposi's sarcoma (idiopathic haemorrhagic sarcoma). Multiple, blue-red plaques and nodules develop on the foot and leg which may ulcerate. The limb becomes grossly oedematous owing to the lymphatic destruction. Lesions may develop elsewhere on the body, including the tip of the nose and the neck.

3.10 HYPERTENSION

In the historical literature there is a description of a hypertensive ulcer known as Martorell's ulcer. This type of ulcer is thought to occur in patients with uncontrolled high blood pressure who present with ulceration on the back of the leg due to arteriolar narrowing. Little research evidence exists to prove whether such an ulcer exists or whether this type of ulcer is due to another cause such as arterial or venous disease.

3.11 TRAUMA

Plate 7 (between pp. 102 and 103) shows a picture of a patient with a traumatic ulcer. This patient had normal venous and arterial circulation and the reason he did not heal remains unclear, although in this case a long delay in seeking treatment may have caused irreparable damage to his microcirculation and the development of underlying osteomyelitis. We do not know.

3.12 IATROGENIC ULCER

The dictionary definition of iatrogenic is 'induced in a patient by a doctor's actions or treatment'. However, this definition can easily be extended to the role of the nurse.

Activity 10 MINUTES

Can you think of any nursing action that could cause an ulcer to develop or an existing one to break down?

FEEDBACK

You may have mentioned:

- removing dressings that are adhering to the wound bed causing the wound to bleed

- using topical agents or dressings that cause an allergic reaction
- cleaning the wound aggressively during cleansing
- causing tissue necrosis through applying bandages tightly over bony prominences.

You may have also made many other suggestions.

● ●

3.13 FACTITIOUS ULCERATION

It is often reported anecdotally that patients deliberately tamper with their ulcers to prevent healing or cause them to recur. However, there is little empirical evidence to suggest that patients with leg ulcers do this. Practical problems such as skin irritation may cause a patient to scratch to alleviate the condition and result in professionals labelling him or her as factitiously causing the leg ulcer. Even if this is occurring, labelling patients in this way does little

to help them with the problem. Brenman & Serafin (1992) discuss the issue of factitious problems in some detail highlighting that Hippocrates recognised this phenomenon in 400 BC.

| Activity | 45 MINUTES |

Make a note of any evidence of your own patients' tampering with their ulcers, or instances when this might be assumed.

Then write a short résumé of what your response to this situation was.

● ●

FEEDBACK

Whatever the circumstances might be, it is important to respond sensitively.

● ●

SUMMARY

In this section you have learned the following things.

- Venous ulceration is the commonest type of ulceration and is predominantly caused by venous hypertension which damages the microcirculation.
- Arterial ulceration is the second largest category of ulceration predominantly caused by atherosclerosis leading to progressive occlusion of the arteries and tissue necrosis.
- The underlying pathophysiology of the patient with a diabetic foot ulcer is complex. Ulceration may result

from neuropathy or ischaemia but is frequently a combination of both, complicated by the risk of infection in the immune-compromised patient.

- Lymphoedema is frequently seen in patients with venous ulceration and complicates the management of these patients.
- The patient with rheumatoid arthritis is prone to ulceration. The aetiology is complex and may involve vasculitis, trauma, and venous or arterial insufficiency.

REFERENCES

Abbott R D, Brand F N, Kannel W B 1990 Epidemiology of some peripheral arterial findings in diabetic men and women: experiences from the Framingham Study. American Journal of Medicine 88: 376–381

Boulton A J M, Kubrusly D B, Bowkder J H, Gadia M, Quintero L C, Skyler J S et al 1986 Impaired vibratory perception and diabetic foot ulceration. Diabetic Medicine 3: 335–357

Boulton A J M, Connor H, Cavanagh P R (eds) 1994 The foot in diabetes, 2nd edn. John Wiley, Chichester

Brenman S, Serafin D 1992 Factitious problems in wound healing. In: Cohen I K, Diegelmann R F, Lindblad W J (eds) Wound healing: biochemical and clinical aspects. W B Saunders, Philadelphia, ch 29

Browse N L, Burnand K G 1982 The cause of venous ulceration. Lancet ii: 243–245

Bryant R A 1992 Acute and chronic wounds: nursing management. Mosby, St. Louis

Bull R H, Gane J N, Evans J, Joseph A E, Mortimer P S 1993 Abnormal lymph drainage in patients with chronic venous

leg ulcers. Journal of American Academic Dermatology 28: 585–590

Callam M J, Ruckley C V, Harper D R, Dale J J 1985 Chronic ulceration of the leg: extent of the problem and provision of care. British Medical Journal 290: 1855–1856

Cawley M I 1987 Vasculitis and ulceration in rheumatic diseases of the foot. Baillière's Clinical Rheumatology 1(2): 315–333

Chant A D B 1990 Tissue pressure, posture and venous ulceration. Lancet 336: 1050–1051

Coleridge Smith P D, Thomas P, Scurr J H, Dormandy J A 1988 Causes of venous ulceration: a new hypothesis. British Medical Journal 296: 1726–1727

Cornwall J, Dore C J, Lewis J D 1986 Leg ulcers: epidemiology and aetiology. British Journal of Surgery 73: 693–696

Cullum N 1994 The nursing management of leg ulcers in the community: a critical review of research. Department of Health, HMSO, London

Dale J J 1995 The aetiology of leg ulceration. In: Cullum N, Roe B (eds) Leg ulcers: nursing management: a research based guide. Scutari, London

Delbridge L, Appleberg M, Reeves T S 1983 Factors associated with the development of foot lesions in the diabetic. Surgery 93: 78–82 du Vivier A 1993 Skin manifestation of disordered circulation. In du Vivier A (ed) Atlas of clinical dermatology, 2nd edn. Gower Medical Publishing, London, ch 21

Edwards A T, Blann A D, Suraz-Mendez V J 1994 Systemic responses in patients with intermittent claudication after treadmill exercise. British Journal of Surgery 81: 1738–1741

Fernando D J S, Hutchinson A, Veves A, Gokal R, Boulton A J M 1991 Risk factors for non-ischaemic foot ulceration in diabetic nephropathy. Diabetic Medicine 8(3): 223–225

Harding Rains A J, Mann C V (eds) 1988 Bailey and Love's short practice of surgery. Lewis, London, p 113

Herrick S E, Sloan P, McGurk M, Freak L, McCullum C N, Ferguson M W J 1992 Sequential changes in histological pattern and extracellular matrix deposition during the healing of CVI. American Journal of Pathology 141(5): 1085–1095

Higley H R, Ksander G A, Gerhardt C O, Falanga V 1995 Extravasation of macromolecules and possible trapping of transferring growth factor in venous ulceration. British Journal of Dermatology 132: 79–85

Japp A J, Tooke J E 1994 Is microvascular disease important in the diabetic foot? In: Boulton A J M, Connor H, Cavanagh P R (eds) The foot in diabetes, 2nd edn. Wiley, Chichester

Mortimer P S 1990 Investigation and management of lymphoedema. Vascular Medicine Review 1: 1–20

Mortimer P S 1995 Managing lymphoedema. Clinical and Experimental Dermatology 20: 98–106

Negus D 1991 Leg ulcers: a practical approach to management. Butterworth Heinemann, Oxford

Pun Y L W, Barraclough D R E, Muirdeu K D 1990 Leg ulcers in rheumatoid arthritis. Medical Journal of Australia 153(10): 585–587

Rayfield E J, Ault M J, Keusch G T, Brothers M S, Nechemias C, Smith H 1982 Infection and diabetes: the case for glucose control. American Journal of Medicine 72: 439–450

Robbins S L 1967 Pathology. Saunders, Philadelphia, p 58

Rose G 1991 Epidemiology of atherosclerosis. British Medical Journal 303: 1537–1539

Ross R 1986 The pathogenesis of atherosclerosis—an update. New England Journal of Medicine 314(8): 488–500

Sneddon I B, Church R E 1983 Practical dermatology, 4th edn. Edward Arnold, London, p 166

Stewart C P, Jain A S, Ogston S A 1992 Lower limb amputee survival. Prosthetics and Orthotics International 16:11–18

Struckmann J 1995 The pathophysiology of venous ulceration. Scope on Phlebology and Lymphology 2(3): 12–15

Young M J, Boulton A J M 1991 Guidelines for identifying the at-risk foot. Practical Diabetes 8(3): 103–105

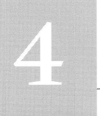

4 Assessment

Introduction

Assessment is a process which is comprehensive, structured and ongoing. It is an essential prerequisite to the effective planning of care. Moffatt et al (1994) highlighted the poor quality of nursing assessment in a study of wound care practice within a community trust. In 34% of patients the underlying aetiology of the ulcer had not been recorded, yet treatment was still proceeding. It is difficult to understand on what basis the treatment decisions were being made. Interestingly, this study also highlighted that 45% of treatment decisions were made by the district nurse alone.

The focus of this section is on the process of assessment. We have divided the process into seven stages:

- preparing
- greeting
- exploring
- observing
- measuring
- summarising
- referring.

Whilst these stages are described separately, there is often considerable overlap between them, especially exploring, observing and measuring. We have used at times a case history drawn from clinical practice to illustrate the complexities of the assessment process. In addition, these issues are further explored in the case studies in Section 6.

LEARNING OUTCOMES

When you have completed this section you should be able to:

- discuss the factors which are important in preparing for a comprehensive assessment of the patient with leg ulceration
- explain the factors involved in initiating a therapeutic relationship with patients and carers
- display the interpersonal skills required to collect information in order to further develop that therapeutic relationship
- describe the process of interpreting the information collected through exploration and observation

- explain how measurement enhances the process of exploration and observation
- outline the process of summarising the assessment, formulating a plan of care and referring to other members of the multidisciplinary team.

4.1 PREPARING

It is hard to say where preparing begins. We have used the word in its broadest sense. It may be that preparing begins with a consideration of the philosophy of your place of work and the writing of guidelines, policies or standards.

There is no doubt that there are many practical considerations which will vary according to where you work, but whether you work in an institutional setting or in the patient's home, you will need to consider the following.

Activity   30 MINUTES

Table 4.1 identifies some of the areas in which you need to make preparation when assessing leg ulcers. Look at each area, then write in the appropriate column some of the considerations which you will need to think about. Some examples have already been given to help you.

FEEDBACK

Documentation

It is the responsibility of any professional group to keep an accurate written account of their practice. These documents should be structured and comprehensive. One way of achieving this is to use a framework such as a nursing model. You may, however, decide to use a multidisciplinary format, in which case other professionals need to be involved in its development and a pure nursing model might not then be appropriate. A newer concept, which encourages patient partnership, is the use of patient-held records. This concept challenges the traditional view

Table 4.1			
Documentation	*Making contact*	*Equipment*	*Other*
Agreed guidelines	Appointment system	Wound swabs	Access to toilets

of the patient as a passive receiver of care. Whatever the design, the most important consideration of all is that the documentation is accurately and regularly completed.

Making contact

Sometimes patients will refer themselves to a nurse whilst others will be referred by other professionals. In either case, an appointment system needs to be in place. In some cases this may consist of a simple telephone call, in others it may involve a more formal system. At times it may be appropriate to send patients preparatory information about what to expect on their first assessment and any requirements such as the production of a urine specimen.

Equipment

In addition to the notes, basic equipment required for the assessment of a patient with a leg ulcer would include:

- hand-held Doppler ultrasound machine with spare battery, headphones and acoustic coupling gel
- sphygmomanometer
- tape measure
- wound mapping equipment or camera if possible
- gloves, aprons, scissors, disposal bags, etc.
- wound swabs
- blood glucose testing strips and glucometer if possible
- sterile dressing packs.

Other considerations

Many patients are assessed and treated in institutional settings such as community clinics, hospital outpatient clinics or wards. If this is the case, a number of structural factors need to be considered, such as:

- a designated clinical area
- ease of access
- reception facilities
- a waiting area

- access to toilets
- refreshment facilities where appropriate
- an efficient transport service
- referral systems to other professionals.

Good preparation provides the basis for a sound therapeutic relationship. Attention to detail helps to create an environment conducive to building relationships. There is nothing worse than the poorly prepared nurse who does not know the patient in front of him or her, who does not have the appropriate equipment to hand, and who is frequently distracted.

4.2 GREETING

The first impression which a patient has on meeting you may affect the whole of the way in which he or she accepts and responds to care. Staff are increasingly working in stressful environments with a pressure on time and resources.

Activity   45 MINUTES

Read the following scenario carefully.

Mrs G., who is wheelchair bound, arrives at the clinic with her husband. This is their first visit. Having battled to push the wheelchair through two sets of swing doors, they arrive at the reception desk.

Mrs G.'s husband asks where to go for the ulcer clinic. The receptionist, barely looking up, points down a corridor.

Mr and Mrs G. arrive at the room with the sign saying 'Ulcer Clinic'. Unsure what to do Mr G. knocks timidly at the door. The door opens and a rather harassed nurse appears and says, 'Yes?' Mr G. explains that his wife has an appointment. The nurse tells them to sit and wait. Mr G. positions the wheelchair in the corridor but is worried that it is causing an obstruction. There seems to be no other alternative.

Mr and Mrs G. sit and wait, Mrs G. nervous and withdrawn, Mr G. becoming increasingly anxious and irritated. Staff go in and out of the clinic; no-one speaks to either of them. 50 minutes later, the door opens and the nurse tells them to come in. Mr G. pushes the wheelchair through the door but is unsure where to go and hesitates. The nurse abruptly tells him to go behind the screens and get his wife ready.

What four practical things could you alter within this health care setting to make the situation less stressful for patients?

FEEDBACK

There are a number of practical things that can be done to improve this situation. Some of the possibilities are easier to achieve than others.

- Mr and Mrs G. have difficulty gaining entrance to the building. Much can be done to assist this. Automatic doors could be fitted and ramps provided for wheelchairs. Hospitals and clinics are now required to provide good facilities for disabled patients.
- Mr G. is forced to ask where the clinic is. Appropriate signposts would help this situation. Receptionist staff are part of the wider team, and should realise how important a friendly greeting is. Training could be requested to improve the situation.
- You may have found yourself in a similar situation to Mr and Mrs G., unsure whether to knock or go into a room. The nurse greeting the couple should have been welcoming in her approach and given clear information as to what would happen. Waiting can often occur in a busy clinical area. Patients are usually very understanding if the situation is clearly explained. During the waiting period, patients and relatives can be given literature to read concerning their visit and treatment. This immediately helps to allay anxiety. A cup of tea is also welcome if appropriate.
- The nurse should immediately be assessing the nonverbal communication occurring. Mr G. is anxious and irritated but Mrs G. is withdrawn. It is easy to notice demanding people but it is also essential for the nurse to recognise how frightened both Mr and Mrs G. are. To professionals, the health care environment seems normal but to patients it may appear frightening. Leg ulcer patients are repeatedly reported to be non-compliant. The therapeutic nurse–patient relationship begins at this initial meeting.

Activity   45 MINUTES

Observe a colleague greeting a patient. Make detailed notes of your observations in terms of what is said, any nonverbal communication and any restriction in the environment, e.g. cramped conditions and time constraints. Make your notes as soon as you can *after* the event before you forget the details of what you saw, then put a tick against those events which you think represented a benefit to the patient and a cross against those which did not.

FEEDBACK

We obviously do not know what you saw but hopefully you were able to spot some elements of practice which either need to be improved or which were examples of good practice. It is common to dwell on the negative aspects of practice but it can be more useful to recognise good practice and understand how this was achieved.

Activity   10 MINUTES

Read the following two scenarios carefully. Compare the two. Are there any advantages or disadvantages in either approach? Which do you feel more comfortable with?

Scenario 1

Mr G. struggles to lift his wife from the wheelchair to the couch. The nurse returns, clutching a Doppler machine, stethoscope and a set of notes. The space is cramped and Mr G. is unsure whether to sit or stand. The nurse appears not to notice this but remains standing at the end of the couch. Mrs G. appears withdrawn, her eyes cast down and her hands tightly knotted together. Mr G. fusses over his wife, correcting her pillow and insisting that she remove her coat. The nurse is clearly irritated by this and suggests that Mr G. should wait outside while she attends to his wife. Mr G. attempts to protest but agrees somewhat reluctantly. The nurse takes a rapid history and fills in the relevant documentation. Mrs G. is only able to answer some of the questions and appears to know little about her previous history. At the end of the assessment, the nurse concludes that Mrs G. has a venous ulcer and that compression therapy is required. Following treatment Mr G. is asked back into the room and told when his wife must next attend clinic. He is handed an educational leaflet and told to phone if there are any problems. He leaves without protest.

Scenario 2

Mr G. is shown into a cubicle with his wife. The nurse asks if he would like help in moving his wife on to the couch. He says that he can manage. The nurse stays nearby in case help is needed.

The nurse returns to the cubicle and introduces herself to Mr and Mrs G. She explains that she will be responsible for Mrs G.'s care and that they can contact her during the day if they are experiencing problems. The cubicle is very small and the nurse offers to move the wheelchair so that they can all sit down comfortably.

The nurse notes that Mr G. continues to look anxious and Mrs G. remains withdrawn and non-communicative. The nurse lays down the notes she has brought to fill in and asks them to tell her what has been happening.

Mr G. takes the lead. He explains that the ulcer has been present for 6 months. During this time he has dressed the ulcer using dressings prescribed by the general practitioner. The nurse asks if he has been offered professional help from the district nurse. He says that he has but that this was not necessary. He continues to give an accurate medical history and describes the drugs which Mrs G. takes. Occasionally he turns for clarification to his wife who nods when prompted. The nurse turns to Mrs G. and asks how she is feeling. She says that she is fine and turns to her husband for reassurance. The nurse suspects that there are other problems they are not yet able to talk about.

The nurse completes her nursing assessment, explaining carefully what she is doing at every stage. At the end of the assessment, it is clear that Mrs G. has a venous ulcer requiring compression therapy. During the dressing procedure, the nurse prompts Mr G. to tell her a little more about the situation and the difficulties of caring for his wife who is now very immobile from osteoarthritis. Initially, he offers no further information. It is only as the nurse turns to leave the cubicle that he blurts out that all is not well.

Mr G.'s eyes fill with tears and with a sense of relief he tells of his wife's rapid deterioration. He suspects that she is suffering from senile dementia and has been living in fear that they will be separated. This has forced him to refuse help for her leg ulcer, but he now has to admit that he can no longer cope.

FEEDBACK

We would anticipate that you feel more comfortable with Scenario 2 which illustrates a holistic approach

to the assessment of Mr and Mrs G. The nurse uses interpersonal skills to show empathy, pick up non-verbal communication, give encouragement and begin to build a therapeutic relationship. As a result, Mr G. is able to share his experiences and fears with the nurse and consequently the assessment is much 'richer', revealing that the leg ulcer was only one problem of many.

We find it difficult to see any advantages in Scenario 1 other than that the clinic appointment system is likely to run like clockwork and the nurse can remain emotionally detached. These have traditionally been, and still may be, important considerations for some nurses but lead to assessments in which much valuable information is withheld or overlooked. These scenarios illustrate two approaches to care described by Kasch & Knutson (1985) as either 'position centred' or 'person centred'.

The position-centred approach

Professions such as nursing and medicine are often power centred. This means that the professional has complete authority over the patient and carer who must comply completely with instructions given by the nurse. Scenario 1 is a good example of this approach.

The person-centred approach

A person-centred approach to nursing is used in Scenario 2. The nurse is able to incorporate a knowledge of the patient and carer's health beliefs and views the patient as an equal.

You can see that the two approaches above produce different information. Drew (1986) makes an interesting observation about the power relationship between nurses and their patients.

> When there is an imbalance of authority and power, as in the patient/care giver relationship, the person who is dependent is vulnerable to the emotional message of the other.
>
> Should we not ask ourselves what is wrong with the way we provide care? Why is clinical competence not enough? Might not impersonal albeit expert care be as negligent as outright technical incompetence?

4.3 EXPLORING

The process of building a therapeutic relationship has already begun. As Mr G. begins to talk more freely, the nurse is able to develop her exploration of the underlying problems. It is interesting to note that, up until now, most of the insight gained by the nurse has come from Mr G. Whilst the couple should not be divided for assessment purposes, the process of exploration should draw out Mrs G.'s experience of living with her leg ulcer. The nurse is now faced with the task of drawing Mrs G. into the conversation.

Activity 15 MINUTES

If you were faced with Mrs G.'s reluctance to speak can you suggest how you might go about drawing her into the conversation?

FEEDBACK

This is a difficult question to answer. Much depends on the characters of Mr and Mrs G. If Mrs G. has become reliant on Mr G. to communicate for both of them, it will be quite a challenge to get her to drop her passive stance. Some practical strategies might include:

• directing the questioning to Mrs G.
• maintaining eye contact with her
• asking open-ended questions rather than those requiring yes or no answers
• becoming an 'active listener' by prompting her, encouraging her to restate things and trying not to use terms she will not understand
• thinking about your tone of voice and the speed at which you speak
• if Mr G. answers the question directed at his wife, acknowledging his answer but shifting the focus back to her as quickly as possible
• if all else fails, trying to find an opportunity to be alone with Mrs G.

Using these techniques, the nurse manages to encourage Mrs G. to talk about the situation she finds herself in. A number of insights into the quality of life for her and her husband begin to emerge as she speaks.

'I can't remember how long I've had this ulcer but it isn't getting any better. I don't really know what caused it but I do remember banging my leg.' Mr G. interrupts and tells the nurse, 'the doctor said it was due to her circulation but he didn't tell us anything else.' The nurse asks him if he has ever been given any more information. He says he has not. Mrs G. continues, 'I hardly get out at all these days. It's just too difficult. Not only can't I walk but I'm afraid people will bang into my leg. I've even stopped having the grandchildren over. I was too frightened to sit them on my knee in case they bang my leg. To

tell the truth, the family don't visit often now. I know they're busy but I think they notice the smell when they come. I'm not myself these days, I keep forgetting things. I find myself bursting into tears for no reason. I'm very tired, the pain from the ulcer keeps me awake at night and I can't be bothered to do things during the day. I've noticed that we don't go out as much as we did. I'm sure people can smell the ulcer; that's another reason for staying indoors.'

Activity 10 MINUTES

Using the scenario above, list ten quality of life issues that Mr and Mrs G. face.

FEEDBACK

You could have mentioned hopelessness, lack of knowledge, isolation, fear of trauma, smell from the ulcer, reduced mobility, pain, depression and worry, tiredness, sleeplessness.

Hopelessness

Mrs G. does not seem very hopeful that her leg ulcer is healing. Roe et al (1995) found in a study of 88 patients that 77% felt that they were improving but that 15% were resigned to having an ulcer.

Knowledge

Mr and Mrs G. do not seem to really understand what has caused her leg ulcer and why it will not heal. This situation is quite common. Roe in the same study found that 20% of patients did not know or could not remember the cause of their ulcer. Mrs G. does not seem to want to know more about her condition and is fairly passive about the situation. 60% of patients in one study did not wish for more information on their ulcer or related issues. Leg ulcer patients as a group appear passive towards their situation. This may be because they have given up hope of healing and have low expectations from those providing care.

Isolation and fear of trauma

Mr and Mrs G. seem to avoid going out because of her fear that her leg may be knocked or that people will notice her leg ulcer. Her family are not visiting as frequently either. A number of authors have shown that leg ulceration leads to increasing social isolation. Hyland et al (1994) found that 38% of patients never shopped in crowded areas, 26% were afraid to sit children on their knee and 34% kept away from cats. Roe et al (1995) found that 80% of patients felt that they were going out less frequently owing to their ulcer, pain or discomfort. 27% noted reduced contact with friends and noted interference in their daily activities.

Smell from the ulcer

Mrs G. refers on two occasions to the smell of her ulcer. She notes that this reduces her social contact with her family and is an embarrassment in public places. Roe found that 49% of patients felt that other people noticed their ulcer and 55% of patients found this upsetting. These patients had a significantly poorer quality of life with higher levels of anxiety and depression. This situation was made worse if patients were unable to leave their homes and became socially isolated. Van Toller (1994) states that the malodour associated with leg ulcers is due to putrescine and cadaverine, both of which induce a gag reflex. He states that the malodorous smell is constantly detectable, unlike pleasant smells, which one quickly gets used to.

Reduced mobility

Mrs G. appears to have reduced mobility, although it is difficult to know whether this is due to fear of further trauma or other problems. She also suffers with severe osteoarthritis. A number of studies have noted that leg ulcer patients are often immobile (Moffatt et al 1992). It is sometimes difficult to know whether this is due to other factors such as arthritis, or to the ulcer itself. Hyland et al (1994) found that 40% of patients had difficulty getting on and off a bus, 30% had difficulty climbing stairs, and 37% had restricted travel due to their ulcer. Moffatt et al (1992) found that 50% of patients had limitations in mobility with 11% of these requiring transportation to a community clinic.

Pain

Mrs G. experiences considerable pain. It is only in recent years that it has been acknowledged that patients with venous ulcers suffer varying degrees of pain. In the Riverside study, Franks et al (1994) found that 80% of patients with venous ulcers experienced pain. Roe et al (1995) found that pain scores were higher in the ulcer group than the control group and that pain increased with ulcer size and reduced arterial circulation.

Depression and worry over ulcer

Mrs G. recognises that her mood has deteriorated and that she finds herself bursting into tears more often. Depression has been consistently noted in the quality of life research of leg ulcer patients. Franks et al (1994) noted that there was a significant reduction in depression, anxiety, hostility and cognition following effective treatment, with changes in depression and hostility related to complete ulcer healing. Roe et al (1995) noted that 90% of patients found their ulcer was a source of worry and that patients with leg ulcers had significantly higher rates of depression than matched controls.

Tiredness/sleeplessness

Mrs G. clearly states that the pain from her leg ulcer disturbs her sleep and leaves her feeling tired, irritable and lacking in energy. A number of studies have highlighted the relationship between pain from the ulcer and lack of sleep. Hyland (1994) found that patients in pain suffered from lack of sleep and during the day were preoccupied with their ulcer and had a generally poorer quality of life. Roe et al (1995) found that 74% of patients had interrupted sleep which in 69% of cases was due to pain.

It is possible to see from only one patient how many quality of life issues are raised. The literature raises other points which we will cover briefly to complete the picture.

Interference with daily activities

Many patients find that leg ulceration affects even simple daily activities. Roe et al (1995) found that 90% had problems in washing or bathing, 82% with dressing and 78% experienced problems with ill-fitting footwear.

Caring for relatives

Little is known concerning the role of leg ulcer patients as carers. However, Roe found that 18% (16 people) in her study were carers, that 10 of these had difficulty caring for their relatives, and this increased their levels of anxiety.

Sex

Only 3% of patients in the Riverside study had an active sex life (Moffatt et al 1992). Roe et al (1995) reported three people in a population of 88. While this might be explained partly by the fact that many ulcer patients are elderly, the issue may be very important in younger patients and the smell associated with the ulcer will almost certainly have a detrimental effect on relationships.

Positive aspects of leg ulceration

Anecdotal accounts of patients wishing to keep their ulcer for secondary gain are common (Muir Gray 1983). However, little is available in the research evidence to support this suggestion. Roe et al (1995), however, found that 10 patients reported positive aspects of leg ulceration. These related to the support services (such as district nurses) that were available and warn us of the dependency that patients may develop if the ulcer does not heal. Mrs G.'s case study highlighted the suffering associated with leg ulceration and the way in which it affects the patient's quality of life. It is only recently that the impact of this aspect of leg ulceration has been recognised.

In addition to the quality of life issues, a detailed exploration should build a rich picture of the background to the patient, family and environment, such as:

- previous medical history including medication
- previous nursing history including treatment
- social circumstances, e.g. occupation, home environment, support services, dependency
- health beliefs
- signs and symptoms and ulcer history
- risk factors
- nutritional status.

The first four aspects are explored in the case studies where it is possible to present a more realistic picture of such complex issues. The last three will be considered in the next part of this section.

Certain medical conditions and risk factors are also linked to the individual types of leg ulcer.

Signs and symptoms and ulcer history

Venous and ischaemic ulcers are associated with characteristic signs and symptoms.

Activity   20 MINUTES

Box 4.1 lists an assortment of signs, symptoms, extracts from medical histories and risk factors. Use the space on the right to identify whether they are venous (V) or arterial (A).

FEEDBACK

The signs and symptoms, medical history and risk factors are grouped correctly in Table 4.2. If you have been able to get most of these right you should be on your way to being competent at making a differential diagnosis between venous and arterial ulceration.

Box 4.1 Signs, symptoms, medical history and risk factors: venous or arterial ulceration?

Ulcer on dorsum of foot	Familial link
Ankle flare	Pain on walking in thigh relieved by rest
Thrombophlebitis	Poor capillary refilling time
Warm leg	Gangrene
Calf pain on walking relieved by rest	Prominent veins
Varicose eczema	Aching heavy legs
Shiny hairless limb	Ulcer in gaiter region
Varicose veins	Loss of calf muscle
Nocturnal pain	Trophic nail bed changes
Atrophe blanche	Transient ischaemic attacks
Fixed ankle joint	High blood cholesterol
Reddish blue foot on dependency	Mild ankle swelling
Hyperkeratosis	Pigmentation
Cerebrovascular accident	Previous arterial surgery
Previous varicose vein surgery or injection sclerotherapy	Absent, diminished pedal pulses
Normal pedal pulses	Pulmonary embolism
Leg blanches on elevation	Dependency oedema
Pain in forefoot and toes at rest	Smoking
Deep vein thrombosis	Cold leg
	Myocardial infarction

Table 4.2 Venous vs arterial ulceration: signs and symptoms, medical history and risk factors

Venous	Arterial
Signs and symptoms	Signs and symptoms
Ankle flare	Ulcer on dorsum of foot
Warm leg	Calf pain on walking relieved by rest
Varicose eczema	Shiny hairless limb
Varicose veins	Nocturnal pain
Atrophe blanche	Reddish blue foot on dependency
Fixed ankle joint	Leg blanches on elevation
Hyperkeratosis	Pain in forefoot and toes at rest
Normal pedal pulses	Cold leg
Prominent veins	Poor capillary refilling time
Aching, heavy legs	Gangrene
Ulcer in gaiter region	Trophic nail bed changes
Loss of calf muscle	Pain in thigh on walking relieved by rest
Mild ankle swelling	Absent, diminished pedal pulses
Pigmentation	Dependency oedema
Medical history and risk factor	Medical history and risk factor
Thrombophlebitis	Cerebrovascular accident
Previous varicose vein surgery	Smoking
or injection sclerotherapy	Myocardial infarction
Deep vein thrombosis	Transient ischaemic attacks
Familial link	High blood cholesterol
Pulmonary embolism	Previous arterial surgery

Risk factors

In Section 1.1 you saw that risk factors are important in showing us how a disease will progress. The following activity explores these issues further.

Activity 45 MINUTES

Read Article 5 in the Reader (p. 135), then answer the following questions.

1. What two roles does a risk factor play?
2. Why is it important to identify a risk factor for disease?
3. How certain is it that obesity is a risk factor for the development of varicose veins?
4. What did the Tubingen study find happened to women in pregnancy?
5. What factors were found to prolong venous ulcer healing?

FEEDBACK

1. A risk factor:
   a. identifies patients who are predisposed to develop the disease
   b. helps predict the progression, severity and outcome of the disease.

2. Identifying a risk factor for a disease helps to plan preventive care targeted at the people who are at greatest risk of developing the condition.

3. This answer is not as straightforward as it seems. Many studies referred to in the paper failed to take account of patients' height. When both height and weight are taken into consideration, height is the more important risk factor owing to the increased hydrostatic pressure. However, many patients who are overweight are also immobile which shows that a combination of risk factors can be most detrimental.

4. The Tubingen study found that in women who had had two or more pregnancies, the risk of developing varicose veins had doubled.

5. It was found that venous ulcer healing was prolonged by old age, large ulcer size, long ulcer duration, reduced general mobility and limited ankle movement. You may have also noted down treatment at home and being male. These were weak risk factors and probably indicate other problems in these patients.

Nutrition and wound healing

Nutrition is recognised as an important consideration in wound healing. Poor nutrition may result in weak scars and failure to heal (McLaren 1992).

Read Article 6 in the Reader (p. 139), then use the content of this article to identify questions which you might use in an assessment of Mrs G.'s nutritional status. Make two lists as follows:

- in the left-hand column write down the questions you would ask
- in the right-hand column write down the reasoning behind your questions.

Your questions should include any peripheral issues which may affect Mrs G.'s nutritional status, such as well-fitting dentures.

FEEDBACK

We have identified a number of questions that we would ask Mrs G, which we have listed in Table 4.3. You may have thought of many more.

Measuring nutritional status

If you thought Mrs G. was protein deficient, you could measure her serum albumin. A normal measurement is in the region of 35–50 g/l. If it is below 35 g/l you may consider using protein supplements. However, it should be remembered that serum albumin measurements reflect the nutritional status 2–3 weeks before they were taken.

Is Mrs G. anaemic? A routine haemoglobin test should be carried out. Iron supplements may be required.

The paper suggests a number of other measurements that can be used in the severely malnourished patient. These are:

- serum transferrin
- total protein and lymphocyte count
- creatinine
- vitamin and mineral status.

It should be stressed that whilst assessment of nutritional status and provision of a well-balanced diet are essential components of holistic care, there will be instances when referral to a dietitian will

Table 4.3 Assessing nutritional status	
Question	Reason for asking question
How much protein is Mrs G. eating each day?	Protein is needed for tissue regeneration. Protein deficiency leads to poor wound healing by prolonging the inflammatory response.
How many calories does she need each day?	Calories are needed to provide energy for tissue defence and wound repair. A normal adult requires 1500–3500 calories a day. 50–60% of the calories should be in the form of carbohydrates. More calories are required during periods of illness and infection. Patients with a large leg ulcer may be losing copious amounts of exudate and will require much higher calorific intake to compensate for this loss.
What carbohydrates and fat does she eat?	Carbohydrates and fats are required for energy. Glucose is needed for wound healing. When glucose is not available, the body uses protein and fat to produce glucose.
Does she take adequate amounts of vitamin C?	Vitamin C is found in fresh fruits and vegetables and is required for collagen synthesis and for epithelialisation. Lack of vitamin C causes the capillaries to become fragile, and old scars may reopen owing to degeneration of the cellular matrix. Vitamin C may increase the effectiveness of leukocytes and macrophages. The recommended daily intake of vitamin C is 60 mg. Supplements of up to 250–500 mg have been recommended but this remains open to debate.
Does she take adequate amounts of vitamin A?	Vitamin A is found in egg yolks and fish liver oils and is required to aid the inflammatory stage of healing. It aids the formation of mucopolysaccharides which act as protective sheaths around collagen.
Does she have an adequate fluid intake?	Adequate hydration is essential, particularly when the patient is taking a high protein diet.
Is she normal or abnormal weight?	Recording Mrs G.'s weight and height are important baseline measurements. These two measurements can be used to calculate a body mass index.
Does she have a good appetite?	A poor appetite may be due to her depressed state or another cause.
Does she find difficulty eating?	If she does, this may be due to ill-fitting dentures, mouth ulcers or broken teeth, etc.
Who cooks for her?	Food which is poorly cooked and presented will affect her appetite.

be indicated for more comprehensive assessment and for advice (McLaren 1992). These will include patients with:

- heavily exuding ulcers
- impaired immune defence mechanisms
- debilitating disease
- eating/swallowing disorders
- malabsorption
- terminal disease
- metabolic disorders.

It is sometimes useful to encourage a patient to complete a food diary for 1 week. This will highlight deficiencies in nutritional intake.

4.4 OBSERVING

As a nurse caring for a patient with a leg ulcer you are involved in a complex process of observing and interpreting what is said, what you see and what remains unsaid. The following continuation of the scenario highlights these issues.

The nurse, having listened to Mr and Mrs G., suggests that it is now time to have a look at the wound. She removes Mrs G.'s shoes and stockings and notices that exudate has collected in the bottom of the shoe. As the nurse begins to remove the dressing, she notes that Mrs G. flinches with pain and draws her leg back. The dressings are saturated with exudate. The dressing has stuck slightly to the wound and the nurse uses a little warmed isotonic saline to help with the removal of the dressing. Mr G. hovers anxiously, commenting that the wound has not improved.

Mrs G. has a large venous ulcer on her medial malleolus which is partially covered with yellow slough but with evidence of granulation tissue. She anxiously comments to the nurse about the smell. The edges of the wound are sharply defined and the skin beneath the ulcer around the ankle is red and macerated. The skin on Mrs G.'s leg is otherwise generally dry and flaky. It is pigmented and the leg feels 'woody' to the touch (induration). There is an area of small dilated venules over the medial aspect of her foot just below the ankle. The nurse palpates the leg and can feel a large dilated vein running down the inner side of Mrs G.'s leg. There is some evidence of oedema. Mrs G. has bunions and her toenails need to be cut. The nurse then turns to Mrs G.'s other leg. She notes that this leg also has skin changes, appears dry and flaky and has evidence of varicose veins. She has restricted ankle movement and reduced calf muscle bulk in both legs. The nurse notices how pale and tired Mrs G. seems. Despite the exudate collecting in her shoe, Mrs G. is spotlessly clean and neatly dressed. The nurse asks what

dressings have previously been used. Before Mrs G. can answer, Mr G. interrupts and lists a number of products that have been used, adding that none of them has worked. The nurse senses some conflict between them regarding previous treatment.

You will notice that as the assessment continues the process of exploration has not stopped. As the nurse observes what is in front of her she continues to explore previous treatments. She also begins to interpret the information and starts to draw conclusions, e.g. that Mrs G. is not quite as demented as the nurse has been led to believe. There is also evidence of intuitive thinking on the part of the nurse in that she senses some conflict in their relationship. Whilst objectivity is seen as a critical component in assessment, the use of intuitive thinking remains more controversial and subject to a long-standing debate.

In contrast to the demanding process of trying to piece together a picture of your patient through combining questioning, observation and intuitive feeling, there is the straightforward requirement to accurately record what is seen.

Activity 20 MINUTES

Use the preceding scenario to note which observations made by the nurse regarding Mrs G.'s leg you would consider important to note down in her care plan. We have thought of 16 points.

FEEDBACK

You should have noted the following:

- the ulcer is large
- it is positioned on the medial malleolus
- it is partially covered with yellow slough
- there is evidence of granulation tissue
- the ulcer is malodorous
- the edges of the wound are sharply defined
- the skin beneath the ulcer is red and macerated
- the skin is otherwise dry and flaky on both legs
- the skin is pigmented and 'woody' to the touch
- there are small dilated venules over the medial aspect of the foot just below the ankle (ankle flare)
- there is evidence of varicose veins and skin changes on both legs
- there is some oedema
- Mrs G. has bunions
- her toenails need cutting
- she has restricted ankle movement and reduced calf muscle bulk in both legs
- the patient experiences pain on dressing removal.

Categorising observations

You need to think about how you are going to document your assessment of the wound. You could, of course, list your observations randomly on blank paper as you have done above but we have stressed the importance earlier of structured comprehensive documentation. This documentation is used not only for your own purposes, but to communicate with other professionals. You might, at some stage, need to design your own assessment form and the categories you have defined could be a starting point for such an undertaking.

Activity   15 MINUTES

Look at your observations. Can you group them or categorise them in any way?

· ·

FEEDBACK

Some possible categories might include:

- skin condition
- wound condition
- exudate
- size and site
- pain
- infection.

· ·

Skin condition

Patients with leg ulceration frequently present with a variety of skin conditions. Your assessment tool should have the facility to record:

- erythema
- wet/dry eczema
- evidence of contact dermatitis
- maceration
- hyperkeratosis
- other skin conditions, e.g. psoriasis.

Wound condition

Your assessment tool should have the facility to record:

- stage of wound healing, i.e.

  —granulation
  —epithelialisation
  —yellow slough
  —black eschar
  —other

- assessment of wound margins, e.g. rolled edges may indicate chronicity.

Exudate

Your assessment tool should have the facility to record colour, amount and odour of the exudate.

Size and site

Your assessment tool should have the facility to record size and site. The issue of wound measurement is dealt with later in this section (p. 52).

Pain

Your assessment tool should have the facility to record:

- the presence of pain
- the nature of the pain
- the site of the pain
- the continuity of the pain, e.g. worse at night or during dressing change
- whether the pain is relieved through analgesia
- any other contributory factors that either enhance or relieve pain.

The assessment of pain is dealt with more comprehensively later in this section (p. 55).

Infection

Your assessment tool should have the facility to record:

- whether clinical signs of infection are present
- whether a wound swab has been taken
- results of microbiological investigation
- use of antibiotic therapy when required.

A wide variety of approaches has been used in the design of assessment forms (Morison & Moffatt 1994). Some professionals use a visual approach with diagrams of legs on to which observations can be recorded. Others use a table format. Both have advantages and disadvantages but it is very difficult to design something which covers all eventualities, e.g. multiple ulcers occurring at different times. Whatever format you choose, it is vital that it is seen as one component of a comprehensive assessment document. If you look at the account so far of the complexities of Mrs G.'s case, you can see how difficult it would be to document this.

Activity   10 MINUTES

What constraints can you identify which would make comprehensive efficient documentation more difficult to develop?

FEEDBACK

There are many constraints which you could have identified. Here are some suggestions.

- Time—both in designing the form and completing it
- Relevance—users need to have ownership and see the relevance of the information collected
- Acceptability—to a wide range of personal or professional preferences and also to formal institutional requirements
- Resources—such as designing, printing, etc.

4.5 MEASURING

The process of measurement enhances exploration and observation and adds an objective dimension to the assessment process.

Scenario continued

Having examined Mrs G.'s leg, the nurse measures the wound with a ruler and records its length and width. The wound is shallow and does not require any measurement of depth. There are no signs of infection and the nurse decides not to take a wound swab. The nurse has noted that the patient's signs and symptoms and the appearance of the leg suggest that Mrs G. has a venous ulcer (see Sect. 3). However, it is now important that the nurse assesses Mrs G.'s arterial circulation to check for the presence of any arterial disease by recording a resting pressure index using Doppler ultrasound.

Mrs G. has been sitting upright on a couch during the nursing assessment. The nurse now asks Mrs G. to lie in a semirecumbent position and explains the procedure to her. As Mrs G. reclines, it is obvious that this new position is uncomfortable and causes her pain from her arthritis. The nurse measures Mrs G.'s resting pressure index (RPI) in both legs. Her index is 1.0 in both legs.

In addition to routine measurements of blood pressure, pulse, respiration, height, weight, blood sugar, urinalysis and ankle circumference, the nurse arranges for blood tests for haemoglobin and rheumatoid factor. The assessment so far has shown that pain is a prominent feature in Mrs G.'s life. In order to assess this aspect more fully, the nurse uses the McGill Pain Questionnaire (Melzack & Katz 1992). All these measurements are carefully documented.

The continuation of the scenario above illustrates the way in which precise measurement enhances the ongoing process of assessment. Measurements can be routine or in response to observations of individual needs.

Self-assessment 5 MINUTES

Why has the nurse arranged for blood tests for:

1. haemoglobin
2. rheumatoid factor?

FEEDBACK

1. You may remember that the nurse thought Mrs G. looked pale and tired. Many patients with chronic ulcers present with anaemia which, if severe, may delay healing.
2. Mrs G. presents with severe osteoarthritis. The blood tests for rheumatoid factor will show if she has rheumatoid arthritis which is associated with other types of ulceration (see Sect. 3).

Wound measurement

Activity 30 MINUTES

The scenario describes the use of a ruler to measure the wound.

1. Do you think this method is sufficiently accurate? Give reasons for your answer.
2. What method of measurement do you use in your work?
3. What are the difficulties in measuring wounds?
4. Now read Article 7 in the Reader (p. 143) and compare the answers you have just given to those discussed in the paper.

FEEDBACK

In addition to the issues raised by Plassmann in Reader Article 7, a complementary technique that is becoming more popular is the use of photography in wound assessment. While this can be a difficult technique to master and to some extent is dependent on the quality of the equipment available, it is nevertheless very useful. Bellamy (1995) has written a practical guide to the use of photography in wound assessment. There is no reason why this technique should not become routine nursing practice given the right resources. The objective benefits of photography extend beyond measurement alone. The progress of healing can be recorded visually. This can also have therapeutic benefits to the patient who sees the progress being made. This process could, of course, be counterproductive in a patient whose wound is deteriorating. In either case, the nurse needs an objective record of the progress of the wound.

. . . .

The use of Doppler ultrasound

It is only during the last decade that Doppler ultrasound has been used as part of a nursing assessment. Williams et al (1993) state: 'The adequacy of the vascular supply is perhaps the single most important factor determining the rate of healing in any wound or ulcer'. Traditionally palpation of pedal pulses was the accepted method of determining the adequacy of vascular supply within a nursing assessment. The use of Doppler ultrasound to record a resting pressure index (RPI) is a valuable and more reliable method of assessing the patient's arterial circulation.

An RPI is a comparison between the brachial systolic pressure and the ankle systolic pressure, and these are usually equal in a patient with normal circulation. It is sometimes referred to as the ankle brachial pressure index (ABPI). Any reduction in the ankle systolic reading indicates reduced flow.

You have probably noticed that as a car passes you, the sound you hear changes in tone. The frequency of the sound you hear changes as the source of the sound moves towards you and then away from you. This is the Doppler principle recognised by Christian Doppler, an Austrian physicist. This principle, in a refined form because it uses very high frequency sound, is the basis for the Doppler ultrasound technique (Williams et al 1993). The early Doppler ultrasound devices were quite large but modern devices now available are small, portable and battery operated. The sound can be monitored either through an internal speaker or headphones. Article 8 in the Reader (p. 148) contains an excellent summary of how Doppler works and its use in assessment.

Guidelines for measuring the resting pressure index are given in Box 4.2.

Box 4.2 Guidelines for measuring the resting pressure index

In this procedure like any other, you should explain to the patient what you are doing.

Stage 1
The patient should be lying as flat as possible and be relaxed and comfortable. Williams et al (1993) recommend that the patient should lie in this position for 15–20 minutes before proceeding further.

Stage 2
- Place the sphygmomanometer cuff around the arm and apply ultrasound gel over the brachial pulse.
- Hold the Doppler probe gently over the brachial pulse until a good signal is obtained. This is generally at an angle of 45–60 degrees between the Doppler probe and the artery. As the artery may not be parallel to the skin, the probe angle may need to be adjusted in order to obtain a good signal.
- Inflate the cuff until the signal disappears, then gradually lower the pressure until the signal returns. This is the brachial systolic pressure (no diastolic reading is recordable with Doppler). In order to ensure that you have an accurate reading, repeat the process at least one more time.

Repeat stages 1 and 2 on the other arm. Take the highest reading regardless of which arm it comes from.

Stage 3
- Place the sphygmomanometer cuff around the leg immediately above the ankle, having covered the ulcerated area with cling film or a dressing.

- Try to palpate the dorsalis pedis, anterior tibial, posterior tibial and peroneal pulses (see Sect. 5).
- Locate (isonate) the same pedal pulses using the Doppler probe and gel. Avoid using excessive pressure which may obliterate the signal. The probe angle is generally 45–60°.
- Locate the probe on the strongest pulse you have found.
- Repeat the procedure using all the other pedal pulses if possible. Barnhorst & Barner (1968) noted that the dorsalis pedis pulse was congenitally absent in 12% of the individuals they studied.
- Take the highest of the readings on the affected limb.

Repeat stage 3 on the other limb even if this is not ulcerated.

Stage 4
- To calculate the resting pressure index: divide the ankle pressure by the brachial pressure (a calculator or pre-printed chart can be used to perform this calculation).
- The pressure index should be calculated separately for each leg.
- A normal resting pressure index is generally greater than 1.0. In a healthy adult an index of 0.9 indicates mild arterial disease. An index of below 0.5 indicates severe arterial disease, possibly with ischaemic rest pain.

Activity   15 MINUTES

Answer the following questions about the recording of the resting pressure index (RPI).

1. Why is it important to lay a patient flat?
2. What would you do if you could feel pedal pulses with your finger but cannot locate them using the Doppler machine?
3. What practical problems might you encounter in the clinical area when attempting to record an RPI?
4. How often do you think you should repeat your measurement of RPI?

FEEDBACK

1. It is important to lay the patient flat in order to eliminate the effects of exercise and stress on the blood pressure.
2. It is likely that there are some very practical reasons why you cannot find the patient's pulse. The Doppler device may not be working. The simplest reason is that the battery is flat. A variety of different probes are available. It may be that you are using the wrong one. If you are in a noisy clinical area, you may need to be listening for the pulses using the headphones.

    It could, of course, be that your technique is not very good, e.g. you have the probe at the wrong angle or you are looking in the wrong place!
3. In the scenario Mrs G. has difficulty lying flat. A number of patients may have this problem. Some will only be able to stay sitting in a chair. If this does happen, the ankle pressure will be falsely elevated. This should be noted in the patient's notes. While the technique is not particularly painful, some patients will experience pain during this procedure. Patients with circumferential ulceration over the site of pedal pulses may be especially difficult to assess. Patients with gross obesity or oedema present a challenge in that they may require a larger size of cuff. It may be difficult to record the brachial systolic pressure in patients with atrial fibrillation. People with severe arterial disease and diminished pulses are especially difficult.
4. The use of the Doppler ultrasound should be considered part of the dynamic process of assessment. All patients with a current ulcer should have their RPI checked at least every 3 months. Any patients who present with a change in signs and symptoms, e.g. increased pain, should be reassessed.

Activity   10 MINUTES

Using the following equation:

$$\frac{\text{Ankle systolic pressure}}{\text{Brachial systolic pressure}} = \text{RPI}$$

calculate the following pressure indexes and state what they indicate. We have completed the first one for you.

Brachial systolic pressure	140 mmHg
Ankle systolic pressure	140 mmHg
RPI = 1.0	

Brachial systolic pressure	180 mmHg
Ankle systolic pressure	150 mmHg
RPI =	

Brachial systolic pressure	140 mmHg
Ankle systolic pressure	132 mmHg
RPI =	

Brachial systolic pressure	160 mmHg
Ankle systolic pressure	80 mmHg
RPI =	

FEEDBACK

1. RPI = 1.0; this is normal arterial circulation.
2. RPI = 0.8; provides evidence of significant established arterial disease.
3. RPI = 0.9; indicates a mild degree of arterial disease.
4. RPI = 0.5; indicates severe arterial disease. The patient may be experiencing ischaemic rest pain.

Certain conditions are associated with abnormal readings:

- Diabetes—calcification of the medial lining of the artery can result in an abnormally high RPI, e.g. above 1.4. When this occurs the vessel becomes rigid and cannot be compressed. Consequently the signal cannot be obliterated. Up to 10% of diabetics may have this condition (Boulton et al 1994).
- Oedema—practical difficulties may be experienced in detecting or obliterating the signal, and this may lead to unreliable findings.
- Atherosclerosis—difficulties may arise due to reduced pulses complicated by the presence of calcification.
- Renal disease—patients may also have calcification of vessels.

Activity   **45** MINUTES

Read Article 9 in the Reader (p. 153), then answer the following questions.

1. What percentage of patients had no detectable pulses in this study?
2. What proportion of patients could have had inappropriate treatment based on the information concerning palpation of their pedal pulses?
3. What independent risk factors were identified in the study as being associated with a lack of pulses in patients with a normal RPI?
4. What proportion of patients had heart failure?
5. What proportion of patients had ulceration of mixed aetiology?
6. What two problems are discussed in this paper relating to patients with intermittent claudication?

FEEDBACK

1. In this study 31% of patients had no detectable pulses for a variety of reasons.

2. Up to 37% of patients could have had inappropriate treatment.

3. A number of factors were noted. These were a history of cardiac failure, a fixed ankle joint, the presence of diabetes mellitus and no history of phlebitis (an unexplained anomaly).

4. 9% of patients in the study had varying degrees of heart failure for which they were being treated.

5. Up to 20% of patients had mixed aetiology with the risk of arterial disease increasing with age.

6. Patients with intermittent claudication may:

   a. have a normal resting pressure index which falls after exercise, indicating early arterial disease
   b. be too immobile to walk far enough to suffer claudication and only present once rest pain is established.

Activity   **40** MINUTES

In order to consolidate your understanding of Doppler ultrasound, read Articles 10 and 11 in the Reader (pp. 158 and 162).

Assessment of pain

On a number of occasions Mrs G. has referred to the pain her leg ulcer is causing. McCaffery (1972) stated

that 'Pain is whatever the patient says it is and occurs whenever the patient says it does'. We have already noted from the quality of life literature that pain was the worst feature of having a leg ulcer.

Activity   **60** MINUTES

Many patients with leg ulcers experience pain. Ask three colleagues and three patients what factors aggravate the pain during treatment and make a list of their comments.

FEEDBACK

We have identified the following factors which aggravate pain during treatment:

- rough technique in removing dressings
- use of adherent dressings that cause trauma on removal
- prolonged time with the wound exposed to the air
- antiseptic solutions
- rough cleansing or debridement of wounds
- excessive pressure applied during wound measurement
- poor bandaging technique causing constriction or slippage of bandage
- wound infection
- rough handling of patient.

These are just a few suggestions that we noted. You may have found others.

Pain assessment tools

Regular formal assessment of pain is not carried out in every clinical area. In the following activity we want you to look at this issue more closely.

Activity   **45** MINUTES

1. Is a pain assessment tool used where you work; if so, which one? Is it consistently filled in by all staff? If not, discuss with two or three of your colleagues why this is so and make a note of your findings.
2. Choose a patient you are treating with a leg ulcer. Explore this patient's experience of pain a little more deeply than perhaps you would normally. Even if you think the patient is not in

pain ask him or her about it. You might be surprised by the answers. Encourage the patient to talk to you by using open-ended questions, e.g. 'What is your pain like?', rather than 'Are you in pain?'.

As soon as you can, write down what the patient has told you. Try not to place your own interpretation of what has been said on to the conversation.

• •

FEEDBACK

Hollinworth (1995) found that nurses frequently failed to assess pain either verbally or by using pain assessment tools, but relied heavily instead on their previous nursing experience and nonverbal cues to understand the patient's pain. The same study found that pain was not assessed or documented during dressing changes. While analgesia was advocated for pain relief, it was not used.

• •

A number of pain assessment tools have been developed. One example is given in Figure 4.1 which shows a simple visual analogue scale on which the patient places a cross to denote the severity of pain.

The most widely used tool is the McGill Pain Questionnaire (Melzack & Katz 1992). This was developed by Melzack in an attempt to measure the subjective experience of pain and is recognised as the leading pain measurement scale (McDowell & Newell 1987).

You may have been surprised about what your patient told you about the pain he or she was experiencing. Charles (1995) recorded patients' comments concerning their experience of living with a leg ulcer. One patient reported: 'The pain was terrible, I couldn't bear it.' Other patients went on to say that they had difficulties making health professionals believe what they had to say. One patient commented: 'They [nurses and doctors] never believed I was in pain.' This supports the argument that nurses are frequently underestimating the pain the patient has. Professionals often have preconceived ideas about the pain the patient should be experiencing. This is linked to the stereotyped view of the underlying pathology—that venous ulcers are not painful. Nurses are also influenced by the coping mechanisms

a patient uses. Patients with what appears to be minimal altered pathology are often considered to have pain of a psychological origin.

Hofman (1996) found in a pilot study of 20 patients that 18 had pain. The site of the severest pain varied in different patients. Six had pain in the wound, six at the peri-wound area and six elsewhere in the leg. In some cases traditional advice given to venous ulcer patients, such as limb elevation, aggravated the pain. Lindholm et al (1993) reported pain to be the most dominating factor for patients with leg ulcers.

The subject of pain in ulceration has been a neglected area of concern until very recently. There has been a long-held belief by professionals that venous ulcers are not painful, although there is no evidence to support this view. Recent work using generic quality of life tools has shown that as many as 80% of venous ulcer patients have pain of varying degrees (Franks et al 1994). Pain, while still not fully understood, should form part of a comprehensive nursing assessment (Rice 1994).

4.6 SUMMARISING AND REFERRING

Summarising is the process of drawing together the exploration, observation and measurements which the nurse has made so far. In many ways the summarising stage is synonymous with the beginning of the planning process. 'Referring' is the process of involving other professionals caring for Mrs G. as a result of your summary.

Summarising

Activity   45 MINUTES

Drawing on the assessment we already have about Mrs G. carry out the following task.

1. Use Table 4.4 to list the factors which need to be addressed in a care plan for Mrs G. under the headings:

   • physical
   • psychological
   • social.

2. Include in your table other professionals whom you think should become involved.

1   2   3   4   5   6   7   8   9   10

Fig. 4.1 A simple pain assessment tool.

Table 4.4	
	Referral
Physical problems	
Psychological problems	
Social problems	

FEEDBACK

Your summary table might look something like Table 4.5.

This last activity illustrates the process of summarising from the nurse's point of view. These issues should be discussed with Mrs G. and goals for treatment agreed on. Some of the points identified are relatively straightforward to address, e.g. choice of dressing or bandage. Other issues are more subtle and difficult to address, e.g. the tension within their relationship. The nurse may gain greater insight as she develops a therapeutic relationship with Mr and Mrs G. over the next few weeks. This illustrates the dynamic process of assessment. If Mrs G.'s ulcer does not heal satisfactorily, the nurse should consider whether referral to a hospital for further investigation may be required.

Referring

In recent years it has been recognised that all leg ulcer patients should have access to a specialist vascular service. Increasingly leg ulcer services are being developed which have an established link between the community and hospital. Other specialist support services include dermatology, diabetology, and plastic surgery.

Table 4.5 Summary of Mrs G.'s assessment

	Referral
Physical problems	
Problems associated with the wound	Discuss with medical practitioner and decide together an appropriate regime
Mrs G.'s current dressing adheres to the wound causing trauma and pain	
Inadequate control of exudate has led to maceration	
Possible history of contact allergy (past dressings have not worked)	If situation does not resolve, referral to a dermatologist might be required for patch testing
The skin is dry and requires rehydration	
No evidence of effective compression therapy in the past	
Toenails need cutting	Referral to podiatrist might be required
Anaemic	Discuss results of blood test with GP
Poor pain control leading to lack of sleep	
Poor general mobility and limited ankle function	A referral to the physiotherapist may be necessary for full assessment of mobility
Psychological problems	
Depression and anxiety	
Compliance—professional help has been offered in the past but refused	
Mr G.'s dominance over treatment issues may affect acceptance of professional advice and treatment	
Smell from ulcer leading to social isolation	
Tension between Mr and Mrs G.	
The level of dementia affecting Mrs G.	Possible involvement of the psychogeriatrician
Social problems	
Little is known at this stage about Mr and Mrs G.'s home environment	It might be appropriate to request a home visit by the district nurse—involvement of an occupational therapist if adaptations to the home are required
Are Mr and Mrs G. receiving all their benefit entitlements, e.g. attendance allowance?	Other support services such as meals on wheels or home carer might be utilised
Social isolation	Refer to social services/day care centre etc.
Inappropriate footwear	Refer to orthotist

Referral criteria

Much of the epidemiological literature relating to leg ulceration (Callam et al 1985, Cornwall et al 1986) highlights that few patients are currently referred to specialist hospital services despite many patients remaining unhealed for years.

Increasingly, health authorities are developing referral criteria to assist nurses in the decision-making process. These require to be developed collaboratively with the professional groups involved. Such criteria are now being used as measurable standards within an audit process. An example of referral criteria designed for this purpose at Charing Cross Hospital is given in Box 4.3.

Box 4.3 Charing Cross Hospital referral criteria

- Referral of any patient with an RPI of less than 0.5—patient to be seen within 1 week of referral
- Patients with an RPI of 0.5–0.8 require referral
- Young mobile patients referred for full investigation and possible vein surgery
- Patients with recurrent ulceration
- Any patient failing to make satisfactory progress within 3 months
- Any patient with an ulcer of unusual aetiology requiring tissue biopsy

Other health authorities have developed similar criteria. These often reflect local availability of resources and expertise, e.g. all diabetics with ulceration, all patients with large ulcers referred to plastic surgery unit for grafting, patients with intractable skin problems referred to a dermatologist for patch testing. Morison & Moffatt (1994) describe some of the more specialist vascular investigations, which include:

- treadmill exercise tests
- segmental pressures
- angiography
- air plethysmography and photoplethysmography
- ambulatory venous pressures
- duplex ultrasonography.

Negus (1991) describes these investigations in greater depth.

Specific tests used in the assessment of the diabetic foot are examined in Case Study 6 (p. 102).

This section on assessment illustrates the importance of a multidisciplinary approach to care. We have used a venous ulcer to illustrate the principles involved in the process of assessment. Regardless of the type of ulcer, these principles remain the same. Obviously patients differ both in terms of the aetiology of their ulcers and their individual needs. Assessment is the cornerstone upon which you build your plan of care. We explore assessment further in the case studies where we look at a number of individuals with different problems.

SUMMARY

In this section you have learned the following things.

- It is important to use a structured approach to assessment.
- Many factors must be considered in initiating and sustaining a therapeutic relationship with the patient and carer.
- A truly holistic assessment involves the collection and interpretation of many types of information, both qualitative and quantitative.
- The nurse often plays a pivotal role in the coordination of care.
- The assessment process makes great demands on your interpersonal skills.
- Accurate recording of measurements and documentation of care is an essential component of effective assessment and a requirement of every practitioner.

REFERENCES

Barnhorst D A, Barner H B 1968 Prevalence of congenitally absent pedal pulses. New England Journal of Medicine 278: 264–265
Bellamy K 1995 Photography in wound assessment. Journal of Wound Care 4(7): 313–316
Boulton A J M, Connor H, Cavanagh P R (eds) 1994 The foot in diabetes, 2nd edn. John Wiley, Chichester
Callam M J, Ruckley C V, Harper D R, Dale J J 1985 Chronic ulceration of the leg: extent of the problem and provision of care. British Medical Journal 290: 1855–1856
Charles H C 1995 The impact of leg ulcers on patients' quality of life. Professional Nurse 10(9): 571–574
Cornwall J, Dore C J, Lewis J D 1986 Leg ulcers: epidemiology and aetiology. British Journal of Surgery 73: 693–696
Drew N 1986 Exclusion and confirmation: a phenomenology of patients' experience with care given. Image Journal of Nursing Scholarship 18(2): 39–43
Franks P J, Moffatt C J, Connolly M, Bosanquet N, Oldroyd M, Greenhalgh R M, McCollum C N 1994 Community leg ulcer clinics: effects on quality of life. Phlebology 9: 83–86
Hofman D 1996 Pain assessment in the management of leg ulceration. Abstract from the Proceedings of the 5th European Conference on Advances in Wound Care, European Wound Management Association. Macmillan, London
Hollinworth H 1995 Nursing assessment and management of pain at wound dressing changes. Journal of Wound Care 4(2): 77–83
Hyland M E, Ley B A, Thomson B 1994 Quality of life in leg ulcer patients: questionnaire and preliminary findings. Journal of Wound Care 3(6): 103–105
Kasch C, Knutson K 1985 Patient compliance and interpersonal style: implication for practice and research. Nurse Practitioner 10(3): 52–54
Lindholm C, Bjellrup M, Christensen O, Zederfelt B 1993 Quality of life in leg ulcer patients. An assessment according to the Nottingham Health Profile. Acta Dermato Venereologica (Stockh) 73: 440–443
McCaffery M 1972 Nursing management of the patient with pain. Lippincott, Toronto
McDowell I, Newell C 1987 Measuring health: a guide on probing scales and questionnaires. Oxford University Press, Oxford
McLaren S M G 1992 Nutrition and wound healing. Journal of Wound Care 1(3): 45–55
Melzack R, Katz J 1992 The McGill Questionnaire: appraisal and current status. In: Turk D C, Melzack R (eds) Handbook of pain assessment. The Guildford Press, New York, ch 10
Moffatt C J 1994 Auditing a leg ulcer service. Nursing Standard 8(Aug 24): 52
Moffatt C J, Franks P J, Oldroyd M, Bosanquet N, Greenhalgh R M, McCollum C N 1992 Community clinics for leg ulcers and impact on healing. British Medical Journal 305: 1389–1392
Moffatt C J, Lambourne L A, Jones A C, Franks P J 1994 Clinical community wound care audit: the UK perspective. In: Cherry G W, Leaper D J, Lawrence J C, Milward P (eds) Conference proceedings, 4th European Conference on Advances in Wound Management. European Wound Management Association. Macmillan, London, p 110
Morison M, Moffatt C J 1994 A colour guide to the assessment and management of leg ulcers, 2nd edn. Mosby, London
Muir Gray J A 1983 Social aspects of peripheral vascular disease of the elderly. In: McCarthy S T (ed) Peripheral vascular disease in the elderly. Churchill Livingstone, London, pp 191–199
Negus D 1991 Leg ulcers: a practical approach to management. Butterworth Heinemann, Oxford
Rice A S C 1994 Pain, inflammation and wound healing. Journal of Wound Care 3(5): 246–248
Roe B, Cullum N, Hamer C 1995 Patients' perceptions of chronic leg ulceration. In: Cullum N, Rose B (eds) Leg ulcers nursing management: a research-based guide. Scutari Press, London
Van Toller S 1994 Invisible wounds: the effects of skin ulcer malodours. Journal of Wound Care 3(2): 103–105
Williams I M, Picton A J, McCollum C N 1993 The use of Doppler ultrasound 1: arterial disease. Wound Management 4(1): 9–12

5 Professional intervention

Introduction

Having made an assessment of your patient you now have to plan and provide effective treatment. This section deals firstly with some general issues such as wound cleansing, infection, skin care and dressings, and secondly with a discussion on the management of specific types of ulcer. Having said this, each patient will present with a unique set of circumstances and for this reason the principles outlined are explored further in the case studies in Section 6.

LEARNING OUTCOMES

When you have completed this section you should be able to:

- discuss the principles of effective wound cleansing
- discriminate between commensal and pathogenic organisms and their involvement in leg ulcer healing
- select an appropriate skin care regimen for each patient
- select appropriate dressings for individual patients
- describe the range of interventions available for the management of venous ulceration including:
  —compression therapy
  —intermittent pneumatic compression therapy
  —skin grafting
  —preventing ulcer recurrence and the role of patient education
- describe the range of interventions, both conservative and radical, available for the management of arterial ulceration
- explain the principles of the management of an ulcer due to both venous hypertension and arterial disease
- discuss the limited options available in the management of ulcers in patients with rheumatoid arthritis
- describe the range of interventions available for the management of foot ulceration in the diabetic patient.

Before you start this section it is useful to have in your mind the priorities of your intervention.

Activity   15 MINUTES

Define what you feel the general priorities of professional intervention should be.

· ·

FEEDBACK

Morison & Moffatt (1994, p. 55) provide us with the following five priorities.

- 'To *correct* the underlying causes of the ulcer. This normally means improving the patient's venous and/or arterial circulation in the affected limb.'
- 'To *create* the optimum local environment at the wound site.'
- 'To *improve* all the wider factors that might delay healing, especially poor mobility, malnutrition and psychological issues.'
- 'To *prevent* avoidable complications such as wound infection, medicament dermatitis, or tissue damage due to over-tight bandaging.'
- 'To *maintain* healed tissue.'

· ·

5.1 WOUND CLEANSING

Historically a wide range of solutions have been employed to clean wounds. Hippocrates suggested tepid water, wine and vinegar. Dealey (1994) describes a 'special balm' used in the Middle Ages which was made by 'boiling young puppies in oil of turpentine and then adding earthworms'. More recently, the First World War led to the development of antiseptic solutions such as Eusol (Edinburgh University solution of lime).

Activity   10 MINUTES

Read Article 12 in the Reader (p. 165).

1. Make a list of the solutions that you currently use to clean wounds.
2. What is the most frequently used solution in your experience?

FEEDBACK

Surprisingly, there is little in the way of empirical evidence related to the cleansing of wounds (Cullum & Roe 1995). In recent years there has been a move away from strong antiseptics as these are thought to delay healing. It is interesting to note that current best practice recommends simple techniques similar to those proposed by Hippocrates, i.e. cleansing wounds with warm water or isotonic saline. There is some debate that we may have gone too far in this respect and that in certain instances, such as a patient with very poor blood supply, antiseptics may play a role in preventing severe overriding infection.

Activity   15 MINUTES

Let us return to basics for a moment. List four things that we are trying to achieve by cleaning wounds.

FEEDBACK

You could have said that in cleansing a wound we are trying to:

1. make the wound socially clean
2. debride the wound
3. prevent secondary infection
4. ensure skin integrity.

We will look at each of these in turn.

Making the wound socially clean

This apparently simple statement is in fact quite complex and could be further divided into the psychological, therapeutic and cultural aspects of cleansing.

In some societies, cleanliness is highly regarded; hence the saying 'cleanliness is next to godliness'. Having a leg ulcer sometimes prevents patients from complying with their cultural norms, which in turn can cause psychological distress. We have already seen that odour associated with leg ulceration reduces patients' quality of life. The cleansing process can be comforting and can remove many of the bacteria on the skin surface which produce the smell. It is generally not necessary to cleanse leg ulcers using the aseptic technique associated with surgical wounds. From the outset the aim in surgical wounds is to remove organisms from the operation site preoperatively and prevent the introduction of pathogens intraoperatively and postoperatively. To this end a strictly controlled technique is used, requiring sterilisation of equipment and use of gloves or a 'non touch' technique. In contrast, chronic wounds such as leg ulcers are usually already heavily colonised with a wide variety of organisms which do not necessarily cause clinical infection (see Sect. 5.2). The emphasis therefore should be on prevention of cross-infection. Effective hand washing and cleansing/disinfection of equipment should be practised according to local policy. One of the dangers of using a 'clean' approach rather than aseptic technique, is that it is correctly perceived as less rigorous and this lack of rigor is extended to the issue of cross-infection.

In practical terms, there is no reason why a patient with leg ulceration should not have a bath or shower. In the community, however, it is becoming increasingly more difficult to organise someone to be available to dress the wound afterwards. Warmed saline is sometimes used to clean wounds and this is a very safe option. Bale & Jones (1997) describe the basic principles of hand washing, wearing of gloves, irrigation and use of sterile dressings in all types of wound, acute or chronic, and make the following recommendation:

> Cleansing of a wound should only be performed when clearly indicated and irrigation with saline or water should be in most cases sufficient. Wounds that are clean, with healthy tissue, do not require cleansing and should be left undisturbed to maintain the optimum environment for healing.

If you are aware that cleansing a wound causes your patient great discomfort, you should consider pre-dressing analgesia. A popular method of cleansing is immersion of the leg in a bucket of warm tap water. The bucket should be lined with a plastic bag which is changed between patients and the bucket disinfected in accordance with universal infection control procedures (Wilson 1995).

Debriding the wound

Soaking the leg in warm water aids the process of debridement. You will find it much easier to remove dead scales and debris if the leg has been soaked for 5–10 minutes. The leg should be gently dried with a piece of non-sterile paper towel. Using a pair of fine-toothed forceps, remove the debris carefully without causing further trauma. Scales and scabs may lead to skin problems and can act as a pressure source beneath compression bandages. The accumulation of necrotic tissue within a wound base can lead to secondary infection.

Preventing secondary infection

Thomas (1990) warns:

> the presence of slough and devitalised tissue will predispose a wound to infection by acting as a bacteriological culture medium and inhibiting the action of leucocytes in controlling invading organisms.

Ensuring skin integrity

The skin has an important barrier function. Any break in the skin may lead to infection. Patients who have their legs bandaged often present with dry, flaky skin which may itch and cause the patient to scratch, causing further trauma. You can improve this situation by adding a little emollient to the warm water (avoid using products which contain lanolin which may cause allergies).

Further research is needed in relation to this area of practice. A number of important questions have yet to be answered, Cullum (1994) states that 'it is clear that we have insufficient evidence concerning when to cleanse, how to cleanse, and when to stop'.

5.2 INFECTION

Leg ulcers are chronic wounds and usually contain many different sorts of bacteria. In order to understand how infection affects your patients you need to appreciate the difference between a colonised wound and one which is clinically infected. To assist you in understanding the difference, let us briefly review some basic microbiological definitions.

Commensals are part of what is known as the normal flora of the body. These are organisms which populate the body and do no harm to their host providing they are not transferred to a site in which they are not normally present.

Pathogens are microorganisms which cause disease. Pathogenic infection is dependent on the susceptibility of the host.

Colonisation refers to the presence of potentially pathogenic organisms in the absence of any signs of infection. Therefore a colonised leg ulcer does not require the same treatment as an infected leg ulcer.

Clinical infection occurs when microorganisms cause adverse effects in the host. Thompson & Smith (1994) provide the following definition of infection:

> invasion and multiplication of micro-organisms in body tissues, which may be clinically inapparent or result in local cellular injury because of competitive metabolism, toxins, intracellular replication, or antigen–antibody response.

Deciding when a wound is clinically infected can at times be very difficult.

Using your general professional knowledge and experience, list four signs of clinical infection.

• •

FEEDBACK

Wilson (1995) lists the following signs of clinical infection:

- inflammation
- pain
- swelling
- heat.

• •

Wound infection is often accompanied by the production of purulent exudate and the patient may also show signs of systemic infection such as a raised temperature. The elderly, in particular, may have a systemic infection in which the clinical signs are less obvious (Gilchrist 1994).

Cutting & Harding (1994) discuss the issue of identifying infected wounds in depth, giving the presence of abscess, cellulitis and discharge as examples of traditional diagnostic criteria. They suggest that in some instances the presence of pus with or without inflammation may often be the only criterion used. They suggest the following additional criteria should be used:

- delayed healing (compared with normal rate for site/condition)
- discoloration
- friable granulation tissue which bleeds easily
- unexpected pain/tenderness
- pocketing at the base of wound
- bridging at base of the wound
- abnormal smell
- wound breakdown.

Cutting & Harding (1994) point out that these criteria have only been tested in relation to open or granulating wounds formed as a result of surgery and that they have not been tested in relation to burns or leg ulcers. This is an interesting statement in that it raises the issue of whether or not specific types of wounds might require different, additional or modified criteria.

There is no doubt that chronic leg ulceration poses us some specific problems; for instance how do we decide whether delayed healing due to infection has occurred, given that each patient presents with a wide range of unique variables to take into consideration which also might cause delayed healing, e.g. in venous ulceration the extent of the underlying venous damage will greatly influence the rate of healing.

A study by Trengrove et al (1996) indicated that wound healing was not delayed by the presence of one specific group of bacteria but when four or more groups of bacteria were involved then delayed healing occurred. They suggest that no one group of bacteria was more detrimental than any other and that the findings support the theory that the number of organisms present in a wound is a more important factor in wound healing than types of organism. It was noted that bacterial flora changes as wound healing progresses but that, with possibly the exception of the skin flora, these changes are not related to changes in healing.

Taking specimens

In order to determine the number and type of organisms causing an infection a specimen needs to be taken.

Activity 10 MINUTES

Describe four methods of taking a wound specimen.

FEEDBACK

Gilchrist (1996) lists the following ways to take a specimen:

- biopsy
- fine needle aspiration
- tape stripping
- irrigation
- aspiration
- cylinder scrub
- contact plate
- velvet pads
- PVC discs
- swabs.

The method used depends on whether a qualitative or quantitative sample is required. Biopsy is considered to be the best method but in practice the swab is the method used most commonly.

Taking a swab

There has been considerable debate over how to take a swab and there is little consensus. Gilchrist (1996) describes the often conflicting advice to be found in the literature on this subject. The issues under debate are:

- whether to clean a wound before taking a swab
- the type of swab to be used
- whether the swab should be pre-moistened
- how many swabs to use
- what motion to use and how hard to press
- how much of the wound to sample
- the type and use of transport medium.

Activity 10 MINUTES

Given the earlier discussion of colonisation in chronic wounds, would you routinely take a wound swab from every leg ulcer patient? Give reasons for your answer.

FEEDBACK

If you routinely swab leg ulcers you will find a range of both commensal and pathogenic organisms. Cullum (1994) cites a number of studies which highlight this point. Schraibman in 1990, for instance, reported taking routine bacterial swabs on 165 occasions from 91 leg ulcers. He isolated 261 different organisms which were colonising the ulcers. 21.5% were *Staphylococcus aureus*; 37.1% were faecal organisms; 11.5% were anaerobes and 18.8% were beta-haemolytic streptococci. Schraibman has also suggested that this latter organism is responsible for delayed healing (Schraibman 1995). A repeated theme in these research reports is that with the exception of beta-haemolytic streptococci, colonisation of leg ulcers does not result in delayed healing. The answer to the question we posed then is that rather than routinely taking a wound swab, you should be looking for signs of clinical infection.

Self-assessment 5 MINUTES

From our discussion so far on infection you will have appreciated that taking routine wound swabs is not appropriate. In what circumstances do you think it would be appropriate?

FEEDBACK

A wound swab should be taken when there are obvious signs of clinical infection and/or any other good reason for suspecting a hidden clinical infection, e.g. wound deterioration or failure to progress (indolent). Care should be taken in patients whose immune system is depressed, such as in those having high doses of corticosteroids who may present with few signs of cellulitis.

Antibiotics

Wound infection should be treated with systemic rather than topical antibiotics which are unlikely to be absorbed (Gilchrist 1994). Even when given systemically, patients are often prescribed short (5-day) courses. They may, however, require longer treatment owing to poor perfusion of the drug into the infected tissues. Infection that fails to resolve should be reassessed and a repeat wound swab taken to check whether the causative organism is still present. In some infections, topical antiseptics in conjunction with antibiotics may be appropriate. Antibiotics may be used more prophylactically in patients undergoing skin grafting to prevent graft rejection from organisms such as beta-haemolytic streptococci and *Pseudomonas aeruginosa*.

Leaper (1994) points out that guidelines based on good empirical evidence regarding the use of antibiotics in open wounds, either for prophylaxis or treatment, are not available. In certain circumstances such as, for example, in the presence of cellulitis, lymphangitis, a spreading necrotising infection or clear indications for prophylaxis, there are clear unambiguous indications for antibiotic treatment. In other circumstances, given the difficulties in making the distinction between colonisation and clinical infection, the decision is much more difficult. Leaper describes the historic overuse of antibiotics which led ultimately to the development of resistant organisms such as *Staphylococcus aureus*. He warns against the persistent use of topical wound treatments which contain antibiotics given that 'their efficacy has not been established' and that there is no evidence that open wounds have to be sterile to heal.

Methicillin-resistant Staphylococcus aureus (MRSA)

This organism is a Gram-positive bacterium which can be found as a commensal in many people. Hosein (1996) states that the organism colonises 30% of healthy humans, usually being found in the nose,

axilla and perineum. Young (1996) describes the first incidence of MRSA in the UK during the 1980s in London from where it has gradually spread. Young states that there are two elements to the organism's mechanism of resistance:

1. an intrinsic ability to resist the activity of the antibiotic
2. the development of acquired resistance by the bacteria through mutation and proliferation in the presence of the antibiotic.

There are now different strains of the organism. Young describes some strains as endemic, found commonly in hospitals, and others as epidemic (EMRSA) which spread quickly and easily, being resistant to a wide range of antibiotics including: bacitracin, erythromycin, gentamicin, penicillin, tetracycline, ciprofloxacin, fusidic acid, kanamycin, and rifampicin.

Whilst the results of a systemic MRSA infection can be severe or fatal, it is possible for the organism to colonise a leg ulcer with little effect on the host. Indeed it may go completely unnoticed. Sometimes colonisation is detected through routine screening but Young advises that 'an aggressive clinical approach is not usually needed'. Young recommends the following approach to management.

Establish a moist wound environment using occlusive dressings. Wound exudate is thought to be bactericidal and occlusion to promote the body's non-specific immune response as well as preventing airborne cross-infection. The dressing chosen should be, as with all dressing choices, appropriate to the individual healing needs of your patient. In addition to being an occlusive dressing it should be waterproof such as a hydrocolloid.

Commence topical antiseptic/antimicrobial therapy using povidone-iodine, chlorhexidine or mupirocin, etc. according to local policy. There is a great deal of debate over this issue and little consensus apart from the fact that topical agents should be used for limited periods only to prevent the development of resistance.

The control of cross-infection is of vital importance in the management of MRSA. Close attention should be paid to the environment in which the patient is treated, hand washing, and disinfection/disposal of equipment.

The treatment of malodorous wounds with metronidazole

The issue of antibiotic resistance also has implications for the use of metronidazole in the treatment of malodorous wounds, given that there seems little empirical evidence to justify its use. Hampson (1996) has undertaken an extensive review of the literature relating to this subject and points out that an understanding of malodour in bacteriological terms has yet to established. The widely held view that the unpleasant odour is the result of the metabolic activity of anaerobic organisms has not yet been proven. Hampson states that the most likely explanation is that the odour is due to 'a complex interaction between anaerobes and aerobes' and suggests that 'any alteration to the aerobe/anaerobe ratio might disrupt the delicate balance required to cause the smell'. Hampson concludes that the justification for prescribing metronidazole is mainly anecdotal.

5.3 SKIN CARE

You will often find that patients with leg ulcers will have problems with their skin. These problems can be fairly minor but sometimes are a major factor in delayed healing. Section 3.2 outlines some of the more commonly encountered dermatological conditions associated with ulceration.

Activity   6 0 MINUTES

Discuss this issue with your colleagues and identify five factors that you agree are common problems. Make a note of how you and your colleagues deal with them.

FEEDBACK

Some of the common problems you may have identified are:

- varicose eczema
- skin irritation
- trauma due to scratching
- folliculitis
- secondary infection
- inappropriate choice of skin care products
  —contact allergy.

Irritation from varicose eczema and dehydration of the skin are common problems you will come across.

The irritation arising from varicose eczema is due to inflammatory reactions and exacerbated by the build-up of the outer epidermis. Patients who have their legs bandaged can suffer dehydration as the result of the accumulation of the outer layers of the epidermis which are shed normally during activities such as washing.

Irritation often leads patients to scratch their legs, causing further trauma. This problem can often be simply dealt with by washing the leg to remove skin

scales (see Sect. 5.1) and applying a topical emollient such as 50% white soft paraffin mixed with 50% liquid paraffin. Care should be taken when choosing emollients to avoid products containing lanolin or creams with a cetylstearyl alcohol base which may lead to allergy. You should remember, when applying any cream to the leg, to work it in using downward movements of the hand.

- Applying cream in the opposite direction could lead to a condition called folliculitis as the hair follicles lie in a downward plane. Folliculitis is an infection/inflammation of the hair follicle usually related to staphylococcal infection.

- Any breaks in the skin can lead to infection. Fungal infections are common in patients with leg ulcers, particularly between the toes. Fungal infection can lead to secondary bacterial infection. In order to identify fungal infection, skin scrapings are taken and sent to the microbiologist. Treatment using antifungal agents may be required for several months.

- Poor wound care practice can lead to skin damage. Inappropriate choice of dressings may lead to contact allergy and delayed healing. Cullum (1994) reports that between 50% and 85% of patients with venous ulceration have contact allergy as a result of treatment. Factors which contribute to contact allergy are:

  —multiple application of wound care products —of which there are many—to broken skin
  —accumulation of products in folds of skin
  —use of an occlusive dressing which increases absorption;
  —failure to recognise the early stages of contact allergy.

The frequent problems caused by topical agents have led to a move towards the use of non-allergenic products wherever possible. If you suspect that your patient has a contact allergy you should immediately stop using the product. Wash the leg with warm water to remove any residual allergen. If there is a very florid reaction, i.e. the patient is distressed, itching and erythematous, a topical steroid may be required. In severe allergic reactions a potent steroid may be required. This may need to be applied daily initially and reduced in frequency and strength over time. When the allergy has completely subsided an emollient can be used. Paste bandaging, particularly with bandages containing ichthammol, can be used to soothe irritable skin. However, the preservatives used in paste bandages can in themselves cause allergy. If the skin problems do not resolve, the patient should be referred to a dermatologist who may undertake patch testing to identify the allergens and to identify other skin problems such as psoriasis which may be complicating the situation. The problem of contact dermatitis will be further explored in Case Study 1 (p. 89).

● ●

5.4 DRESSINGS

There is now a huge range of dressings to choose from, ranging from the simple protective cover to those designed for highly specific situations. The factors which will influence your choice of dressing are both numerous and complex. Thomas (1990) states that there is:

> no single dressing suitable for the management of all types of wound, and few dressings are ideally suited for the treatment of a single wound during all stages of the healing process.

Activity   **30 MINUTES**

Discuss the statement above by Thomas (1990) with a colleague. Think about it in the context of leg ulcers. Do you agree with what has been said or not? Note down your reasons for either agreeing or disagreeing. What are the consequences of such a statement for clinical practice?

● ●

FEEDBACK

Making generalised statements about wounds is difficult to do. The statement by Thomas implies the uniqueness of each individual wound and there is no doubt that each patient with a leg ulcer presents with a unique set of complex circumstances. But just imagine the consequences if we consider it to be true. Do you have access to every type of dressing? Some are available in hospital clinics but not in the community. Who decides at what stage of healing a particular wound is? In many leg ulcer patients different parts of the wound are at different stages of healing; for instance, the wound may be essentially sloughy with some small areas of granulation and evidence of epithelialisation around the edges.

This is an important statement but by including it we do not mean to imply that dressings have little benefit in wound healing. There is considerable anecdotal evidence to support the use of modern dressings. Issues such as patient comfort and relief of pain may be the most important in management and may help your patient in terms of compliance with other treatments such as compression.

This situation is compounded by the fact that whilst there has been quite a lot of research related to dressings, much of it to date lacks rigour. The following statement appears at the end of an extensive review of the research into topical applications by Cullum (1994): 'The research evidence provides little in the way of direction for those making clinical decisions'.

The effectiveness of a given dressing has to be evaluated in the context both of the underlying aetiology and the treatment regime as a whole. In the case of venous ulcers treated with effective compression, for instance, Blair et al (1988a) and Callam et al (1992) indicated that there was little difference in healing rates despite the use of different dressings. Given the wide range of complex variables to be controlled in this type of research, it is arguable that we will never be in a situation where we can categorically compare one dressing against another.

So where does all this leave you as a practitioner who must make choices over dressings? For a start you will be working within the limitations of what is locally available; you will have to work within a budget and some dressings are very expensive; you will have to consider how frequently dressings will be changed and by whom and you will have to consider the acceptability of a particular product to the patient. Above all, you will have to balance your own experience of what works with your knowledge of available research.

● ●

The following four activities use different types of wounds as a basis for discussing some of the factors which influence your choice of dressing. They are derived from a classification of wounds by Thomas (1990) and are as follows:

- black and necrotic
- yellow and sloughing
- clean with significant tissue loss (granulating)
- clean and superficial (epithelialising).

Black and necrotic wounds

Activity   **10 MINUTES**

A patient has a wound on his heel which is approximately 10 cm^2 in area. The wound contains a hard black plug of dead (necrotic) tissue called an 'eschar'. There is a thin red line around the plug which indicates that it is about to lift. There is virtually no discharge. There are no signs of underlying clinical infection.

This wound obviously needs debriding. The simplest and quickest method would be surgical excision but this can also be achieved with a dressing. This type of wound is typical of some arterial ulcers or pressure sores.

What dressings facilitate debridement and how do they achieve this?

FEEDBACK

You should have said that dressings which facilitate debridement are hydrocolloids and hydrogels and enzymatic preparations.

Hydrocolloids and hydrogels

The underlying principle of these dressings is occlusion. They are used to seal the wound and keep it moist. The eschar is rehydrated and this enables the natural process of autodebridement to occur (autolysis). A hydrogel dressing in itself is not impermeable; it enables rehydration but must be used in conjunction with a suitable secondary moisture-retaining dressing.

The concept of moist wound healing dates back to the 1960s when Winter (1962) found that wounds in pigs covered with an occlusive film epithelialised twice as fast as those left exposed. Hinman & Maibach (1963) confirmed this finding using human volunteers. The experimental wounds in both these studies, however, were very small and superficial and whilst the principle of moist wound healing has been generally accepted, the findings were never intended to be extrapolated to all wounds regardless of type.

There was concern at the time that the moist environment created by occlusion would lead to an increase in bacterial growth and clinical infection. Subsequent studies have shown this fear to be largely unfounded (Varghese et al 1986, Gilchrist & Reed 1989, Hutchinson 1990, 1992).

Enzymatic preparations

These contain proteolytic enzymes, e.g. streptokinase and streptodornase, and are occasionally used to debride wounds. Hard eschar must be scored or the solution injected with great care under the eschar to allow the enzyme to penetrate the tissue. Research concerning its effectiveness is limited.

Yellow and sloughing wounds

Activity   15 MINUTES

The wound you have to dress is situated on the medial malleolus and has a surface area of approximately 50 cm². It is covered with thick yellow slough and the patient complains of both pain and odour. A moderate amount of exudate is produced which requires the dressing to be changed three times per week. There is no sign of underlying infection. This type of wound is typical of a chronic non-healing venous leg ulcer.

1. Summarise the problems that need to be addressed.
2. What dressing would be most appropriate in dealing with each problem?

FEEDBACK

1. You should have said that the problems are:
   a. debridement of slough
   b. control of pain
   c. excessive exudate requiring frequent dressing
   d. odour reduction.

2. a. Debridement of slough can be treated as outlined in the previous activity with a hydrocolloid, hydrogel dressing (often used in conjunction with a semipermeable film dressing) or enzymatic debrider. The use of biosurgical techniques involving sterile maggots is gaining popularity at present. Paste bandaging is often used in venous ulceration.
   b. Control of pain is also achieved in situations where the wound is kept moist. Dressings which dry out and/or adhere to the wound will increase the amount of pain experienced by patients.
   c. Excessive exudate requiring frequent dressing can be controlled by a wide variety of products which absorb fluid. These include simple dressing pads, alginates, hydrocellular dressings (including foams) and polysaccharide bead dressings.
   d. Odour reduction can be achieved through the use of activated charcoal dressings. However, these are not available in the community. In certain cases the odour can be reduced by using a hydrogel containing metronidazole. We might choose to dress this wound with a hydrocolloid dressing covered by a charcoal dressing, if available, providing it can be changed frequently enough to prevent maceration.

The hydrocolloid dressing should contain moderate exudate if effective occlusion is achieved, but during the debridement process it is normal to see an increase in exudate and the wound may appear larger as necrotic tissue is removed. In practice, venous ulcers of this type are commonly treated with compression therapy. This will cause the wound to debride effectively and using a simple non-adherent dressing and compression bandaging has been shown to reduce pain (Morison & Moffatt 1994). The bandages themselves absorb exudate and to some extent reduce odour, though this may remain an outstanding problem. A charcoal dressing can be placed between bandage layers if required.

Granulating wounds

Activity   **10** MINUTES

The wound you have to dress is situated on the lateral malleolus and has a surface area of approximately 15 cm^2. The wound surface has a bed of healthy granulation tissue with a moderate amount of exudate produced which requires the dressing to be changed twice weekly. There is no slough remaining in the wound. The surrounding skin is well hydrated and there is no evidence of maceration or signs of allergic reaction. This is typical of a healing venous ulcer. What dressings would promote continuing progress in this wound?

FEEDBACK

The most important factor you should note from the above description is that the wound is healing and that you should interfere with this process as little as possible. It would be important not to apply any product to this wound which would either cause an allergic reaction or delay healing. You may, in some instances, have no choice but to change the dressing regime. For instance, there is some evidence that occlusion may cause hypergranulation (proud flesh) (Thomas 1990).

There are a number of ways of dealing with hypergranulation.

- Change to a more permeable dressing. Although the mechanism for this is unclear, hypergranulation is thought to be due to overhydration and overstimulation.
- A pad can be applied over the primary dressing to provide local pressure.
- In exceptional cases local application to the wound of corticosteroid cream or a silver nitrate pencil (75%) may be required under medical supervision.

Epithelialising wounds

Activity   **10** MINUTES

The wound you have to dress is situated on the lateral side of the foot. The patient is a diabetic with reduced sensation and on removing the dressing you note a little dry exudate on the dressing. Most of the wound has been covered with epithelium except for a small 'island' of approximately 1 cm^2 remaining unhealed. What are the main considerations in dressing this wound in the last stages of healing?

FEEDBACK

The first consideration again is for you to interfere as little as possible. One example of a dressing which would be appropriate would be a low-adherent dressing with a protective backing.

Because of the patient's reduced sensation you have to continue dressing this wound even when it appears to have completely epithelialised in order to provide some protection to the new delicate epithelium. The patient is unlikely to know if further trauma is occurring especially from footwear, given the position of the wound.

The individuality of patients has to be reiterated. We have presented four relatively straightforward scenarios. We have shown the importance of site in the final activity but this is only one of many variables to be taken into account. Others include: the degree of mobility; whether the patient wants to dress his or her own wound; the cosmetic appearance; whether it will interfere with maintaining personal hygiene; and whether the wound is infected. A number of writers have attempted to define the characteristics of the 'optimum dressing' (Turner 1982, Thomas 1990). Box 5.1 shows Thomas's criteria.

Box 5.1 The characteristics of the optimal dressing (Thomas 1990)

A dressing should ensure that the wound remains:

- moist with exudate but not macerated
- free from clinical infection and excessive slough
- free of toxic chemicals, particles or fibres released by the dressing
- at the optimum temperature for healing to take place
- undisturbed by frequent and unnecessary dressing changes
- at an optimum pH value.

For a more detailed exploration of the range of modern wound dressings, refer to Flanagan (1997).

Another useful recent source is that of Bale & Jones (1997, p. 56) who have developed a table outlining the range of products available and an indication of their use.

Morison & Moffatt (1994, pp. 77–81) provide a useful algorithm which guides the practitioner through the process of choosing a dressing.

5.5 VENOUS ULCERATION AND COMPRESSION THERAPY

As we have seen, over 70% of leg ulcers are caused by venous disease with ulceration developing as a result of chronic venous hypertension. Currently, the most effective treatment for venous ulceration is compression therapy. Whilst historically there are a number of references to the use of bandages in the treatment of venous ulceration, it is not clear when practitioners, on any great scale, began to use bandages specifically to apply pressure rather than as a means of holding the dressing in place. If you look at the chronology in the Reader (Article 4, p. 129), you will notice that the earliest reference to the use of bandages is probably Majno in 1975 BC. Certainly Hippocrates in the 4th century BC describes the use of bandages in treating leg ulcers and recognises the skill in applying them. Bandages were used routinely by the Greeks and Romans. Often ancient practitioners achieved healing but misunderstood the effect that the bandaging was having. In many instances their intention was to drive out 'evil humours' which would cause madness and death. It is only recently that researchers have begun to understand the principle behind compression therapy. Vin (1995) speaks of the 'relaunching' in the 20th century of the compression method arising from the introduction of zinc paste boots by Unna in the 19th century. Despite considerable work in the latter part of this century (Sigg 1963, Meyerovitz & Nelson 1964, Stemmer 1969, Sigel et al 1975, Raj et al 1980, Blair et al 1988b, Sockalingham et al 1990, Callam et al 1992, Duby et al 1993), effective compression bandaging is still not consistently applied to patients with venous ulceration. In a study by Cullum (1994), as few as 25% of venous ulcer patients were receiving compression therapy.

How compression works

Compression therapy seeks to provide graduated compression with the highest pressure at the ankle and the lowest at the knee. If the same tension is maintained during the application of the bandage the natural increase in circumference of most legs will achieve this. In order to understand how graduated

Box 5.2 Laplace's Law

Sub-bandage pressure (SP) is proportional to
$$\frac{T \times N \times 4630 \text{ (constant)}}{C \times W}$$

SP = pressure extended by the bandage
N = the number of layers of bandage
T = the tension of the bandage
C = the circumference of the limb
W = the width of the bandage

compression works, you need to be familiar with Laplace's Law (Box 5.2).

You can see that all of the criteria contributing to sub-bandage pressure have practical implications when applying compression. We will return to them later in this section.

The physiology of compression therapy

Compression therapy:

• reduces the distension in the superficial veins and counteracts the high pressure (venous hypertension) (Sigg 1963)
• restores damaged valve function in some patients (Sarin et al 1992)
• encourages and enhances blood flow in the deep veins (Sigel et al 1975)
• reduces the volume of blood by 62% in the standing position
• facilitates the action of the calf muscle pump by providing a skin against which the muscle can expand; restriction of the muscle directs pressure inwards on to blood vessels, thereby increasing venous return
• forces fluid into both the venous and the lymphatic system, thus reducing oedema
• reduces the symptoms of venous disease such as aching limbs and pain from the ulcer
• increases the healing rate of venous ulceration (Blair et al 1988b, Callam et al 1992, Duby et al 1993)
• improves skin condition; some studies report increased removal of fibrin during compression therapy (Vin 1995).

We have used the term 'compression therapy' deliberately in preference to compression bandaging even though it will be clear to you by now that bandaging is the most common method of applying compression.

Activity 5 MINUTES

Suggest two other methods of applying compression to a limb.

FEEDBACK

You could have suggested elasticated stockings and shaped tubular bandages. We will look at these next.

Compression stockings

Provided the patient has been given the correct size, elasticated stockings are a safe alternative to bandages. They can be full length but generally below-knee stockings are the most frequently used. There are three classes of compression stocking. These are described in Table 5.1. They are unsuitable in patients with a high level of exudate and are often used after initial compression therapy with bandages.

Table 5.1 Classes of compression stocking		
Class	Pressure applied	Recommended use
I	14–17 mmHg	Varicose veins Mild oedema
II	18–24 mmHg	Moderate/severe varicose veins Prevention of ulcer recurrence
III	25–35 mmHg	Gross varicose veins Post-phlebitic limb Recurrent ulceration Lymphoedema

Tubular bandages

Shaped tubular bandages are able to apply low levels of compression but are often below the level required to be clinically effective. Straight tubular bandages are more frequently used. These are incapable of applying graduation and often result in tight bands around the ankle and the accumulation of oedema in the foot.

Assessment considerations

Compression is a powerful therapy which if applied injudiciously can cause a great deal of damage which in some instances may result in amputation of a limb (Callam et al 1987). Therefore, before applying any type of compression to a patient's leg there are a number of factors to be taken into account during assessment.

Activity   15 MINUTES

The headings below represent three categories covering the factors which might cause damage to a patient with a leg ulcer. Suggest at least two such factors for each category.

Previous and current medical problems

Limb/mobility

Patient acceptability

FEEDBACK

Some of the factors you should have identified are as follows.

Factors relating to previous and current medical problems

* Patients with significant arterial disease should not be having compression therapy. It is generally agreed that high compression can be safely used if the patient's resting pressure index is greater than 0.8.
* Patients with rheumatoid arthritis and diabetes mellitus may have a venous ulcer and require compression. However, this must be used with great care because of the possibility of underlying microvascular disease.
* Some patients present with mixed venous and arterial ulceration. Following arterial reconstruction patients may be treated with compression therapy for the venous component of the ulcer. These patients must be supervised very carefully for any signs of the graft blocking.
* Compression therapy should not be used to reduce the oedema from heart failure. The effect would be to put even greater strain on the heart.

Factors relating to the limb and mobility

* The shape of the limb can pose certain problems for the safe application of compression therapy.

(A)

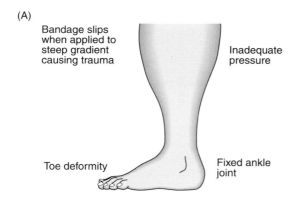

Bandage slips when applied to steep gradient causing trauma

Inadequate pressure

Toe deformity

Fixed ankle joint

(B)

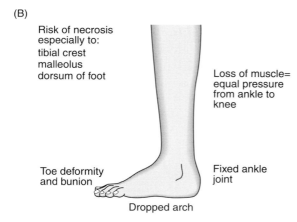

Risk of necrosis especially to:
tibial crest
malleolus
dorsum of foot

Loss of muscle= equal pressure from ankle to knee

Toe deformity and bunion

Fixed ankle joint

Dropped arch

Fig. 5.1 Leg shapes and factors to be identified during assessment: (A) the inverted 'champagne bottle' leg; (B) the thin leg with reduced calf muscle.

The two shapes shown in Figure 5.1 are typical examples in patients with venous ulcers. The diagrams show factors which must be identified during assessment.

• The degree of general mobility is an important consideration in choosing between bandage types. This will be affected by factors such as obesity and arthritis. Practical consideration should be given to footwear, e.g. adequate size, ulcer position, level of exudate, etc.

Factors relating to patient acceptability

Problems with compliance are frequently reported with leg ulcer patients. The nurse needs to find out whether the patient will tolerate the bandage and may need to consider options, such as whether the outer bandage can be removed at night or increasing pressure over a period of time, if the patient finds the treatment uncomfortable. A patient who has had an unsatisfactory experience of compression therapy may be unwilling to try again. This may have been due to poor bandage application and/or inappropriate choice of bandage.

Activity 30 MINUTES

In the light of your own professional experience, suggest three factors which influence whether or not compression therapy is used, and three factors which influence whether or not it is used effectively.

FEEDBACK

Factors which influence whether compression therapy is used or not include the following.

• Availability of bandages—some of the bandages used to apply compression are not available through prescription in the community.
• Fear of using compression—this often results from poor assessment and an inability to ensure that the patient has a good blood supply.
• Understanding that compression is the most effective component of treatment of a venous ulcer rather than the dressing.
• Acceptability to patients—they have to have confidence in the technique and appreciate the relevance to them.
• Availability of training and a policy to support its use on all suitable patients.

Factors which influence the effectiveness of compression therapy include the following.

• Poor knowledge of the properties of bandages.
• Inappropriate choice of bandage leading to pressure damage or inadequate pressure being applied.
• Problems with application such as excessive layers and overextension of the bandage at mid-calf level leading to a tourniquet effect.
• Patients who will not comply with the required level of compression for effective treatment.
• Bulky bandages causing patients to have problems with footwear.
• Use of compression therapy on patients for whom it is contraindicated, e.g. in cases of severe arterial disease.

The science of bandaging

There are a number of terms used to describe the function of elastic bandages (Thomas 1995). In order to understand the scientific principles behind bandaging, you need to understand these terms.

Activity   10 MINUTES

Link the list of bandaging terms to the appropriate definition in Table 5.2 by drawing connecting lines between them.

Table 5.2 Terms used to describe the function of elastic bandages: link each term with its definition

Term	Definition
Power	The ability of a bandage to extend and return to its original length
Conformability	The change in length when subjected to a given force
Extension	The force required to bring about a specific extension in bandage length
Elasticity	The direct application of pressure
Compression	The ability of a bandage to follow the contours of a limb

FEEDBACK

Your lines should have created the definitions given in Table 5.3.

Table 5.3 Terms used to describe the function of elastic bandages

Term	Definition
Power	The force required to bring about a specific extension in bandage length
Conformability	The ability of a bandage to follow the contours of a limb
Extension	The change in length when subjected to a given force
Elasticity	The ability of a bandage to extend and return to its original length
Compression	The direct application of pressure

Power

You can determine the difference in power between bandages by simply noting how much effort is required to extend the bandage. Very powerful bandages, such as traditional blue line bandages, require greater effort and will apply much higher pressure to a limb than a bandage that requires little effort to extend it.

Conformability

This can be a very important factor in treating venous leg ulceration. Many patients have champagne-bottle-shaped legs and more conformable bandages will accommodate this. Generally bandages of lower power are more conformable.

Extension

Most bandages are applied at a 50% extension, i.e. the bandage is fully extended and relaxed back by 50%. Nelson (1995) suggests that nurses often change their extension of the bandages as they go up the limb which can lead to a tourniquet effect. The bandage should remain at the same extension all the way up the limb. The reduction in pressure will occur as the circumference of the limb increases (Laplace's Law).

Elasticity

Many of the traditional bandages were not truly elastic as they were made of natural fibres. These bandages were incapable of maintaining pressure for any length of time. Bandages containing elastomeric fibres are capable of sustaining compression.

Studies report that elastic bandages achieve significantly higher healing rates than non-elastic (Callam et al 1992). While both types aim to apply graduated compression, there are differences in the way they achieve this.

Elastic bandages aim to apply continuous pressure irrespective of patient movement and position. Their elasticity allows them to 'give' when the muscle beneath contracts and to then return to the original extension. After 1 week there is little change in the pressure applied (Blair 1988b, Sockalingham et al 1990). Elastic bandages are currently the most popular in the UK.

Inelastic or 'short stretch' bandaging

Graduated compression can also be applied using inelastic or short stretch bandaging. This method of bandaging is particularly popular in other parts of Europe. These bandages are made of cotton and are applied to the limb at between 90–100% extension. This applies a rigid inelastic cuff around the calf which will not yield when the calf muscle contracts. These bandages require the patient to exercise and when the calf muscle expands there is a steep rise in the sub-bandage pressure. While at rest the pressures are relatively low. The low resting pressure is considered safer in patients who have a degree of arterial disease with reduced perfusion, particularly at night. These bandages rapidly lose their pressure on application. As a result of reduction in oedema they may need to be reapplied in the early stages of treatment.

Multilayer bandaging systems use weaker, more conformable elastic bandages and rely on the build-up of layers to achieve the desired level of compression (Blair et al 1988b, Callam et al 1992, Moffatt & O'Hare 1995).

Compression

Stemmer (1969) recommended that a pressure of between 35 and 40 mmHg was required at the ankle to reverse the effects of chronic venous hypertension. Many of the new bandages and bandage systems aim to apply this level of pressure. As yet we do not know whether this is the optimum pressure. When pressure exceeds 60 mmHg compliance becomes a major problem. It may be that in time it will be possible to prescribe a level of compression appropriate to each underlying aetiology. A classification system has been developed which describes four groups of compression bandages and their recommended use in clinical practice (Table 5.4).

The classification in Table 5.4. is based on the assumption that bandages are applied in a spiral with 50% overlap ensuring two layers of bandage at any point on the limb. If you refer back to Laplace's Law (p. 70), large limbs may have less pressure applied at the ankle than would result from the same bandage applied to a small limb. This highlights the importance of reading manufacturers' instructions which give ranges of limb circumferences within which the stated pressure will be achieved.

Multilayer bandaging systems include cohesive and adhesive bandages which adhere to themselves as well as applying compression. They keep the bandages in place and provide extra durability.

Bandaging technique

Regardless of the appropriate choice of compression method, practical bandaging skills and identification of any limb abnormalities are critical to the effective use of compression. Magazinovic et al (1993) noted that few nurses had an understanding of the principles behind bandaging and as a consequence made inappropriate choices.

Figures 5.2–5.5 illustrate the safe application of bandages.

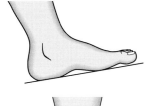
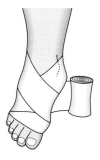
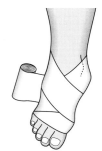

- Flex the foot slightly to avoid excessive layers around the ankle.
- Ensure the bandage is applied from the base of the toes to avoid oedema.
- Avoid excessive figure-of-eight turns around the ankle.
- Check for foot deformities, such as bunions. Avoid excessive pressure over these areas.
- Ensure that the patient has good ankle movement when the bandage is applied.
- Ensure that the patient wears suitable footwear.

Fig. 5.2 Bandaging the foot.

Table 5.4 Classification of compression bandages		
Type	*Level of compression*	*Recommended for*
3a	Light; 14–17 mmHg	Varicose veins Mild eczema
3b	Moderate; 18–24 mmHg	Moderate varicose veins Prevention of ulcer recurrence Treatment of mild oedema
3c	High; 25–35 mmHg	Treatment of venous ulceration and oedema
3d	Very high; 35–50 mmHg	Very large limbs with chronic venous disease and oedema

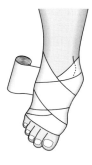

- A spiral application should always be used for strong, single-layer, elastic bandages.

- Patients and carers can be taught this technique.

- The bandage should be applied up to the tibial tuberosity, ensuring that the patient can bend the knee.

- The bandages should be applied at 50% overlap.

- The extension of the bandage should not increase up the limb.

- Care should be taken to avoid applying extra layers. Excessive bandage should be cut off and, if bandages need joining, this should be with minimal overlap.

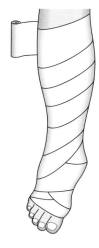

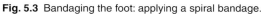

Fig. 5.3 Bandaging the foot: applying a spiral bandage.

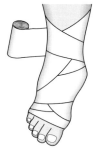

- The foot is bandaged using a figure-of-eight around the ankle.

- The bandage is then continued in a figure-of-eight up the limb.

- This is a useful technique for bandaging disproportionate limbs.

- It helps prevent bandage slippage.

- It is more difficult to apply.

- A figure-of-eight application applies greater pressure than the same bandage applied in a spiral

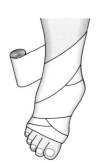

- This is the technique used to apply layer 3 of the 4-layer bandage system (Blair et. al. 1988)

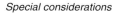

Special considerations
- Any vulnerable points such as the tibial crest should have extra padding to prevent pressure necrosis.

- Inverted 'champagne bottle' shaped legs may require extra padding to the gaiter region to prevent bandage slippage.

- A spiral technique applies less pressure than the application of the same bandage using a figure-of-eight technique.

- Bandages should always be applied according to the manufacturer's insructions. Certain bandages have symbols to guide correct bandage extension, e.g., a rectangle which converts to a square when the bandage is extended by 50%

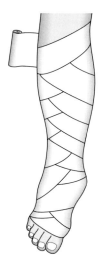

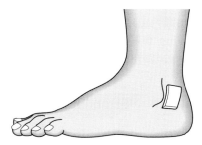

Fig. 5.5 Bandaging the foot: ulcers lying behind the malleolus.

- Ulcers lying behind the malleolus may have insufficient pressure applied by bandages.
- A foam or cotton wool pad can be applied over the primary dressing to increase local pressure and aid ulcer healing.

Fig. 5.4 Bandaging the foot: a figure-of-eight technique.

Choosing bandages

It is very important that you are able to choose an appropriate compression system based on your assessment of the patient. In order to do this you need to know the advantages and disadvantages of the different approaches to compression. The factors to be considered are often complex and to assist you in understanding this process we have provided the following scenarios which illustrate five typical situations together with a rationale for the choice of compression method used.

Activity   5 MINUTES

Scenario 1: Mrs A.

The patient is a 65-year-old woman whose assessment shows she has a normal arterial circulation (RPI = 1.0) and a venous ulcer on the medial malleolus. Previous medical history reveals two episodes of deep vein thrombosis and no obvious varicosities. She is moderately fit and has good ankle movement. She is cared for by the community nurse at home who obtains bandages on prescription. She finds the pain manageable and that it is relieved by exercise and elevation. She is of average weight and her ankle circumference is 23 cm.

What compression method do you think Mrs A. requires?

FEEDBACK

We have chosen an elastic bandage class 3c (see Table 5.4) which applies a pressure of 25–35 mmHg. This is recommended for patients with established venous ulceration. The ankle circumference is within the range specified to achieve this pressure using this class of bandage. If her ankle was significantly larger the same bandage would apply less compression because of the reduction in pressure as the leg circumference gets larger (Laplace's Law).

Activity   5 MINUTES

Scenario 2: Mr B.

The patient is a 40-year-old man whose assessment shows that he has a good arterial circulation (RPI = 1.1). He has developed a venous ulcer on his lateral malleolus, having sustained a deep vein thrombosis following a rugby injury. He is very active and his job involves him walking throughout the day. Although he attends the hospital outpatients' clinic regularly where he is given new bandages, he reapplies the bandage himself whenever necessary.

What compression method do you think Mr B. requires?

FEEDBACK

We have chosen an inelastic (short stretch) bandage which is useful in patients who are very active because the calf muscle action is enhanced. Mr B. wanted to apply his own bandages and his lifestyle may necessitate frequent reapplication. Short stretch bandages are not available on prescription but Mr B. was able to obtain his from the hospital clinic. You may have chosen a class 3c elastic compression bandage or a class 3 elastic stocking (see Table 5.1) which would have been quite appropriate. This highlights that there is often more than one treatment option.

Activity   5 MINUTES

Scenario 3: Mrs C.

The patient is a 77-year-old woman whose assessment shows that she has minimal arterial disease (RPI = 0.9). She has severe underlying venous disease involving both deep and superficial veins. She is immobile, spending long periods of time in a chair. She has a large ulcer with copious amounts of exudate. She is cared for by the community nurse at home. She has thin ankles and wide calves.

What compression method do you think Mrs C. requires?

FEEDBACK

We have chosen a multilayer bandage system which is capable of applying 40 mmHg. The reason for not using a single class 3c elastic compression bandage is primarily because of the shape of her leg. A single bandage will not conform as well as a multilayer system. The padding layer evens out discrepancies between ankle and calf allowing the bandage to stay in place. The padding layer will also absorb exudate. Even though multilayer systems are not available on prescription, the evidence supporting their effectiveness has encouraged many health authorities to purchase them for use on their patients (Moffatt & O'Hare 1995).

Activity 5 MINUTES

Scenario 4: Mrs D.

The patient is an 85-year-old woman whose assessment shows that she has some arterial disease as well as venous hypertension (RPI = 0.6). She has varicose veins and complains of pain at night. Her ulcer is superficial but the surrounding skin is irritable, causing her to want to scratch it to relieve the discomfort. The ulcer produces a moderate amount of exudate. She is immobile owing to arthritis.

What compression method do you think Mrs D. requires?

FEEDBACK

We have chosen an inelastic (short stretch) bandage applied over a paste bandage. The first reason for this is that Mrs D.'s arterial status contraindicates the use of medium or high compression even though her ulcer is of mixed origin. Secondly, the paste bandage will keep the surrounding skin moist and help maintain the minimal amount of compression. Inelastic bandages by themselves rapidly lose their pressure. There are a number of ways of combining bandages to achieve reduced compression. These should be used with care and are modified according to the patient's signs and symptoms and change in resting pressure index. Compression should never be applied on someone with a resting pressure index of 0.5 or below and/or if there is any doubt about the significance of the arterial disease.

Activity 5 MINUTES

Scenario 5: Mrs E.

The patient is a 45-year-old woman whose assessment shows that she has normal arterial circulation (RPI = 1.0). She has varicose veins and is awaiting surgery. She works unsocial hours and therefore finds it difficult to attend for professional treatment.

Her ulcer is small and on the lateral malleolus with minimal exudate. She is adamant that she wants to care for herself as much as possible.

What compression method do you think Mrs E. requires?

FEEDBACK

We have chosen to prescribe Mrs E. a class III compression stocking which is capable of applying up to 35 mmHg pressure and can be renewed on prescription by her GP. Whilst hosiery is more frequently used to prevent ulcer recurrence, it is an ideal choice for Mrs E. who is very independent and has the manual dexterity to apply a class III stocking. You could have chosen a class 3c elastic bandage instead. However, she prefers the ease with which a stocking can be applied and the cosmetic effect.

Self-assessment 10 MINUTES

1. What level of compression is currently recommended for patients with varicose veins?
2. List at least four factors to be taken into consideration when bandaging a patient's foot.
3. List six factors that can increase the pressure applied by an elastic bandage.
4. What level of compression is currently recommended for patients with chronic venous ulceration?
5. List at least six effects that graduated compression has on venous function.

FEEDBACK

1. The level of compression currently recommended for patients with varicose veins is up to 20 mmHg (3a).

2. Factors to be taken into consideration when bandaging a patient's foot include:

   a. good foot position
   b. avoiding excessive layers
   c. avoiding overextension of bandage around the ankle
   d. pressure over bony prominence
   e. ankle function
   f. footwear.

3. Factors that can increase the pressure applied by an elastic bandage include:

   a. increased bandage extension
   b. choice of bandage
   c. bandage width
   d. increased bandage overlap
   e. small limb circumference
   f. increased number of layers.

4. The level of compression currently recommended for patients with chronic venous ulceration is 40 mmHg. (3c)

5. Effects that graduated compression has on venous function include:

   a. reduction of venous hypertension
   b. restoration of valve function
   c. encouragement and enhancement of blood flow in deep veins
   d. decrease in blood volume
   e. facilitation of calf muscle pump action
   f. reduction in oedema
   g. reduction in venous symptoms such as aching limbs
   h. increase in venous ulcer healing
   i. improvement in skin condition.

Compression in clinical practice

In reviewing the role of compression in healing venous ulcers, it can be seen that it is important to understand the science and the art of bandaging. It is only then that compression therapy can be used effectively. Recent research has shown that bandaging technique can be improved by training, in particular through the use of electronic monitors which measure sub-bandage pressures (Nelson 1995). The study went on to show that improvement was maintained when the subjects were retested after 2 weeks. It would be interesting to see whether improvement in bandaging skills is sustained over longer periods. The last decade has seen major improvements in the healing of previously intractable venous ulcers. Compression is likely to remain the cornerstone of treatment for the foreseeable future.

Intermittent pneumatic compression therapy

Intermittent pneumatic compression was originally developed for the prevention of deep vein thrombosis but is now often used to treat chronic venous ulceration and patients with lymphoedema.

An especially designed boot is applied to the limb and connected to a pump. The boot inflates applying pressure cyclically. The pressure settings can be varied and the machine can be used by patients and families.

The system is particularly useful in patients who cannot tolerate compression and is also useful in patients with severe oedema. Intermittent pneumatic compression has been shown to improve venous return, reduce oedema and increase tissue perfusion. However, Hazarika & Wright (1981) have warned that this technique may not be suitable for patients who fear the electrical equipment involved.

Intermittent pneumatic compression should never be applied to patients with severe arterial disease or with an acute deep vein thrombosis.

Skin grafting

Skin grafts are frequently used to treat large ulcers. A number of techniques exist. These include split thickness meshed grafts and pinch grafts (Leaper 1995). Pinch grafting is now performed by nurses in a number of settings and involves taking pinches of skin from an anaesthetised area of the thigh. The grafts are placed on a granulating ulcer bed. Postoperative care of skin grafts involves ensuring that the patient rests and elevates the limb. Compression bandages are generally applied to the limb and the graft left untouched for a week. Patients will often receive prophylactic antibiotics to prevent graft rejection brought about by organisms such as haemolytic streptococci and *Pseudomonas aeruginosa*.

Developments in the skin grafting techniques

As well as the more traditional approaches to skin grafting which have been described, there are new developments which involve tissue expansion. Keratinocyte grafts involve growing sheets of keratinocytes in a laboratory, having taken a small donor area from the patient. These are then grown into a sheet and reapplied in the form of a graft and are particularly useful in burn patients. Allografts are taken from another individual and xenografts are taken from one species and given to another. Allografts have been shown to stimulate wound healing, although the grafts themselves are eventually rejected. Research continues into the development of composite grafts which can be reconstituted from dermal and epidermal components and dermal equivalents which can form the tissue matrix. These developments may form the next generation of products for use in chronic wound repair.

Venous surgery

Increasingly, skin grafts are combined where possible with venous surgery to correct the underlying venous abnormality. Injection sclerotherapy and saphenofemoral or saphenopopliteal ligation may be performed when the venous ulceration is due to primary varicose veins. There is increasing interest and research into the repair of deep veins and valves in patients with very severe venous diseases. However, currently only 2% of patients will benefit from this type of surgery (Wilson & Burnand 1994).

Recurrence of venous ulceration

The epidemiological information on recurrence of venous ulceration is sparse. The Lothian and Forth Valley study (Callam et al 1985) found that two-thirds of patients had experienced two or more episodes of ulceration and that 21% had experienced more than six episodes. A re-ulceration rate of 69% was found in a dermatology clinic at 1 year after healing (Monk & Sarkany 1982). In a community study which contained an active prevention programme, 26% of venous ulcers had recurred at 1 year and 31% by 18 months (Moffatt & Dorman 1995). Until recently very little work had been undertaken to identify which patients were at greater risk of their ulcer recurring. In the community study by Moffatt & Dorman (1995) a number of factors were found to increase the risk of the ulcer recurring. These included:

- a positive history of a deep vein thrombosis
- a previously large ulcer (greater than 10 cm).

Issues such as poor general mobility and reduced limb mobility were not associated with an increased risk of recurrence, although they can make the process of ulcer healing slower.

Even though evidence is sparse, many practitioners agree that the most effective tool in preventing venous ulcer recurrence is the use of graduated compression hosiery after healing. The difficulties surrounding the use of this hosiery are many and complex. Elderly patients or their carers must be educated not only in the method of application but, just as importantly, in understanding the importance of continuing with the treatment even though the ulcer has apparently healed. This represents quite a challenge for nurses.

Activity   60 MINUTES

Read Article 13 in the Reader (p. 170) and then devise a patient education leaflet to help patients to understand the important 'do's' and 'don'ts' related to wearing their hosiery. Use uncomplicated 'friendly' language and address the patient in the first person.

Start your leaflet with a short introduction which stresses why the patient has been given hosiery and the importance of wearing it.

FEEDBACK

Our leaflet would contain the information presented in Box 5.3.

Your leaflet might be longer than ours and that is all right but one of the difficulties in giving out written information is the danger of giving out so much that the patient just will not read it.

Having said this, the patients will almost certainly require instruction on how to put on their hosiery. You would probably teach this through demonstration, but again a leaflet such as the one in Figure 5.6 would be very useful.

Box 5.3 Patient information leaflet

Introduction
It has probably taken you some time to get rid of your ulcer and, now you don't have to wear those bandages any more, it's quite easy to forget to take care of yourself. If you don't wear the stockings you have been given, every day, you could soon have another ulcer. Even though your ulcer has healed, the veins in your leg are still not working normally. It is the pressure your stocking gives that helps improve your circulation. Here are some do's and don'ts to help you.

Do's
- Do ask for help if you have difficulty in either putting on your stockings or taking them off again.
- Do be careful when putting on or taking off your stockings as your skin is still delicate and can easily be damaged.
- Do keep your leg clean and keep your skin supple by using a cream or ointment.
- Do remove your stockings at night.
- Do let your GP or nurse know if your leg swells up, feels or looks different in any way, or if you get a scratch or cut.

Don'ts
- Don't use creams or ointments which contain lanolin. You could cause an allergy or irritate your skin. Ask the advice of your nurse if you are not sure.
- Don't forget to put your stockings back on every morning if you have taken them off for the night.
- Don't wear shoes which are too tight for you.
- Don't forget what it was like to have an ulcer.

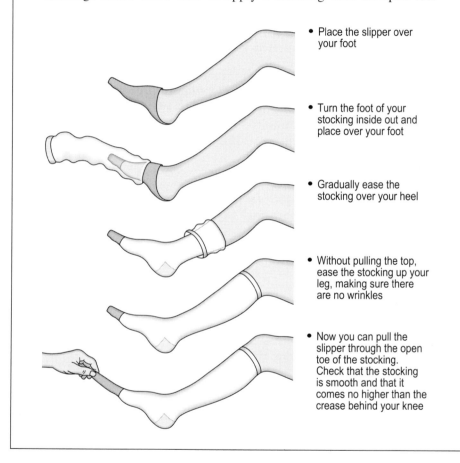

Compression stockings

In order to provide firm support and stop your legs becoming swollen, your stockings should feel firm and be worn every day. You can take them off at night but you should put them on again first thing every morning before your legs become swollen.

Because they need to be firm-fitting, your stockings will take a little longer to put on than ordinary stockings or socks. Regular use of a moisturising cream will help you get them on and keep your skin in good condition. The drawings below show how to apply a stocking with an open toe.

- Place the slipper over your foot

- Turn the foot of your stocking inside out and place over your foot

- Gradually ease the stocking over your heel

- Without pulling the top, ease the stocking up your leg, making sure there are no wrinkles

- Now you can pull the slipper through the open toe of the stocking. Check that the stocking is smooth and that it comes no higher than the crease behind your knee

Fig. 5.6 (A) Patient leaflet on compression hosiery.

Activity   20 MINUTES

Have a second look at the article on hosiery (Reader Article 13, p. 170) and make a new list of 'do's' and 'don'ts'. This time it should be in the form of some guidelines for yourself—some 'do's' and 'don'ts' for clinical practice.

FEEDBACK

We won't repeat the content of the article but hopefully your list includes some advice on issues such as:

- assessing the patient's suitability for compression stockings

Whenever you can, raise your legs.

Get your legs as high as you can. Don't sit upright with your legs hanging down.

The best position would be with your legs level with your chest. Perhaps you could lie on a sofa with your legs on a pillow on the arm.

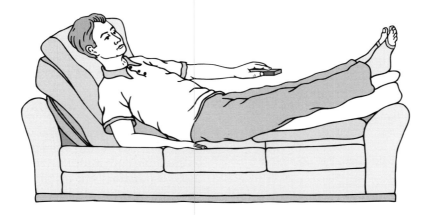

If your legs feel tight or they ache, this is probably because you have not been moving much. Go for a walk or at the very least do the following foot exercises.

- Point your toes toward the floor and then bring your foot back as far as you can. Repeat this exercise at least ten times.

- Move your toes in a circular motion, making as big a circle as you can. You can try this exercise in both a clockwise and anticlockwise direction. Repeat this exercise at least ten times.

Whatever you do, don't take your stockings off.

Fig. 5.6 (B) Patient leaflet on compression hosiery.

- choosing the appropriate product
- identifying areas at risk of pressure damage
- giving advice and support to patients
- giving advice to GPs concerning the information required on a prescription for hosiery, e.g. size, class, length, etc.

5.6 MANAGEMENT OF ARTERIAL ULCERATION

Arterial ulcers present us with complex problems and the prognosis can be very different from that of a patient with a venous ulcer. For the patient who presents with very severe ischaemia, the outcome is

Box 5.4 The outcome of critical ischaemia (Vowden & Vowden 1996)

60% will undergo vascular reconstruction or transluminal angioplasty.
20% will have primary amputation.
20% will have temporary treatment.

At year 1
25% will have had an amputation.
55% will still have legs.
20% will have died.
70% of above-knee and 85% of below-knee amputations have some mobility.
20% only, gain full mobilisation.
31% of amputees will be dead.

At 2 years
Between 15 and 50% of those who have had initial amputations will have had a second amputation.

At 3 years
56% of all amputees will be dead, the higher the amputation the worse the prognosis.

bleak. The European Working Group on Critical Limb Ischaemia (1992) defined 'critical limb ischaemia' as:

> Persistently recurring rest pain requiring regular analgesia for more than two weeks with an ankle systolic blood pressure ≤ 50 mmHg and/or a toe systolic pressure of ≤ 30 mmHg or ulceration or gangrene of the foot and toes.

Box 5.4 presents the findings reported by Vowden & Vowden (1996) from their review of the literature.

Patients often present with complex medical and/or psychological problems. The emphasis of management is usually to improve the underlying aetiology. For this reason a multidisciplinary approach is vital.

Options for dealing with the cause of the ischaemia

Arterial reconstructive surgery

A number of surgical techniques can be used to revascularise different parts of the leg, e.g. aortobi-femoral graft, femoropopliteal bypass and femoro-peroneal bypass. The type of operation varies according to the site of the obstructed vessel. The principle of bypass surgery is the same regardless of site, i.e. to create a new route, using autologous vessels (using the long or short saphenous veins from the same patient) or an artificial prosthesis, to 'bypass' the occluded vessel.

Percutaneous transluminal angioplasty

Percutaneous transluminal angioplasty can also be used for local occlusions. A balloon catheter is inserted in the artery, under X-ray control, which is inflated to shear or split the atheromatous plaque within the vessel. A new innovation, which acts in a similar way, uses a laser to remove plaque through heat vaporisation.

Lumbar sympathectomy

This has been used traditionally to dilate the arteries in the leg but is now thought to have little value in patients with diabetes and those with severe ischaemia (Bryant 1992).

Pharmacological agents

Bryant (1992) discusses the use of pharmacological agents such as vasodilators, rheological agents, anti-coagulants and antiplatelet agents and concludes that vasodilators are of limited use; that the rheo-logic agent pentoxifylline (Trental) has been shown to improve the microcirculation; that anticoagulants are rarely indicated; and that antiplatelet drugs may have a part to play in modifying the development of plaque.

Activity   15 MINUTES

Given the above discussion of ways of dealing with the underlying cause of ischaemia, what do you think are the three priorities of nursing management?

● ●

FEEDBACK

The nurse can do a great deal to help the patient by providing: effective wound management; control of symptoms; and reduction of risk factors through effective patient education.

● ●

Effective wound management

Effective wound management in the patient with an arterial ulcer involves the principles discussed in subsections 5.1–5.4. However, there are some specific issues you should be aware of.

• Debridement should be used with caution. In the presence of an adequate blood supply debridement may promote healing. This can be achieved through surgical means, autolysis, or chemical debridement. The latter may cause sensitivity and, if the blood supply is inadequate, hyperaemia and tissue necrosis. Patients presenting with dry gangrene should not be debrided until the underlying vascular status is ascertained. If debridement is undertaken in a poorly vascularised foot, the resulting open wound may become infected and lead to greater tissue loss.

- Promoting a moist wound environment should also be done with care because of the danger of bacteria causing overwhelming infection in the patient whose blood supply is inadequate to provide sufficient oxygen. The wound should be observed frequently because deterioration can be rapid. However, a recent study showed that keeping the wound occluded significantly reduced the level of pain experienced (Gibson et al 1995).

- Compression therapy should never be used in a patient with a resting pressure index of less than 0.5.

Control of symptoms

Control of symptoms such as pain and oedema are significant problems for patients with arterial disease. Effective pain control with opiates is frequently required. Control of oedema is difficult. Whilst you should encourage elevation of the legs, this should never be above the level of the heart as this will reduce the effect of gravity on tissue perfusion. This is different from the advice you would give to a patient with venous ulceration, where high elevation helps venous return to the heart.

Reduction of risk factors

This can be important in preventing further deterioration. Patients should be advised to stop smoking, reduce weight, modify their diet and prevent further trauma to their limbs. This will often involve helping patients' families adjust to a modified lifestyle. Achieving these goals may be difficult, demanding and often unsuccessful.

5.7 MANAGEMENT OF MIXED AETIOLOGY ULCERATION

When caring for a patient with an ulcer of combined arterial and venous origins it is essential that you have identified the significance of the arterial disease during your assessment because this factor will determine whether or not you can use compression therapy. Full compression can be applied safely to patients with an RPI greater than 0.8. You will remember from Section 5.6 that compression should never be applied to patients with an RPI of less than 0.5. A reduced level of compression can be applied to patients with an RPI of 0.6 and 0.7 but the exact level of compression will depend on the severity of their symptoms and ability to tolerate bandages. Generally no more than 25 mmHg pressure should be applied.

In some circumstances vascular surgeons may correct the underlying arterial problem and, providing the RPI is above 0.8, full compression can be used postoperatively with careful supervision. If the patient shows any sign of deterioration the RPI should be remeasured and if necessary compression discontinued. Similarly, arterial angioplasty is increasingly used to improve the blood supply.

Activity   20 MINUTES

Review your own patients. Make a note of:

1. how many have ulcers of mixed aetiology
2. what types of compression therapy are being used and what is the greatest priority in making decisions about these patients.

FEEDBACK

1. The literature suggests that 10–20% of patients have ulceration of mixed aetiology. The older they become the higher the chance of their having concurrent arterial disease.
2. In deciding on reduced compression one of the most important factors will be the patient's ability to tolerate compression. Consideration of the patient's signs and symptoms is the greatest priority and should not be ignored.

5.8 MANAGEMENT OF ULCERS IN PATIENTS WITH RHEUMATOID ARTHRITIS

Managing a patient with an ulcer associated with rheumatoid arthritis can be challenging. Careful assessment must identify the underlying aetiology (see Sect. 3). If the patient has a venous component, compression therapy may be required. This must be very carefully applied to avoid any trauma as the skin in these patients is often delicate owing to prolonged use of steroids. Attention to skin hygiene is important as these patients are especially prone to infection. Care should be taken to ensure that the compression therapy does not limit ankle movement as this may compromise their already limited joint function.

Skin should be kept supple by using emollients and protected from trauma.

If the underlying origin of the ulcer is arterial, care is as described in Section 5.7. However, these patients may present with microvascular disease which causes local tissue ischaemia and ulceration. This type of ulceration is frequently very painful and produces copious amounts of exudate. Analgesia frequently involves the use of opiates, particularly prior to dressing changes. Wound management should address the problem of exudate and the primary dressings should not be allowed to adhere as this will increase pain. Despite the severity of the ulceration, skin grafting procedures frequently fail owing both to the accumulation of oedema as patients cannot elevate their limbs and to high doses of steroids which delay wound healing. Graft failure is particularly pronounced during an exacerbation of the disease. Because of the debilitating nature of the disease, appetite is often poor. This, together with protein loss from high exudate levels, can lead to delayed wound healing and anaemia.

The complexities of managing a patient with rheumatoid arthritis are explored in Case Study 9 (p. 109).

5.9 MANAGEMENT OF DIABETIC ULCERATION

The management of ulceration in the patient with diabetes represents one of the most difficult aspects in the general field of leg ulceration; so much so that your first priority, if possible, should be prevention of ulceration. Caputo et al (1994) describe the central role peripheral neuropathy plays, it being present in '80% of diabetic patients with foot lesions'. They go on to state that 'in most cases, ulceration is a consequence of the loss of protective sensation'.

Neuropathy is often compounded by the presence of arterial disease and infection.

Once ulceration has occurred, the patient has a potentially limb-threatening, if not life-threatening, condition.

Activity   50 MINUTES

We have described the origin of diabetic ulceration in some detail in Section 3, and Case Studies 6 and 7 (pp. 102–107) explore some of the practical issues involved. Rather than repeat ourselves in this section we would like you to try to summarise the management of diabetic foot ulceration by completing an algorithm devised by Caputo et al (1994) (Fig. 5.7). Then check your answers by reading their excellent

summary entitled *Assessment and Management of Foot Disease in Patients with Diabetes* (Reader Article 14, p. 175). We have filled in the treatment for the simplest type of ulcer. You will note that, regardless of the severity of the ulceration and treatment, all the pathways end at the same box. Think in terms of the long-term goals of management.

FEEDBACK

You probably found this activity quite demanding. We make no apologies for this because the consequences of inappropriate or inadequate treatment of this type of patient can be so devastating for the patient, family and yourself.

5.10 COMPLIANCE AND PATIENT EDUCATION

Wise (1986) describes the concept commonly termed the 'social ulcer'. There are repeated anecdotal references in nursing to a group of patients who are perceived to deliberately delay the healing of their ulcer. They are said to do this because they are seen to be predominantly elderly and isolated and to enjoy the social contact associated with the care of their ulcer, either with health care professionals or, if they attend a clinic, with their fellow patients. There is no doubt that anyone who has observed a busy leg ulcer clinic will have sensed a camaraderie or even 'club-like' atmosphere. For this reason some institutions have begun to explore the concept of a 'well ulcer clinic'. Ruane-Morris et al (1995) describe the formation of healed ulcer groups (HUGs) which consist of a group of 6–8 patients with an RPI of 0.8 or greater, who have a healed ulcer. These groups undertake a five-session programme designed to promote self-care and the 'maintenance of healthy legs'. The recurrence rates in these groups seems to support the validity of these groups, although a randomised controlled experimental model has not been used to evaluate the findings. Whether or not patients deliberately interfere with their ulcer is a different matter from the general issue of compliance with treatment. There is perhaps a danger in being too judgemental in our attitude to patients. How many of us practice what we preach? For example, as health professionals we know the dangers of smoking, yet many of us make an active decision to take the risk because the consequences seem so remote and impersonal, i.e. 'it won't happen to me'. It is hard to imagine why someone who has

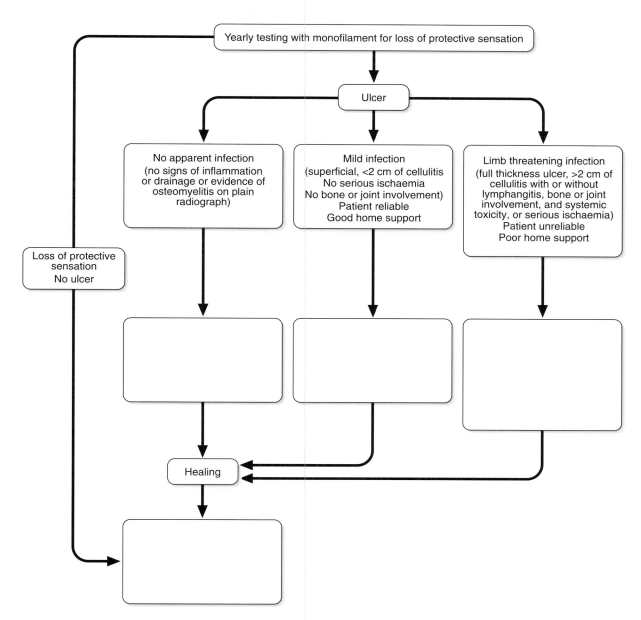

Fig. 5.7 Management of diabetic foot ulcers.

had a leg ulcer for months or even years could possibly not comply with recommended preventive measures, but it happens. Travers et al (1990) reported that 60% of patients in a study of 32 women found that the cosmetic appearance of their hosiery was unacceptable and that 54% did not wear it at all.

Throughout this pack we have made a number of references to health promotion, patient education and to the relationship between health care professionals, patients and carers. It is essential that a relationship of trust and partnership is developed. Patients are more likely to take ownership of their problems if they have been actively involved in decisions about their treatment and have faith in those

caring for them. For example, it may be that you want to apply high compression to someone with a venous ulcer but who is concerned that the bandage will increase the pain. You may have to compromise and accept that the level of compression will have to be increased slowly and that healing will take a little longer than you might like. The alternative, if you expect the patient to passively comply, might be that you will never be able to get him or her to accept an effective level of compression.

How we communicate with patients is also important. Porritt (1990) emphasises the importance of patient-centred communication to building a successful relationship. McCleod-Clarke (1988) states

'It will always be easier to tell someone what to do or give prescriptive advice rather than facilitate or assist them in making their own decision'.

Think about the above quotation and identify at least four skills you think an effective facilitator requires.

FEEDBACK

The skills required by someone who seeks to become a good facilitator are both numerous and subtle. Your list should have included some of the following.

- Listening to patients actively.
- Empathising with patients.
- Encouraging patients to talk.
- Answering patients' questions.
- Mutually deciding goals.
- Using clear, unambiguous language.

- Sensing and responding to mood and nonverbal cues.
- Focusing on issues.
- Helping to clarify issues.
- Re-enforcing learning.
- Just being there.

The last of these may at first seem ambiguous but Wilson-Barnett (1988) describes an exploration of the effect of psychiatric nurses on patients, which suggests that the presence alone of a trusted practitioner is enough in itself to provide comfort to patients.

As an educator of patients you will need to acquire these kinds of personal characteristics and, in addition, you will have to take into account countless practical considerations when attempting to educate your patients. Can they hear what you are saying? Can they see what you have written? Do they speak the same language as you do? Are they literate? Are they numerate? And ultimately, do they have the cognitive ability to understand what you are trying to communicate? An in-depth exploration of the issues of patient compliance and health education is extremely complex and beyond the scope of this pack.

SUMMARY

In this section you have learned the following things.

- There is a dearth of empirical research on wound cleansing, though current trends are toward simple methods which avoid antiseptics and recognise the important social elements of cleansing.

- Leg ulcers are often heavily colonised with microorganisms, but antibiotic treatment is only indicated when the signs and symptoms of clinical infection are present.

- Skin care is an important priority in maintaining skin integrity and preventing skin problems relating to varicose eczema irritation and contact allergy.

- Dressings must be matched to the stage of wound healing. Choice of products will be influenced by many external factors, such as availability and lifestyle.

- Compression therapy is the cornerstone of management for venous ulceration and lymphatic disorders. For compression to be effective the practitioner must understand the scientific principles that underpin its use as well as the problems of practical application.

- A number of alternative techniques are used in the treatment of venous ulceration. These include:

—intermittent pneumatic compression
—skin grafting
—venous surgery.

- Strategies for prevention of recurrence are important and should include appropriate use of compression hosiery and patient education.

- The prognosis for patients with arterial ulceration can be bleak. Interventions include:

—arterial reconstructive surgery
—percutaneous transluminal angioplasty
—lumbar sympathectomy
—pharmacological agents.

- Treatment for arterial ulceration should include control of infection and pain, and reduction of risk factors.

- Management of mixed ulceration is highly dependent on the patient's signs and symptoms. Compression therapy should be used with caution.

- Ulceration in patients who have diabetes represents one of the most difficult challenges for the practitioner. The complicated risk factors surrounding the patient with diabetes will contribute to delayed healing. Priorities include relief of pressure, treatment of infection, rigorous debridement, effective wound management and risk factor reduction.

- The effectiveness of treatment strategies depends largely on cooperation and effective patient education.

REFERENCES

Bale S, Jones V 1997 Wound care nursing. A patient-centred approach. Baillière Tindall, London

Blair S D, Backhouse C M, Wright D D I, Riddle E, McCollum C N 1988a Do dressings influence the healing of chronic venous ulcers? Phlebology 3: 129–134

Blair S D, Wright D D I, Backhouse C M, Riddle E, McCollum C N 1988b Sustained compression and healing of chronic venous ulcers. British Medical Journal 297: 1159–1161

Bryant R A 1992 Acute and chronic wounds: nursing management. Mosby Year Book, St. Louis

Callam M J, Ruckley C V, Harper D R, Dale J J 1985 Chronic ulceration of the leg: extent of the problem and provision of care. British Medical Journal 290: 1855–1856

Callam M J, Harper D R, Dale J J, Ruckley C V, Prescott R J 1987 A controlled trial of weekly ultrasound therapy in chronic leg ulceration. Lancet 2(8552): 204–206

Callam M J, Ruckley C V, Dale J J, Harper D R 1987 Hazards of compression treatment of the leg: an estimate from Scottish surgeons. British Medical Journal 295: 1382

Callam M J, Harper D R, Dale J J, Brown D, Gibson B, Prescott R J, Ruckley C J 1992 Lothian and Forth Valley Leg Ulcer Healing Trial part one, elastic versus non-elastic bandaging in the treatment of chronic leg ulceration. Phlebology 7(4): 136–141

Caputo G M, Cavanagh P R, Ulbrecht J S, Gibbons G W, Karchmer A W 1994 Assessment and management of foot disease in patients with diabetes. New England Journal of Medicine 331(13): 854–860

Cullum N 1994 The nursing management of leg ulcers in the community: a critical review of research. Department of Health, HMSO, London

Cullum N, Roe B 1995 Leg ulcers: nursing management: a research based guide. Scutari, London

Cutting K F, Harding K 1994 Criteria for identifying wound infection. Journal of Wound Care 3(4): 198–201

Dealey C 1994 The care of wounds: a guide for nurses. Blackwell Scientific Publications, Oxford

Duby T, Hofman D S, Cameron J, Doblhoff-Brown D, Cherry G, Ryan T 1993 A randomised trial in the treatment of venous leg ulcers comparing short stretch bandages, four layer system and a long stretch paste system. Wounds: A Compendium of Clinical Research and Practice 5(6): 276–279

Gibson B, Harper D R, Nelson A E, Prescott R J, Ruckley C V 1995 Comparison of a hydrocolloid and a knitted viscose dressing in the treatment of arterial leg ulcers. Abstract from 5th European Conference on Advances in Wound Management, Harrogate

Gilchrist B 1994 Treating bacterial wound infection. Nursing Times 90(50): 55–58

Gilchrist B 1996 Wound infection 1. Sampling bacterial flora: a review of the literature. Journal of Wound Care 5(8): 386–388

Gilchrist B, Reed C 1989 The bacteriology of chronic venous ulcers treated with occlusive hydrocolloid dressings. British Journal of Dermatology 121: 337–344

Hampson J P 1996 The use of metronidazole in the treatment of malodorous wounds. Journal of Wound Care 5(9): 421–426

Hazarika E Z, Wright D E 1981 Chronic leg ulcers: the effect of pneumatic intermittent compression. Practitioner 225: 189–192

Hinman C D, Maibach H 1963 Effective air exposure and occlusion on experimental human skin wounds. Nature 200: 377–378

Hosein I K 1996 Wound infection 2. MRSA. Journal of Wound Care 5(8): 386–388

Hutchinson J J 1990 The rate of clinical infection in occluded wounds. In: Alexander J W, Thompson P D, Hutchinson J J (eds) International forum on wound microbiology. Excerpta Medica, Princeton, pp 27–34

Hutchinson J J 1992 Influence of occlusive dressings on wound microbiology: interim results of a multicentre clinical trial of an occlusive hydrocolloid dressing. In: Harding K G, Leaper D L, Turner T D (eds) Proceedings of the 1st European Conference on Advances in Wound Management. Macmillan Magazines, London, pp 152–155

Leaper D 1994 Prophylactic and therapeutic role of antibiotics in wound care. American Journal of Surgery 167(1A)(suppl A Symposium: Wound infection and occlusion—separating fact from fiction): 15S–19S

Leaper D 1995 The management of venous ulcers—the medical and surgical options. Journal of Wound Care 4(10): 477–481

McCleod-Clarke J 1988 Communication: a continuing challenge. Nursing Times 84(23): 24–27

Magazinovic N, Phillips-Turner J, Wilson G V 1993 Assessing nurses' knowledge of bandages and bandaging. Journal of Wound Care 2(2): 97–101

Meyerovitz B R, Nelson R 1964 Measurement of the velocity of blood in lower limb veins with or without compression. Surgery 56(3): 481–486

Moffatt C J, Dorman M C 1995 Recurrence of leg ulcers within a community ulcer service. Journal of Wound Care 4(2): 57–61

Moffatt C J, O'Hare L 1995 Venous leg ulceration: treatment by high compression bandaging. Ostomy/Wound Management 41(4): 16–25

Monk B M E, Sarkany I 1982 Outcome of treatment of venous stasis ulcers. Clinical Experimental Dermatology 7: 397–400

Morison M, Moffatt C J 1994 A colour guide to the assessment and management of leg ulcers, 2nd edn. Mosby, London

Nelson E A 1995 Improvements in bandaging technique following training. Journal of Wound Care 4(4): 181–184

Porritt L 1990 The challenge of listening: how to read the music of the message. In: Porritt L Interaction strategies: an introduction for health professionals, 2nd edn. Churchill Livingstone, Edinburgh

Raj T B, Goddard M, Makin G S 1980 How long do compression bandages maintain their pressure during ambulatory treatment of varicose veins. British Journal of Surgery 67: 122–124

Ruane-Morris M, Thomson G, Lawton S 1995 Supporting patients with healed leg ulcers. Professional Nurse 10(12): 765–770

Sarin S, Scurr J H, Coleridge-Smith P D 1992 Mechanism of action of external compression in venous disease. In: Raymond-Martinbeau P, Prescott R, Zummd M (eds) Phlebology. John Libbey, Eurotext, Paris

Schraibman I G 1990 The significance of beta haemolytic streptococci in chronic leg ulcers. Annals of the Royal College of Surgeons (England) 72: 123–124

Schraibman I G 1995 Antibiotic policy on leg ulcer management. In: Negus D, Jantet G, Coleridge-Smith P D (eds) Phlebology 95 Proceedings of the XII World Congress Union Internationale de Phlébologie. Springer Verlag, Berlin, vol 2, p 941

Second European Consensus Document on Chronic Critical Limb Ischaemia 1992 European Journal of Vascular Surgery 6(suppl A): 1–32

Sigel B, Edelstein A L, Savitch L, Hasty J H, Felix W R 1975 Type of compression for reducing venous stasis. Archives of Surgery 110: 171–175

Sigg K 1963 Compression with compression bandages and elastic stockings for prophylaxis and therapy of venous disorders of the leg. Fortschrifthiche Medizan 15: 601–606

Sockalingham S, Barbanel J C, Queen D 1990 Ambulatory monitoring of the pressure beneath compression bandages. Care Science and Practice 8(2): 75–79

Stemmer R 1969 Ambulatory–elasto-compressive treatment of the lower extremities particularly with elastic stockings. Kassenarzt 9: 1–8

Thomas S M 1990 Wound management and dressings. Pharmaceutical Press, London

Thomas S 1995 Bandages used in leg ulcer management. In: Cullum N, Roe B (eds) Leg ulcers: nursing management: a research based guide. Scutari, London, pp 63–74

Thompson P D, Smith D J 1994 What is infection? American Journal of Surgery 167(1A)(suppl A Symposium: wound infection and occlusion—separating fact from fiction): 7S–11S

Travers J P, Harrison J D, Makin G S 1990 Post operative use of compression stockings in preventing recurrence of varicose veins. Royal Society of Medicine—Venous Forum: London

Trengrove N J, Stacey M C, McGechie D F, Stingemore N F, Mata S 1996 Qualitative bacteriology and leg ulcer healing. Journal of Wound Care 5(6): 277–280

Turner T D 1982 Which dressing and why? Nursing Times 3: 71–75

Varghese M C, Baun A K, Carter, D M, Caldwell D 1986 Local environment of chronic wounds under synthetic dressings. Archives of Dermatology 122: 52–57

Vin F 1995 The physiology of compression: clinical consequences, precautions and contra-indication. In: Negus D, Jantet G, Coleridge-Smith P D (eds) Phlebology 95 Proceedings of the XII World Congress Union Internationale de Phlébologie. Springer Verlag, Berlin, vol 2, pp 1134–1137

Vowden K R, Vowden P 1996 Peripheral arterial disease. Journal of Wound Care 5(1): 23–26

Wilson J 1995 Infection control in clinical practice. Baillière Tindall, London

Wilson N M, Burnand K G 1994 The post-thrombotic syndrome. Current Practice in Surgery 6: 16–24

Wilson-Barnett J 1988 Lend me your ear. Nursing Times 84(23): 51–53

Winter G D 1962 Formation of the scab and the rate of epithelialisation of superficial wounds in the skin of the young domestic pig. Nature 193: 293–294

Wise G 1986 The social ulcer. Nursing Times 82(21): 47–49

Young T 1996 Methicillin resistant *Staphylococcus aureus*. Journal of Wound Care 5(10): 475–477

FURTHER READING

Bale S, Jones V 1997 Wound care nursing. A patient-centred approach. Baillière Tindall, London

Flanagan M 1997 Wound management. (Access to Clinical Education Series) Churchill Livingstone, Edinburgh

Morison M, Moffatt C J 1994 A colour guide to the assessment and management of leg ulcers, 2nd edn. Mosby, London

6 Case studies

The following case studies represent a view of some typical leg ulcer patients. They are all based on the experience of real people.

The patient with a leg ulcer is seldom uncomplicated in terms of assessment and treatment. In order to deliver high quality holistic care, each person must be viewed as unique.

These case studies are designed both to show some of the complexities of caring for people with leg ulcers and to provide an insight into a variety of different professional perspectives.

LEARNING OUTCOMES

When you have completed this section you will be able to:

- identify key factors involved in making nursing assessments in each of the cases described
- plan appropriate care for each of the cases described
- explain the particular nature of patient experiences and their consequences for assessment, planning and intervention
- describe the roles of a wide range of professionals who comprise the multidisciplinary team.

CASE STUDY 1: EVELYN GOLDING —SIMPLE VENOUS ULCER

Scenario

The following scenario puts you in the role of a district nurse making a first visit to a patient with a leg ulcer. She has been previously treated by another district nursing colleague on a daily basis but owing to reorganisation she is now part of your case load.

You make your first visit to Mrs Golding to reassess her chronic leg ulcer. You ring the doorbell and wait a long time for her to answer. Mrs Golding is a frail 84-year-old and evidently she has great difficulty in walking. She lets you in and shuffles slowly back into the living room. You are hit by a wave of heat and the overwhelming smell from her leg ulcer. The room she lives in is cluttered and dirty. Mrs Golding sits in a large armchair near a gas fire and her large black cat returns to sit on her lap. You

struggle to find somewhere to place your bag and have to clear papers from a chair in order to sit down. Looking round the room you notice a bed in the corner of the room covered with debris and there are the half-eaten remains of meals on wheels packs. You note your own revulsion at what you see and wish that you could leave.

Mrs Golding looks pale, tired and uninterested. As you tell her that you will be taking over her care, she nods without question. On being asked about the background to her leg ulcer she replies, 'I have had this ulcer for 6 years and it's getting worse all the time. Sometimes I think I would be better if they took it off.' She looks away, her eyes filled with tears. You prompt her to tell you about herself: 'I lost my husband 10 years ago, he had been ill for a long time. Since then I've lived here alone. My two children are both married. My son has a good job and he is away a lot with his job and my daughter lives in Wales; she has two children but I don't get to see them very often. They have their own lives to lead. To tell you the truth my daughter says that with my leg like this, it isn't healthy for the grandchildren to visit.'

As you listen you sense her sadness and feel helpless to intervene. Prompted by the uncomfortable situation you decide to examine her leg. You explain what you are going to do and with some difficulty clear a space for the equipment and place a plastic bag over the foot stool. You ask Mrs Golding if you can remove the cat from her lap and she unwillingly agrees, but he returns while you are changing the dressing. You remove a sodden outer dressing and a light bandage to reveal a dirty large ulcer on her left leg. You remove a layer of antibiotic tulle gras and the surrounding skin is red and excoriated. There is evidence of skin changes. She winces with pain when you remove the dressing and avoids looking at the ulcer. The offensive smell makes you draw back involuntarily. Sitting down to regain your composure you ask more about her previous medical history. She tells you that she had a hysterectomy when she was 65 years old. Following her operation she had swelling in her left leg and was given a straight tubular bandage to control this, but no further investigations were carried out. On returning home she noticed that the skin became discoloured and the swelling persisted. She tells you she has a great deal of pain in both hips and on examination you find that she has little movement in either ankle. She takes no medication other than the occasional paracetamol, which has little effect. The pain, which seems to be worse at night, has led her to give up going to bed as it involves so much effort. You perform a resting pressure index measurement using Doppler ultrasound which gives a reading of 0.95 on the left leg and 0.9 on the right. Her blood pressure is 150/90 mmHg, and her blood glucose level 3.7 mmol/l. Examination of the nursing notes reveals that her weight is approximately 82 kg and her height 1.5 m. Numerous different dressings have been used, and the application of paste bandages and hydrocolloids appears to have caused the leg ulcer to deteriorate. There is no evidence that compression therapy has been used and the notes do not indicate the cause of the ulcer.

Self-assessment   5 MINUTES

What four factors indicate that Mrs Golding has a venous ulcer?

FEEDBACK

The following four factors indicate a likely diagnosis of venous ulceration.

1. Resting pressure indexes of 0.9 and 0.95 would indicate normal arterial flow in a woman of this age (see Sect. 3).
2. Skin changes in the gaiter region caused by haemosiderin deposits (see Sect. 3).
3. The position of the ulcer in the gaiter region (see Sect. 3).
4. The swelling and skin changes indicating the possibility of an undiagnosed deep vein thrombosis following hysterectomy.

Contact dermatitis in venous ulcer patients

Mrs Golding is typical of many patients with venous ulceration who experience skin problems. The following activity explores these issues further.

Activity   40 MINUTES

1. Read Article 15 in the Reader (p. 182).
2. Is there any indication in the scenario that Mrs Golding has a history of contact dermatitis?

3. Make a note of any issues in the article which have implications for the care of Mrs Golding.

FEEDBACK

Contact sensitivity is a commonly associated problem in patients with venous ulceration. The article suggests that 50–69% of patients suffer with contact sensitivity problems. This situation is often exacerbated when there is concurrent eczema. Contact dermatitis is a form of exogenous eczema caused by irritants or allergens. Sensitivity may occur shortly after exposure to the allergen or perhaps many years after using the substance. While the dermatitis may be limited to the exposed area it is possible for it to spread to other areas of the body (see Sect. 4).

The scenario indicates that she has a history of contact dermatitis. She has erythema in the gaiter region and complains of irritation, pain and swelling.

It is likely that Mrs Golding is allergic to the antibiotic tulle gras dressing used; this is one of the most potent sensitising agents. There is also a danger of increasing the risk of multiresistant organisms when using topical antibiotics. The dressing is unable to adequately deal with the local infection and the organisms develop resistance to the antibiotics.

Mrs Golding's history raises the possibility of other allergies, in particular to paste bandages. Following this treatment the leg ulcer deteriorated. This may be due to the preservative parabens used in paste bandages (Cameron 1995). There is now a new paste bandage which does not contain parabens and is claimed to have a very low allergy rate (Powell et al 1994). There is also a suggestion that Mrs Golding may have been allergic to a hydrocolloid dressing. The allergy rate to hydrocolloid dressings is thought to be low but Mrs Golding may have been allergic to the adhesive backing. It has been suggested, however, that these types of occlusive dressings provide an ideal environment for sensitisation (Cameron 1995). What is thought to be an allergic response to hydrocolloid dressings may be maceration and excoriation due to either the dressing not being changed frequently enough or the dressing being too small for effective occlusion.

If for any reason you consider Mrs Golding has a contact allergy, you should discontinue the treatment immediately. The leg should be washed with warm water or saline to remove any residual allergen. You should document your actions carefully and discuss the situation with Mrs Golding's GP. If the GP agrees, you may wish to use a steroid cream or ointment for a short period of time. If you are uncertain whether to use a cream or ointment it is probably preferable to choose an ointment-based steroid in case Mrs Golding is allergic to the ingredients used in the cream (cetylstearyl alcohol). It is wise to reduce the strength of the treatment before discontinuing. It is also important to remember that steroid creams or ointments can in themselves cause allergy (Hannuksela & Salo 1986).

Given that Mrs Golding may be allergic to some of the products that have been used previously, you should choose a bland, non-sensitising dressing that will cause no further harm (Blair et al 1988). The pre-existing eczematous condition will require the use of an emollient to reduce dryness. Avoid using creams or ointments containing lanolin or cetylstearyl alcohol, or which are perfume based. A useful treatment for Mrs Golding might be 50% white soft paraffin and 50% liquid paraffin. It might be useful to refer Mrs Golding for patch testing to find out the product she is allergic to. Remember that allergies can occur at a later date following patch testing. The successful treatment of the allergy has direct consequences for the rate of healing (Cameron & Powell 1992).

Mrs Golding has a chronic venous ulcer and requires an effective compression regime. There is no evidence that compression has been tried on Mrs Golding. If her oedema is not controlled her venous ulcer will never heal.

Choosing a compression regime

The most important component of Mrs Golding's treatment will be the provision of the right kind of compression (see Sect. 5). The following activity illustrates how you go about choosing an effective regime.

Activity   15 MINUTES

Before deciding on a particular bandaging regime you should assess her limb to identify any specific problems that might influence your decision. Write down the problems which you think you should take into account.

FEEDBACK

You should have noted the following.

- Copious amounts of exudate and skin in poor condition.
- Fixed ankle joint.
- Limited general mobility.

- Failure to go to bed at night or elevate the limb.
- No previous use of compression therapy. Is this due to a problem of compliance with treatment?
- Depression and apathy towards treatment.

Having decided on an appropriate skin care regime, it is now essential to choose an appropriate bandage that Mrs Golding will find comfortable and which will aid venous ulcer healing. Remember when choosing a primary dressing that this wound is covered with slough and produces copious exudate. Your dressing must be able to absorb exudate and prevent further deterioration of the ulcer or surrounding skin.

Self-assessment   10 MINUTES

What is the most appropriate compression bandaging regime for Mrs Golding? Can you suggest three alternatives? Are there disadvantages to any of them? To review the full range of bandages and their clinical use, please return to Section 5.

FEEDBACK

You may have chosen a single elastic bandage such as Setopress or Tensopress. These bandages aim to apply 40 mmHg of pressure at the ankle. They can be rewashed and are available on prescription—an advantage as Mrs Golding is being treated in the community. An elastic bandage may be useful in Mrs Golding's case as this type of bandage applies the same pressure at rest and during exercise. Mrs Golding is very immobile and may benefit from sustained compression. A disadvantage of single elastic bandages is the danger of applying excessively high pressures if the bandage is overextended or if the limb is very thin. You would need to consider how to protect Mrs Golding's leg by use of padding.

Another alternative is to consider the use of a multilayer bandage system containing elastic bandages (Blair et al 1988). Multilayer bandage systems rely on the concept of applying pressure through the use of layers of bandage. The advantage of this system in Mrs Golding's case is that the bandages are very absorbent and conform well to abnormal limb shapes. Like single elastic bandages, multilayer bandages apply 40 mmHg pressure which remains constant until the bandages are removed. These bandage regimes have been successfully used in large community studies. A disadvantage of these bandages is that they are not available on prescription and must be purchased by health authorities. Although these bandages are not excessively bulky, you would need to check that Mrs Golding's footwear is suitable.

Another type of bandaging regime involves the use of short stretch bandages. These bandages are made of 100% cotton. Short stretch bandaging is used extensively in other parts of Europe but there is an increasing interest in the UK. Short stretch bandages apply a relatively inelastic structure around the calf which will not yield when the calf muscle expands. This has the effect of causing a steep rise in sub-bandage pressure during exercise and relatively low pressures at rest.

One of the main advantages of short stretch bandaging is its relative safety. It has been suggested that these bandages are safer in patients with an arterial component because of the low pressures at rest. Mrs Golding has a normal arterial circulation so this may be less of an issue in her case. Mrs Golding's immobility may reduce the potential benefit of these types of bandage.

Case study outcome

Mrs Golding's compression regime began with a four-layer bandage system. Her skin improved rapidly following a short course of steroid cream. Her ulcer took nearly 9 months to heal and her skin required careful attention during this time. At each home visit emollients were applied to prevent skin dehydration. When her ulcer healed she was fitted with a class II compression stocking. Owing to Mrs Golding's immobility a nurse still visits weekly to reapply the stocking and examine her legs. Within 2 months Mrs Golding had improved sufficiently to visit her daughter. This has proved very therapeutic for her and her mood has become more optimistic. She says that the relief of pain has made a great difference to her life; she is now sleeping well at night and going to bed. Her mobility remains a problem and she is still largely housebound and waiting to have a hip replacement which, it is hoped, will improve this situation. As her mobility and quality of life have improved she has begun to take a greater interest in her flat, which is considerably cleaner and less cluttered.

CASE STUDY 2: MR PETER SMITH
—COMPLEX VENOUS ULCER

Scenario

The following scenario places you in the role of out-patient nurse in a district general hospital. Mr Smith is referred to a busy surgical clinic with a non-healing ulcer. The referral letter from Mr Smith's GP says that Mr Smith has tried various treatments but that he will not comply with any of them. The doctors with whom you work ask you to assess him.

You invite Mr Smith into a consulting room. He rises from his chair and angrily tells you that he hopes his visit will be quick as he must get to work. You try to reassure him. He asks why you are assessing him and says that he wanted to see a doctor. You explain your role and ask him to sit. His aggression makes you feel uneasy.

You ask Mr Smith to tell his story.

He tells you that this is the third bout of ulceration. You note that he is only 43 years old. He tells you that following a rugby injury he noted that his leg swelled during the day and that the skin became discoloured. You ask more about his injury. He apparently suffered a lot of soft tissue damage and extensive bruising at the time of the injury but this was never investigated.

Mr Smith tells you that he works in a large accountancy firm that requires him to work long hours and to travel to work by train. You sense Mr Smith's depression and frustration with the situation and prompt him to tell you more. Mr Smith is married with two teenage children. He tells you that the pressures of his career and his leg ulcer are placing a great strain on the family. He is near to tears and explains that because of the smell of his ulcer and his restlessness at night he and his wife now sleep in separate rooms. His children are unsympathetic with their father's condition. He tells you that his leg ulcer dominates his life and that he knows that he is bad tempered. During travel to work people have commented on the offensive smell and he is unable to socialise with clients at work as he should. He tells you that his job is now at risk and that he is afraid that he will not be able to keep up the payments on his large mortgage.

You question him about his previous reluctance to comply with treatment. He becomes angry, stating that coming for treatment requires him to take time off work that he cannot afford. He tells you that the treatments increase the odour but that he tries to control it by showering twice daily and applying large absorbent pads to cope with the exudate. Mr Smith secures the dressing with tape and avoids bandages which he tells you increase the skin irritation. You question Mr Smith about his understanding of the cause of the ulcer. He reports being told that it was due to poor circulation but he cannot be more explicit. On further questioning it appears that Mr Smith does not understand the rationale behind the treatments used. He rather anxiously tells you that he has little belief that the medical treatment will work.

You ask Mr Smith if you can examine his leg. He has a large ulcer in the gaiter region with surrounding pigmentation and dry, scaly skin (Plate 8, between pp. 102 and 103). The ulcer is sloughy with areas of granulation. On examination, Mr Smith's resting pressure index is 1.0 on both legs. His blood pressure is 150/100 mmHg and he weighs 95.5 kg. All other investigations are within normal limits and he has no other relevant medical history. He complains of aching pain in his legs at the end of the day, which is relieved by resting.

Quality of life for leg ulcer patients

You should now be aware that there is considerable suffering and reduction in quality of life for leg ulcer patients. Some of these issues are explored in more detail in this case study.

Self-assessment 5 MINUTES

1. List the ways in which Mr Smith's quality of life is affected.
2. Which do you consider is the most significant disruption to Mr Smith's quality of life?

FEEDBACK

It is difficult to prioritise when assessing and planning treatment for Mr Smith as many of the factors are interrelated. The offensive smell from his ulcer is certainly a dominant factor which affects his life in a number of ways:

- his personal/sexual relationship with his wife understandably causes him great distress
- his relationship with colleagues and clients is impaired to the extent that he cannot function effectively at work
- getting to work is in itself a traumatic experience because of the attitude of his fellow travellers
- his relationship with his children has been affected.

Whilst treating the odour as the main priority might help considerably in improving Mr Smith's quality of life, it is more important to address the cause rather than the effect. If the ulcer can be effectively treated then the odour is no longer an issue. However, treatment of the cause is impeded by several factors including:

- his inability to take time off work
- his need to shower twice a day

- his dislike of bandages
- his lack of belief in the effectiveness of the interventions.

Assessment of quality of life is often neglected. You will notice we have dealt with it first because for this patient it has a greater impact on his life than any other aspect of his leg ulcer.

Activity 30 MINUTES

Use your reflections on Mr Smith's quality of life to compile a detailed assessment for him. If possible, use a structured framework such as a nursing model to help your assessment of his problems, and make sure that planned interventions are thorough, comprehensive and prioritised.

FEEDBACK

The assessment in Box 6.1 shows how you might have undertaken this activity. There are many nursing models or other frameworks to choose from but we have used the Roy Adaptation Model as our theoretical framework (Roy & Andrews 1991).

While you may work in an outpatient clinic that has an ulcer service it is more likely that, once Mr Smith has had all his investigations, he will need to be re-referred to the primary health care team.

Involving the multidisciplinary team

Before discharging Mr Smith it would be useful to speak to both his GP and his district or practice nurse. This will give you more information concerning his non-compliance with treatment as well as providing you with an opportunity to plan his discharge. During the liaison you should try to establish a treatment programme that Mr Smith will comply with and which has the least impact on his job. This may require an appointment very early in the morning or alternatively, late at night. Lack of communication between hospital and community will simply increase his anxiety. Practical measures must be considered. If you are discharging Mr Smith on a particular dressing, is it available in the community? You may wish to give him supplies of the dressing to ensure continuity of care. A very important factor in his successful discharge will involve

---

Box 6.1 Mr. Smith's assessment form

BEHAVIOURAL ASSESSMENT

Adaptive model	Stimuli	Focal; Contextual; Residual
Physiological		
• Exercise and rest	Large (20 cm) malodorous leg ulcer in gaiter region —sloughy + areas of granulation	
• Nutrition	Surrounding skin dry, scaly and discoloured	
• Elimination	Sleeplessness	
• Fluid and electrolytes	Age = 43	
• Oxygen and circulation	Weight = 15 stone—normal diet	
• Regulation	BP = 150/100	
	Urinalysis—negative	
	Blood tests—normal	
	Ankle circumference 24 cm	
	RPI: left = 1.0; right = 1.0	
	Aching pain and oedema at the end of the day relieved by resting	
	Recurrent: three episodes following rugby injury—possible damage to deep venous system	
	Diagnosis = complex venous ulcer	
Role		
	Cannot afford time off because of economic and professional pressures, e.g., job at risk and large mortgage	
	Difficulty in socialising with colleagues and clients because of odour	
	Travelling to work is traumatic owing to odour; people have commented	
Interdependence		
	Children are unsympathetic	
	Mr and Mrs Smith sleep in separate rooms because of odour	
	Financial worries	
Self-concept		
Physical self	Needs to shower twice daily because of odour	
	Pressure of work, fear of redundancy	
Personal self	Possible clinical depression	
	Angry and aggressive	
Interpersonal self	Mistrust of professional intervention	
	Non-compliant with treatments in the past	
	Lack of knowledge of his own condition	
	Lack of belief that ulcer will heal	

---

him having trust in those caring for him and that there is agreement concerning the best treatment programme.

Patient education

How do you educate Mr Smith? One of the most important factors will involve developing an empathic relationship with him. You can see from the scenario that he is deeply distressed and has developed a distrust of professionals. If you are really to help him, you have to try to understand what it is like to be in his position.

Try to create a therapeutic environment for teaching him. The following points are worth considering.

1. Provide privacy and prevent interruptions.
2. Demonstrate that you are really interested by actively listening and sitting near him.
3. Avoid being judgemental.
4. Allow him time to talk, and use open-ended questions.
5. Acknowledge his difficulties, openly praise and encourage him, but do not patronise him.

Mr Smith is clearly an intelligent person and you may have to address a number of the following questions, all of which may affect his compliance with treatment.

1. How much does Mr Smith know about his condition?

2. Does he understand the rationale for the treatments being used?
3. What adaptations to his lifestyle will he agree to?
4. How much inconvenience to his lifestyle can he tolerate? And how will this influence the treatment regime chosen?

You might like to use patient education leaflets to reinforce your education of Mr Smith, but do not forget that careful explanation is more effective than a written leaflet and that he will need constant reassurance and encouragement to comply with these changes.

Case study outcome

Mr Smith has continued to find life extremely difficult. His firm asked him to reduce his hours but is also allowing him to work at home whenever possible. He was very angry with this situation initially, but in practice he has benefited from the reduction in pressure. Unfortunately his marriage ended in divorce and his wife gained custody of the children.

Mr Smith is continuing to treat his own ulcer with supervision by the practice nurse and his GP. Further investigations revealed that he has had a severe deep vein thrombosis in his femoral vein which means that he is likely to have repeated bouts of ulceration.

The treatment regime that Mr Smith found most suitable involved using a hydrocolloid dressing and a class III compression stocking (see Sect. 5). Although the exudate level was high for a few weeks, this quickly subsided once the compression was being used and he only needed to renew his dressing twice a week. His ulcer healed in 14 weeks but unfortunately recurred twice during the following year despite the continued use of compression. However, each time, Mr Smith quickly sought professional advice, which perhaps indicates an increase of trust in those caring for him.

CASE STUDY 3:
ELIZABETH O'CALLAGHAN
—MIXED VENOUS—ARTERIAL ULCER

Scenario

The following scenario puts you in the role of a practice nurse working in a large fund-holding practice with five doctors and three practice nurses. You are given the lead in the surgery to develop a leg ulcer clinic. Mrs O'Callaghan is one of the first patients to present to your clinic.

Mrs O'Callaghan attends for her first visit to your clinic for reassessment of her leg ulcer. She has cancelled three previous appointments but has never given a reason for this. As she enters the room you are struck by her tired appearance and difficulty in walking. She sits down and you ask her to tell you about herself.

Mrs O'Callaghan tells you that she is 82. She retired at 65 owing to her husband's increasingly poor health and since then much of her time has been spent looking after him. A diagnosis of Alzheimer's disease was made a year ago and since then he has become increasingly confused, particularly at night. You ask her if she has any help and she quickly replies that she does not require any. Later, when consulting the practice records, you find that help has been offered in the past but refused. During the interview she never mentions any family support but the notes reveal that she has two children who visit infrequently. Mrs O'Callaghan tells you that she gave up smoking 4 months ago having smoked 30 cigarettes a day for 45 years. You ask her what made her give up and she tells you that she can no longer afford it. You note that Mrs O'Callaghan is neatly dressed and wearing trousers which hide a raised shoe. When you come to examine her leg you find that she has a shortened limb due to polio as a child.

She tells you that it is increasingly difficult to walk and that she has taken to using a stick. You ask her if this is the reason why she failed to attend her previous visits. She replies that it was not but does not offer a reason. On further discussion about her pain you note that her walking distance has decreased. She describes the pain as 'twinges' in her buttocks, but she has not discussed this with her doctor.

She tells you that she developed a small fairly insignificant lesion on her right leg 4 years ago. After a few months of it not healing she sought advice from her GP. Various treatments have been tried but the wound is increasing in size and depth. Her doctor has diagnosed a mixed arterial and venous ulcer. When you record her resting pressure index, you find the readings are 0.7 on her right leg and 0.75 on her left leg. Her blood pressure is 170/100 mmHg and she complains of dizziness in the mornings. Her current medication is 1 aspirin daily and temazepam, 10 mg, at night.

When you examine her leg you note a number of changes in the surrounding skin (see Plate 9, between pp. 102 and 103). Her ankle is fixed and she has a bunion on her right hallux valgus.

Can you identify six factors in the case study which indicate that Mrs O'Callaghan has an ulcer of mixed pathology, i.e. arterial and venous origin.

FEEDBACK

You should have been able to pick up some of the following indicators:

Arterial

1. A history of smoking.
2. Pain on walking and decreased walking distance indicate intermittent claudication but this could be due to other causes such as arthritis or spinal damage.
3. Reduced resting pressure index on both legs (RPI: 0.7 right and 0.75 left).
4. High blood pressure and dizziness which may indicate widespread arterial disease (currently treated by the use of aspirin).

Venous

1. Reduced calf muscle function owing to shortened limb and fixed ankle joint.
2. From looking at Plate 9 it is evident that she has skin changes associated with venous disease, i.e. pigmentation of skin in gaiter region.
3. Position of the ulcer on the medial malleolus.

Activity   15 MINUTES

Given the factors above give an outline of the subsequent management of Mrs O'Callaghan by identifying:

*   what further investigations are required
*   which members of the multidisciplinary team should be involved.

FEEDBACK

*   This type of patient would normally be referred to a vascular consultant to confirm the diagnosis and advise on treatment.
*   Further investigations would include:

    —Doppler studies, segmental pressures, treadmill tests, duplex scanning depending on available resources
    —blood tests to test for rheumatoid and antinuclear factor to eliminate possible autoimmune disorders; full blood count and estimation of haemoglobin levels.

It is clear that Mrs O'Callaghan would benefit from a wide range of support. As a practice nurse you are in an ideal situation to coordinate this but you should discuss your plans with the GP who will review Mrs O'Callaghan's medical condition/medication and arrange referral to a vascular consultant. It might also be an idea to discuss the situation with the district nurse who could provide support for both Mrs O'Callaghan and her husband. However, there is much you can do yourself, such as checking that full benefits such as attendance allowance are being paid and that household aids have been supplied. Other people you might want to involve include:

*   social services who could arrange home carer support
*   a podiatrist who could treat Mrs O'Callaghan's bunions and assess her footwear
*   an orthotist who could review her footwear
*   a physiotherapist who could provide exercises to improve ankle function.

Providing respite care

Mrs O'Callaghan is very tired. She might welcome respite care for her husband but she has previously refused help and you need to draw on all your skills to find out why this was.

Self-assessment   10 MINUTES

What reasons could you suggest which might prevent Mrs O'Callaghan from accepting respite care?

FEEDBACK

Your suggestions might include the following points.

1. She might feel guilty.
2. She might feel that no-one else could care for her husband as well as she does.
3. She might feel that he could die while he is away.
4. She might know that he would be very unhappy in institutionalised care.
5. She may never have come to terms with the fact that he is ill.
6. The case study suggests that her children provide little support. We do not know why this should be but their attitude may influence Mrs O'Callaghan's ability to accept help.
7. Her previous experience with professionals may have influenced her ability to accept help.

These are just a few possibilities; further skilled assessment would reveal others.

Deciding on appropriate treatment

Referral to a vascular consultant might take some time, and in the interim Mrs O'Callaghan will need her ulcer to be dressed. Look at the photograph of her leg (Plate 9, between pp. 102 and 103) and answer the following questions.

Activity   15 MINUTES

1. Refer back to Section 5.4 on dressings (pp. 67–70) and make some suggestions as to what type you would use.
2. What criteria would you take into account when deciding what dressing to use?

FEEDBACK

1. You could have suggested that a hydrocolloid or hydrogel dressing would be an appropriate choice.

2. The following factors represent the basic criteria you should have identified. The dressing should:

   - create a moist environment which will help reduce pain (it should keep the wound moist but not macerated)
   - prevent secondary infection
   - cause no further harm to the wound or surrounding skin which is already slightly macerated
   - provide optimum acidity
   - not require frequent replacement
   - be cosmetically acceptable.

Case study outcome

Mrs O'Callaghan was persuaded to undergo further investigations at the hospital. These revealed that she had significant venous disease. She had an incompetent long saphenous vein and although surgical correction was considered it was decided that this would not be beneficial to her because of her fixed ankle and poor calf muscle pump function. Arterial investigations revealed that she also had widespread arterial disease with peripheral vascular disease in both lower limbs and carotid stenosis. Mrs O'Callaghan has regular follow-up appointments to monitor her arterial disease but no further intervention has been undertaken to date.

Because of Mrs O'Callaghan's mixed aetiology, gentle compression was considered appropriate. A bandage applying approximately 18–24 mmHg (3B)

was used with a hydrocolloid dressing. She tolerated this approach well and the ulcer healed after 10 months. Her resting pressure index was recorded monthly and there was no further deterioration. She benefited also from a new pair of surgical shoes as it was felt that the pain she was experiencing was partly due to an abnormal gait.

Mrs O'Callaghan's children began to offer more support when they realised their mother was ill. Both came to stay with her during the year, providing her with much needed rest. Whilst she attended the leg ulcer clinic for treatment a volunteer looked after her husband. Mrs O'Callaghan has benefited greatly from this support and now feels less socially isolated.

CASE STUDY 4: ALBERT HANSON —ARTERIAL ULCERATION

Scenario

The following scenario places you in the role of a staff nurse working in a care of the elderly day care unit. Albert Hanson, 82 years of age, is referred for assessment by a geriatrician as he is increasingly unable to cope at home. He lives with his 80-year-old wife whose health is also failing. On his arrival you become his named nurse and note that he has a leg ulcer on the lateral aspect of his left leg.

Mr Hanson appears disorientated on arrival in the unit and continually asks for his wife. The ambulance driver who has brought him to hospital tells you that he was not ready when she called and that the council flat where he lives is extremely dirty.

You sit down and talk to Mr Hanson. He is unable to give you any previous history and does not appear to know where he is or why he has been referred. You gently reassure him and consult the referral letter for further information. His general practitioner has provided a comprehensive summary of his previous medical history. The letter says that until 10 years ago Mr Hanson was working full time in a factory. He has six children all of whom live long distances from their parents. Mr Hanson smoked heavily for as long as he can remember and still smokes when given the option. During the last 10 years Mr Hanson has suffered two coronary thromboses and has angina induced by exercise. His confusion has been worsening and he has had several transient ischaemic attacks when he has lost movement in his left arm. General examination revealed that his blood pressure was 180/100 mmHg and his pulse was 85 beats per minute and irregular. The letter indicated that he has lost weight. He currently weighs 58 kg and is 1.8 m tall. The letter also reveals that his current medication includes

75 mg aspirin, temazepam 30 mg nocte, digoxin 0.25 mg daily. The letter does not indicate who supervises his medication.

Examination of Mr Hanson's leg reveals a 'punched-out' ulcer on the lateral aspect of his left leg (Plate 10). He sits with his legs drawn up and appears in pain when lying supine. The area around the ulcer is erythematous and his toes and forefoot appear cyanosed, both feet are very cold and no pedal pulses are palpable.

You are asked to decide on an appropriate treatment regime for Mr Hanson's ulcer. Unfortunately your unit does not have access to a portable Doppler ultrasound machine.

You decide to contact the home carer responsible for Mr Hanson. This reveals that the couple are becoming increasingly confused and at risk. Recently the gas was found turned on in the flat. Mr Hanson is becoming incontinent of urine. Both dislike interference in the home and are often hostile. Accommodation in a sheltered housing unit was found but the couple refused to move. The couple receive meals on wheels and district nursing visits. Discussion with the district nurse reveals that she suspects that Mr Hanson removes the dressing soon after she leaves because on one occasion she returned to collect something she had forgotten and found him undoing the dressing. The district nurse tells you that she monitors the medication.

Self-assessment　　　　**10 MINUTES**

What factors in the case study indicate that Albert Hanson has an ulcer resulting from peripheral vascular disease. Try to suggest at least six.

· ·

FEEDBACK

You should have been able to pick out some of the following indicators.

1. He smokes heavily.
2. He has had coronary thromboses in the past.
3. He has angina.
4. He is disorientated and this might be due to atherosclerosis in his brain.
5. He has hypertension.
6. There is a high incidence of peripheral vascular disease in manual workers.
7. He has transient ischaemic attacks.
8. Atrial fibrillation stimulates thrombosis.
9. He has pain when supine and sits with his legs drawn up.

10. His forefoot and toes are cyanosed and cold.
11. His ulcer has a 'punched-out' appearance with surrounding reactive hyperaemia (see Plate 10, between pp. 102 and 103).

· ·

Cardiovascular risk factors

Activity　　　　**60 MINUTES**

Read Section 4 on arterial risk factors (p. 47) and use this information together with what you have learned from this case study to create an assessment tool which you can then try out, firstly on yourself and subsequently on three colleagues or friends. Remember that if you ask people about their risk factors you may need to provide them with help and support if required.

· ·

FEEDBACK

Looking at the results of your survey of four people, you may be able to spot certain patterns, such as some risk factors being more common than others. Patterns of risk factors may be shaped by lifestyle or cultural factors.

· ·

Appropriate and inappropriate interventions

Activity　　　　**30 MINUTES**

1. From the range of interventions below, choose those which are appropriate for Mr Hanson and provide a brief rationale for your choice. Note any difficulties likely to be encountered in undertaking them.
2. Note down any interventions which should not be used and explain why.

Range of interventions

- Clean the wound with acetic acid.
- Clean with normal saline.
- Apply a light cotton bandage over a hydrocolloid bandage.
- Apply a four-layer bandage.
- Apply a single-layer high compression bandage.
- Apply a paste bandage and light cotton bandage.
- Tell him to stop smoking.
- Organise referral for vascular investigation.

FEEDBACK

The most important intervention involves arranging vascular investigations as you do not yet have enough information with which to clearly determine the underlying aetiology.

It would be a good idea if you could persuade Mr Hanson to give up smoking, but if he has smoked for the last 50 years, and continues to do so despite having two heart attacks during the last decade, it is unlikely that you will be successful, particularly as he is now confused as well.

The wound can be cleaned quite adequately with normal saline. Strong solutions such as acetic acid are not only unnecessary but may harm tissue and are rapidly inactivated in the presence of pus and wound debris.

The wound needs to be dressed. The scenario identifies that Mr Hanson removes his dressing once his district nurse has left. It might be useful to consider using a paste bandage to stop him interfering with the wound. Since you do not know the type of ulcer you are treating, you should use a light cotton bandage over the paste bandage. Under no circumstances should you apply a single high compression or multilayer compression bandage, as the information you do have suggests that Mr Hanson has severe arterial disease and the application of high compression will reduce his peripheral perfusion further which in turn could lead to gangrene.

Whilst there are many indicators that Mr Hanson is suffering from vascular disease, without further investigations we cannot be certain. The decisions made about dressing treatment are really holding measures until all the information is available. Although arterial reconstructive surgery may be recommended, it may be inappropriate considering Mr Hanson's complex physical and social needs. Conservative measures such as those suggested above may become the main strategy for care. The prognosis will depend on the severity of the disease which may be intractable.

Involving the multidisciplinary team

We have seen that Mr Hanson has a number of social problems. For instance, both he and his wife are becoming increasingly confused and they have refused rehousing.

Activity   20 MINUTES

What members of the multidisciplinary team could be enlisted to help, and what would be the nature of their intervention?

FEEDBACK

The help of the following team members could be enlisted.

1. Social services will perform a home assessment to determine the degree of risk and 'package' of care required to keep Mr and Mrs Hanson at home.
2. The geriatrician will make a comprehensive assessment of medical and psychosocial needs, such as weight loss, angina, heart arrhythmia, incontinence and confusion.
3. The GP retains primary responsibility for this family and clearly from the scenario knows them well.
4. The district nurse will dress the ulcer and continue to provide ongoing support to the family. In addition to monitoring compliance with treatment, he or she can provide advice and arrange for aids such as a commode or incontinence pads.

Case study outcome

The situation with Mr Hanson continued to deteriorate. He was found at home, by the district nurse, lying on the floor unconscious. His wife was extremely distressed as she was unable to contact help or lift him up.

They were both admitted to an acute care of the elderly ward and Mr Hanson was found to be suffering from pneumonia. Investigations revealed severe arterial disease. His resting pressure index in the ulcerated limb was only 0.3, and was 0.6 in the other leg. Owing to his overall condition no vascular interventions were undertaken.

During the admission Mrs Hanson became increasingly confused and it was soon evident that the couple would not be able to return home. Four weeks after the admission he died following a cerebrovascular accident. His wife was eventually placed in a long-stay care of the elderly unit, suffering from increasing confusion due to senile dementia.

CASE STUDY 5: MARY PURCELL
—ACUTE EMBOLISM

Scenario

This scenario places you in the role of staff nurse on an acute surgical ward. Mrs Purcell has been admitted with an acute arterial embolism which requires a femoropopliteal bypass operation. Mrs Purcell is a 70-year-old lady who prior to admission had developed severe pain in her right leg. The leg became pale, cold (perished) and on admission no pulses were present. She was developing paraesthesia and had little movement in her foot or leg. Mrs Purcell has a history of atrial fibrillation and reported that she was experiencing pain on walking. She had reduced the distance she walked to compensate for this. She tells you that she smokes 10 cigarettes a day.

On admission Mrs Purcell was accompanied by her daughter who was obviously anxious. She demands to see a doctor and paces up and down, spending a great deal of time making calls to her office on a portable telephone to the annoyance of other patients. This clearly distresses Mrs Purcell who weakly pleads with her daughter to sit down. You try in vain to pacify her. The doctor is delayed in the operating theatre and this aggravates the situation.

Mrs Purcell is taken to the operating theatre following a duplex scan and angiogram and a femoro-popliteal bypass is performed. Prior to surgery an area of gangrenous tissue is apparent on the dorsum of the foot. Following surgery this area develops into a deep ulcer, seen in Plate 2 (between pp. 102 and 103).

Postoperatively her daughter remains demanding and insists that the area of tissue loss is due to negligence. Staff on your ward are intimidated by her and you note that Mrs Purcell is often ignored or avoided by the nurses. She seems withdrawn and depressed. She has little interest in the progress she is making and refuses to eat. While she has many visitors, she seems relieved when they leave. When her family visit her you note that there are frequent arguments which centre around the plans for Mrs Purcell's discharge. Her daughter insists that she should come to live with her but is extremely anxious as to how she will cope because of her demanding career. She busily finds out about agencies which will provide home care. On talking to Mrs Purcell you find that she does not want to live with her daughter but would rather return to her own home. You discover that prior to Mrs Purcell's admission her daughter only visited her infrequently and you suspect that she feels guilty for this and is now trying to make amends. Mrs Purcell asks you to persuade her daughter to allow her to go home and you promise to try.

The surgery was successful and her arterial circulation has improved, her resting pressure index is 0.8 on the affected limb and 0.9 on the other. The surgeons are anxious to debride the wound and apply a skin graft. The ulcer is deep and surrounded by erythema. You are asked for your advice on the treatment regime that should be used. The consultant has recommended daily saline soaks to debride the wound. Wound swabs reveal a group G haemolytic streptococcus.

Self-assessment   10 MINUTES

There are six signs which indicate acute arterial occlusion. Can you identify them?

FEEDBACK

The following signs and symptoms occur in a classic ischaemic limb. Note that they all begin with the letter P—which makes them easier to remember.

1. Pain—is very severe and relief may be gained by hanging the limb over the side of the bed to increase perfusion. Its important to note in this scenario that Mrs Purcell had been experiencing intermittent claudication and reduced walking distance. Patients with diabetes or elderly confused patients may have less severe pain despite the severity of the disease.
2. Pallor—occasionally with severe embolus the leg becomes a marble white colour but more commonly the leg has a mottled blue colour.
3. Pulses—are absent in this patient indicating severe disruption to the arterial circulation.
4. Paraesthesia—is variable but Mrs Purcell has no sensation in her leg. This, when coupled with the lack of pulses, suggests a serious vascular occlusion requiring immediate intervention.
5. Paralysis—Mrs Purcell has very little movement in her foot and leg. Failure of dorsiflexion of the foot indicates severe arterial occlusion.
6. Perished (coldness)—Mrs Purcell's leg is cold to the touch, again indicating a reduction in blood supply.

A limb in this state may progress to gangrene within 24–48 hours. Other medical factors which indicate arterial disease are a history of smoking and atrial fibrillation which precipitate thromboembolism.

Debridement

Activity   15 MINUTES

1. Critically evaluate the method of debridement prescribed by the consultant.
2. Can you offer any alternative regimes?

FEEDBACK

1. The method he has chosen is known as 'wet and dry debridement'. Its action consists of the

application of a wet gauze dressing to the ulcer bed which is allowed to dry. When the dressing is dry it is removed along with dead tissue which has adhered to the gauze. This method, however, removes viable healthy tissue along with the slough and is extremely painful as well as potentially delaying wound healing.
2. The 'wet and dry' method offers no advantage over less painful methods such as those outlined by Morison & Moffatt (1994), such as enzymatic treatment, hydrocolloid dressings, hydrogel dressings or polysaccharide beads or paste. See Section 5 (p. 61).

Infection

Self-assessment   5 MINUTES

What are the implications of the presence of group G haemolytic streptococcus in a patient undergoing skin grafting?

FEEDBACK

Both *Streptococcus pyogenes* and *Pseudomonas aeruginosa* are associated with graft rejection. *Pseudomonas aeruginosa* is also associated with more invasive infection which can ultimately be fatal.

Dealing with conflict

Activity   15 MINUTES

How would you deal with the claim of negligence made by Mrs Purcell's daughter?

FEEDBACK

Your impression is that the daughter's attitude is due to her own previous lack of support for her mother. The stress of the situation, together with the pressure of her busy professional life, may have caused her to 'off load' her anger on to you and your colleagues. Nevertheless claims of negligence are increasing and can lead to litigation if proved. You should consider the following.

- Always be honest.
- Ensure that documentation is up to date, comprehensive and relevant.
- Discuss the situation with the medical team.
- Inform your line manager.
- Ensure that Mrs Purcell is not treated as an unpopular patient but given the same standard of care as any other patient.
- Provide support within the nursing team.
- If possible try to build a relationship with the daughter, do not be drawn into argument but rather explain calmly what is happening and why. This type of interaction would also provide an opportunity for her to express her anxiety and to ask questions.

Case study outcome

Following discussion with the multidisciplinary team it was decided that surgical debridement was the best option for Mrs Purcell. She was given a course of antibiotics to eliminate the streptococcus bacteria from her wound prior to surgery and, after debridement, given a full thickness skin graft.

Mrs Purcell remained on bed rest for a week following the procedure and the graft was successful. She experienced pain from the donor site on her thigh. The initial dressing of paraffin tulle, applied in the operating theatre, was replaced by a hydrogel dressing which gave her immediate relief and prevented any further trauma to the wound bed.

Mrs Purcell's daughter continued to be demanding but her anxiety gradually diminished as it became evident that her mother was progressing well. The accusations of negligence and threats of litigation ceased but the staff nevertheless remained anxious and cautious in their interactions with her.

The following weeks were difficult; Mrs Purcell remained adamant that she wanted to return to her own home. As her physical strength improved so did her determination not to be dominated by her daughter. Eventually they compromised; her daughter paid for a private nurse to attend daily during the first month at home and her mother stayed with her at weekends.

Despite the successful healing of the wound, the long-term prognosis remains uncertain. Mrs Purcell continues to smoke, even though she has had the possible consequences explained to her. It is quite likely that this will lead to occlusion of the arterial bypass graft and make her arterial disease worse. She finds it hard to accept that she can play a part in prolonging her own health, despite the experience she has just been through.

CASE STUDY 6: ALAN PATTERSON
—DIABETIC NEUROPATHIC ULCERATION

Scenario

This scenario places you in the role of a nurse working in a diabetic clinic. This clinic has a multidisciplinary team and encourages all diabetics within the area to attend. Mr Patterson attends for his routine appointment and you note a discoloured area on his second and third toe.

Mr Patterson, who is 55 years old, tells you that the area is not painful and that he noticed it a few days previously. As he had been gardening he thought that he must have dropped a tool on his foot but he cannot remember doing so.

On examination, it is found that Mr Patterson has reduced sensation in both feet. He is unable to detect the vibration when a 128 MHz tuning fork is applied to his foot. On closer examination, a number of reddened areas are evident (see Plate 11, between pp. 102 and 103). His shoes appear narrow and he tells you that they are a smaller size than he normally wears because his normal shoes feel too loose. His skin is dry and his foot is warm to touch. He complains that the skin on the plantar surface of his foot has been cracking and you note an absence of sweating.

His investigations reveal that his blood glucose level is 18 mmol/l. On further questioning it appears that his diabetic control is erratic with periods of high blood sugars. He attends his appointments regularly but visits a chiropodist infrequently despite the calluses developing on his feet. He appears to have reduced joint mobility in his toe joints. Mr Patterson has suffered retinopathy for which he has undergone laser therapy to stabilise the situation. Mr Patterson takes no medication other than his insulin which he injects twice daily. Other investigations include the recording of a resting pressure index which was 1.4 on the affected leg and 1.2 on the other leg.

As usual Mr Patterson is accompanied by his wife and they, as on other occasions, have brought some chocolate for you and your colleagues. Mrs Patterson looks more worried than usual and tells you that she has been reading some of the literature he was given but has been unable to persuade him to take the precautions recommended.

Mr Patterson is extremely cheerful and appears to have little insight into his condition. On questioning it is found that he has been given literature and advice on foot care in the past but has not adhered to this.

Mr Patterson is seen by the diabetic consultant and admitted straight to the hospital ward for intravenous antibiotics.

Self-assessment   5 MINUTES

List at least six of the factors which indicate that Mr Patterson has diabetic neuropathic foot problems which will almost certainly result in ulceration.

FEEDBACK

Your list should have included the following:

- absence of pain
- reduced sensation, e.g. ability to wear smaller shoes without discomfort
- inability to detect vibration
- reddened areas
- skin dry and warm to touch
- skin on base of foot cracking and absence of sweating; these indicate possible autonomic nerve involvement
- reduced joint mobility
- previous retinopathy
- elevated resting pressure index 1.4 in affected leg; this suggests calcification of the vessels
- elevated blood glucose level
- callus formation on feet.

Predisposing factors in diabetic foot ulceration

Self-assessment   5 MINUTES

Without looking back at Section 3.4, can you describe the three factors that are generally held to predispose to diabetic foot ulcers.

FEEDBACK

The three factors are:

1. neuropathy
2. peripheral vascular disease
3. infection.

Neuropathy and the diabetic foot

Mr Patterson has presented with some obvious signs of neuropathy, e.g. his inability to detect the vibration from a tuning fork. Even though he is not completely compliant, it would have been much better

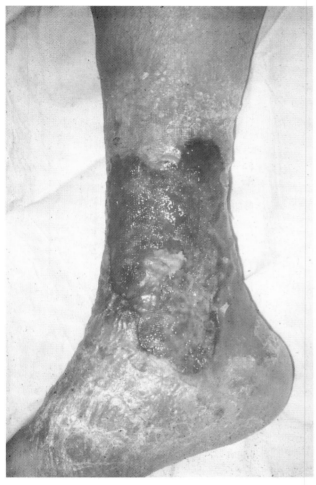

Plate 1 Mrs Golding's ulcer.

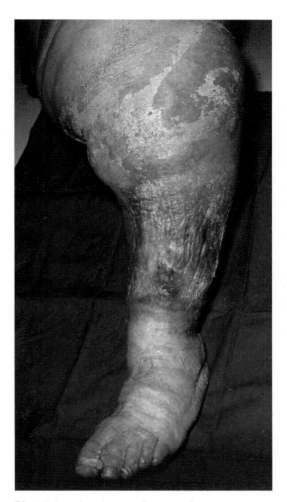

Plate 3 Lymphoedema and venous disease.

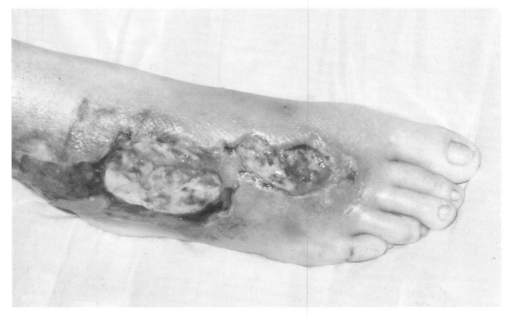

Plate 2 Mrs Purcell's ulcer.

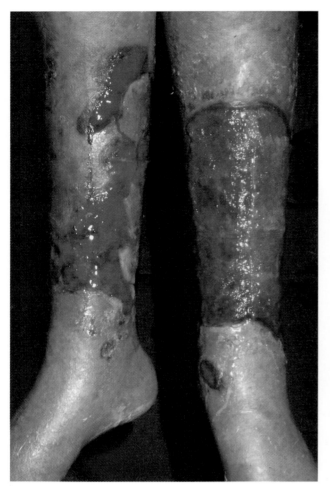

Plate 4 Mrs Fraser's ulcer.

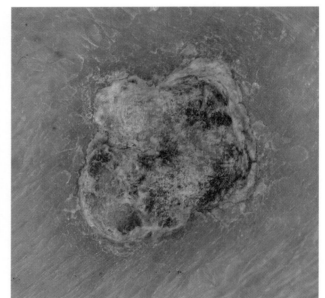

Plate 6 Mr Powers' ulcer.

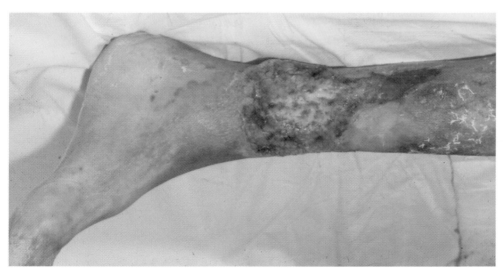

Plate 5 A venous ulcer which has undergone malignant changes.

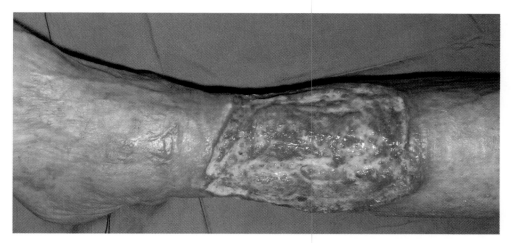

Plate 7 Mr Salmon's ulcer.

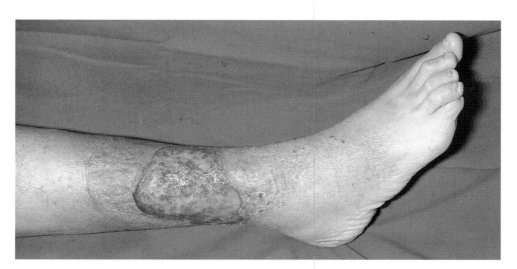

Plate 8 Mr Smith's ulcer.

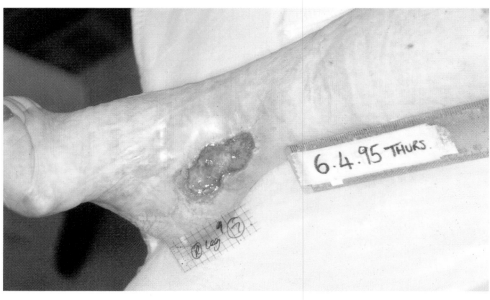

Plate 9 Mrs O'Callaghan's ulcer.

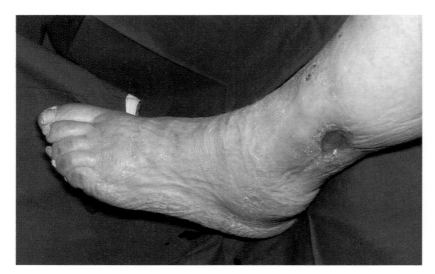

Plate 10 Mr Hanson's ulcer.

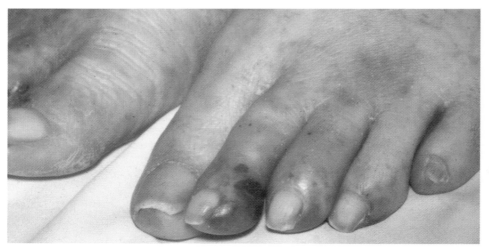

Plate 11 Mr Patterson's ulcer.

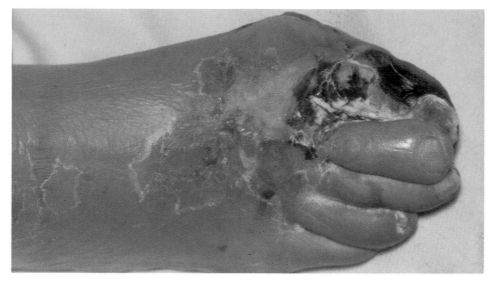

Plate 12 Mrs Tillett's ulcer.

for everyone concerned to have detected the likelihood of him developing foot problems much earlier.

Assessing for sensory, motor and autonomic neuropathy

Activity 10 MINUTES

Review the description of the changes which occur to the neuropathic foot in Section 3.4. What practical means do you think you could use to assess sensory, motor and autonomic nerve damage in the 'at-risk' foot? Make three lists using the headings 'sensory neuropathy', 'motor neuropathy' and 'autonomic neuropathy'.

FEEDBACK

Your lists should have included the following points.

Sensory neuropathy

It would be quite a reasonable assumption to note that patients with sensory neuropathy have no pain (hypoaesthesia). Patients present with a loss of pain and sensation which can sometimes be described as being like 'walking on cushions'.

However, some patients, often in the early stages of neuropathy, do have pain (hyperaesthesia). There is an increased sensitivity to hot and cold as well as touch. It is often described as 'burning pain' and is more severe at night.

Testing for altered sensation

1. Sharp pain—a pin can be used to detect sensitivity to sharp pain. This is best achieved by beginning in an area where there is reduced sensation and moving to an area of normal sensation.
2. Blunt pain—a blunt instrument such as a pen can be used to detect blunt sensation.
3. Touch—this can be simply tested by using cotton wool or by more sophisticated methods such as Semmes Weinstein monofilament.
4. Hot and cold sensation—test tubes of hot and cold water can be used to detect appreciation of temperature changes.
5. Vibration—as seen in the scenario, a 128 MHz tuning fork can be used to assess vibration. The tuning fork is first placed over the sternum in order that the patient knows what to expect. The ability to detect vibration may be lost in very elderly patients.

Motor neuropathy

Testing altered motor function

1. Examine the foot to detect atrophy of the intrinsic muscles, particularly near the toes.
2. Check for foot deformities such as hammer or clawed toes; hallux valgus; bunionette; crowded toes; prominent metatarsal heads and arch deformities such as pes cavus, Charcot's joint (rocker bottom deformities).
3. Check joint mobility at the ankle and toes. This is frequently reduced in diabetics. It is also worth asking the patient to place the palms together in the 'prayer sign'. If the palms do not meet this would indicate restricted mobility.
4. Check under the sole for areas of callus formation. Check beneath the callus for very small blackened areas; these are subkeratotic haematomas and in 50% of cases indicate that a perforating ulcer has already developed.
5. Check all of the foot, particularly areas where there is friction or pressure, for signs of pressure damage, infection or gangrene.
6. Check the patient's footwear and socks for rough linings, use of insoles, foreign bodies and correct fit (too tight, or inadequate depth to accommodate toe deformity). Many patients with diabetes with sensory neuropathy report that a normal-size shoe feels loose owing to reduced sensation.
7. Check nails for thickening and deformity. In severe cases of neuropathy the nail may atrophy. Nail bed infections are common and may lead to cellulitis of the foot.

Autonomic neuropathy

Testing for altered autonomic function

1. Check the overall skin condition to identify autonomic involvement where skin becomes dry, thickened and hard. This leads to cracks and fissures particularly at the heel, allowing bacterial entry.
2. Check for absence of sweating.
3. Check temperature of the foot. A warm red foot is suggestive of autonomic neuropathy with bounding foot pulses and distended foot veins. This should not be confused with an ischaemic foot which is cold to the touch. The severe symptoms associated with an ischaemic foot may be masked by the presence of neuropathy. A study in Manchester found that 40% of its patients had both peripheral vascular disease and neuropathy (Boulton et al 1994).

4. Check for oedema. This is common in patients with peripheral vascular disease and rarely occurs in patients with neuropathy.

Risk factors

A number of risk factors predispose the diabetic patient to develop foot ulceration. These include:

1. a history of previous foot ulceration
2. increased age
3. duration of diabetes
4. neuropathy with or without peripheral vascular disease
5. foot deformity leading to increased foot pressures
6. concurrent retinopathy and nephropathy
7. being a non-compliant patient
8. male sex
9. living at home.

Self-assessment   5 MINUTES

Why has Mr Patterson been admitted to the ward so quickly? Why is he being given intravenous antibiotics before his infection is verified?

FEEDBACK

The diabetic patient with an infection poses a very different problem from many other leg ulcer patients, such as those with venous disease. There is substantial evidence that infection in diabetic patients with foot ulcers is associated with considerable morbidity and mortality (Boulton et al 1994).

Dealing with denial and patient compliance

Activity   5 MINUTES

Your impression is that Mr Patterson does not take his position seriously and this is supported by what his wife has said to you. Tick any of the following steps which would help you to deal with this situation.

1. Show him photographs of gangrenous feet.
2. Introduce him to another patient, i.e. a good role model.
3. Introduce him to a diabetic nurse specialist.

4. Enlist his wife's ongoing help to give him some more educational leaflets.
5. Initiate a multiprofessional team case conference.

FEEDBACK

It is essential to develop a multiprofessional approach to this patient's care but it is most important to foster understanding and cooperation in Mr Patterson. You might get Mr Patterson to take his position more seriously by showing him shockingly graphic photographs but there is an ethical dilemma in this choice of action. It may well be that once hospitalised he will see fellow patients with similar conditions or even with amputated limbs. You cannot prepare Mr Patterson for such eventualities but you should do all you can to educate him. He has already been given educational material to read, with little effect; it is doubtful whether more of the same will change his behaviour.

It may be that enlisting the help of a diabetic specialist nurse who is more experienced in this field would help. He or she would also be able to provide continuing support for Mr Patterson and his family in the community. Mr Patterson's wife could be a strong and important ally. While she obviously appreciates the gravity of the situation, the degree to which she can influence him depends on a number of complex interpersonal and possibly cultural factors.

This scenario suggests that Mr Patterson has a number of problems related to his diabetes. A proactive rather than reactive approach is required. Calling a case conference would be a good starting point. The team could include a physician, vascular surgeon, GP, chiropodist, orthotist, dietitian and the local district nurse.

Case study outcome

Mr Patterson's infection improved following his antibiotic therapy. He required local debridement of necrotic tissue from both toes. These were then allowed to heal by secondary intention. Mr Patterson stayed in hospital for 6 weeks, during which time his condition stabilised. Further investigations revealed that he had arterial disease in both limbs, although this was still at an early stage. An orthotist carefully assessed him and built a pair of orthopaedic shoes for him to wear. These provided complete pressure relief from all areas at risk, especially his toes.

Mr Patterson was discharged into the care of the community nursing service. The diabetic specialist nurse liaised with his district nurse to ensure optimum diabetic control was achieved. His wounds took 4 months to heal and he had no further recurrences.

Initially Mr Patterson seemed to realise the severity of his situation and complied well with his treatment. However, as his condition improved he became less compliant, particularly regarding his diet. His pleasant, jovial manner and gratitude for the help he was receiving made it more difficult for health care professionals, as he appeared to understand and be willing to comply with advice. Over the next 5 years his condition worsened and he finally died of a myocardial infarction, aged 62 years.

CASE STUDY 7: ANN TILLETT—
DIABETIC NEUROISCHAEMIC ULCERATION

Scenario

This scenario places you in the role of staff nurse on a ward. Mrs Ann Tillett is admitted for surgical investigations with a gangrenous toe on her right foot.

Mrs Tillett is a 52-year-old lady who is accompanied to the ward by her husband and daughter. Her hospital notes reveal numerous previous admissions with conditions relating to her diabetes. Mrs Tillett developed diabetes at the age of 10 and has been on insulin since then. During this time she has had poor diabetic control, with elevated blood sugars. The hospital notes indicate that she smokes heavily and has done so for 30 years. Previous diabetic complications include: hyperglycaemic coma, two failed pregnancies at term and diabetic nephropathy. Over the last 2 years Mrs Tillett has noted changes in the sensation of her feet, complaining of a burning pain in both feet at night. Three weeks ago she noted a small lesion on her great toe, which she dressed with a plaster. The situation rapidly deteriorated and she presents with a gangrenous great toe and an area of gangrene on her hallux-valgus (see Plate 12, between pp. 102 and 103).

On examination her foot is cold and swollen. Foot pulses are impalpable. The area of gangrene is nearly dry but a small amount of exudate is seeping from the area. You try to measure a resting pressure index but are unable to obliterate the signal. You are surprised that Mrs Tillett is not in greater pain considering her condition.

When talking to her husband, you establish that the damage to her toe occurred when she wore tight shoes with a rough lining. He tells you that she is afraid that she will die and that the situation is placing a great strain on the rest of the family. He has tried to help her stop smoking but this has failed and led to many family arguments. His story correlates with the hospital notes which suggest Mrs Tillett is non-compliant with treatment and fails to attend her routine appointments. He looks angry and upset and tells you that he is glad she has been admitted and asks that she is not sent home.

Following the investigations, Mrs Tillett has a distal amputation of her great toe for peripheral vascular disease. The consultant is anxious to discharge Mrs Tillett home and asks you to prepare for her discharge. Because of the complications of her home situation, you are asked to arrange a case conference to decide a way forward.

Self-assessment   10 MINUTES

What factors indicate that Mrs Tillett has an ulcer resulting from a combination of neuropathy and ischaemia? Make two lists, one indicating the neuropathic factors and the other, the ischaemic factors.

FEEDBACK

Your lists should be along the following lines.

Neuropathic factors

1. Burning pain in the foot at night.
2. Trauma due to tight shoes (lack of sensation).
3. Absence of pain.

Ischaemic factors

1. Heavy smoker.
2. Gangrenous toe.
3. Cold limb.
4. Swelling.
5. Impalpable pulse.
6. Inability to obliterate signal when taking resting pressure index (calcification of vessels).

Teamwork

Caring for diabetic patients is something you will seldom do alone. You are likely to be one of a team.

Activity   10 MINUTES

Listed below are a number of people and services that can be enlisted in the formation of a 'diabetic foot care team':

- diabetologist
- diabetic nurse specialist
- chiropodist or podiatrist

- diabetic clinic
- orthotist
- local self-help groups.

Make a list of the professionals or services which are available in your area. In order to do this you may have to do some investigating. Your local health centre may be able to help you or perhaps the Family Health Service Authority.

FEEDBACK

Hopefully you have been able to identify at least one of the professionals or services listed.

Activity **60 MINUTES**

1. Choose one of the professionals you identified and make an appointment to talk to either the professional concerned or, in the case of the clinic, one of the people involved in running it.
2. It is a good idea to prepare yourself before the meeting, so make a list of the questions you must ask.
3. Write a short report of your visit including answers to questions such as those above as well as anything that you have found out from your visit that might influence or impact on your care of Mrs Tillett.

FEEDBACK

Questions you might have asked include the following?

- What is the prevalence of people with diabetic foot ulcers in their locality?
- What service do they provide?
- What are the constraints on practice, e.g. resources?
- What is the degree of compliance with treatment?
- Is there any charge for their service and, if so, who pays?
- Are there any new developments?
- To what extent do they collaborate with other professions and services?

Case conferences

As part of your preparation for Mrs Tillett's discharge you have been asked to arrange a case conference. This is quite a demanding task and requires careful planning if it is to be successful.

Activity **20 MINUTES**

Draw up an action plan for the case conference. Your plan should describe in detail how you would go about organising it. Decide who you would invite, where you would hold it, who would be the most appropriate person to lead the discussion and whether or not you would invite the patient and her husband.

FEEDBACK

In addition to the members of the team identified in the previous activity you would need to ensure the presence of Mrs Tillett's GP, a representative from the vascular team, a community nurse, social services, and perhaps a dietitian. Given the psychosocial problems evident in the case you might also like to involve a clinical psychologist.

The venue might seem a relatively unimportant fact to consider but it needs to be conveniently sited to encourage full attendance. It would need to be large enough, private and, if possible, have refreshments available. Make sure that both the details of the venue as well as time of the conference are publicised well in advance and ask those involved to confirm whether or not they will attend.

While traditionally a case conference would be led by the medical personnel, there is no reason why you should not volunteer. The choice of person should ideally be based, not on tradition, but on merit, i.e. the person who is best suited to coordinate Mrs Tillett's care.

Having the case conference is a pointless exercise if you do not involve Mr and Mrs Tillett in the decision-making process. You have to be sensitive to the effect such a meeting might have on the family. You should make every effort to ensure that they are not intimidated by the proceedings and that their needs, opinions and feelings are expressed and valued. Priorities can often centre around resource issues rather than patient need; the challenge facing the team is to provide an appropriate care programme within available resources. This aim is in line with current health service reforms which, in theory, place the patient at the centre of the service.

Activity **15 MINUTES**

Put yourself in the role of leader of the case conference. Write an agenda for the meeting and notes to guide you through the meeting which identify the issues which need to be resolved. When you have completed your plan consider all the options available to you for each issue.

* *

FEEDBACK

Your notes should have included most of the following issues to be addressed. The list is not exhaustive, you may have identified others.

1. Poor diabetic control. To tackle this problem effectively it is necessary to understand the underlying reasons. These may include dietary factors, issues of compliance, patient/family education, and medication. Mrs Tillett's long-standing diabetes puts her increasingly at risk of complications related to the disease, irrespective of the issue of compliance. While good diabetic control may reduce such complications as retinopathy and nephropathy there is little evidence that arterial disease involving the large arteries is reduced by good control. It seems likely from this scenario that Mrs Tillett has significant arterial disease.
2. Current vascular status. The presence of gangrene indicates reduced peripheral arterial circulation. To rely on the raised resting pressure index alone in this case would not be helpful in identifying the extent of the arterial disease. It seems likely that the vessels are calcified and that this caused the problem in obliterating the signal when attempting to measure her resting pressure index (see Sect. 5).
3. General medical condition. Mrs Tillett needs regular vascular follow-up and a complete medical review. She will probably require district nursing assessment, both of her general condition and in order to determine an effective wound care regime.
4. Non-compliance. In the past Mrs Tillett has not complied with treatment or turned up for appointments. Her most recent experiences may have impressed on her the need to take her problems seriously but the underlying reasons should be explored at the conference. Expanding her knowledge of the underlying causes of her problems may in itself help.
5. Her husband's anger and fear; the underlying marital stress; possible depression and denial; and the pressure on her family. These may all be areas in which the psychologist can help. We do not know much about the family's living conditions and this requires more assessment. It may be that the provision of some home aids might be a starting point in reducing the stress levels.

6. The current neuropathy would necessitate a review of appropriate footwear.
7. Smoking. It is never easy to persuade someone who has smoked heavily for many years to stop smoking, but in this case it is important to try.

* *

Case study outcome

Mrs Tillett was discharged home 4 weeks after admission. Although her amputation site was not healed, it was felt by those caring for her that a long stay in hospital would prove detrimental to both Mr and Mrs Tillett. An occupational therapist did a home assessment; this revealed that a number of adaptations and home aids were required. Home carers were provided daily for the first 4 weeks after discharge and the couple were put on the waiting list for sheltered accommodation.

District nurses visited on a daily basis to dress Mrs Tillett's foot and provide support. Mr Tillett, in particular, found the visits very helpful; it was clear that he was afraid the situation might get out of control again.

Mrs Tillett was readmitted 4 weeks after discharge for another angiogram and a balloon angioplasty. This was felt to be the most appropriate intervention as the distal distribution of the arterial disease made reconstructive arterial surgery impossible. The treatment was successful and she returned home again 1 week later.

Mrs Tillett's wound healed after 3 months. The family started family therapy under the supervision of a clinical psychologist. They were able to explore their complex problems, including Mrs Tillett's denial of the situation.

While the long-term prospects for Mrs Tillett are not good, the quality of her life and that of her family has been considerably improved. This case study particularly emphasises how a holistic, multiprofessional approach to care is essential. The peripheral issues Mrs Tillett was facing were more difficult for her to cope with than her medical condition.

CASE STUDY 8: FREDERICK SALMON —TRAUMATIC ULCERATION

Scenario

This scenario places you in the role of a nurse working in a vascular unit. Mr Salmon is a 67-year-old gentleman who is referred to your unit by his GP with a large ulcer of unknown origin on his left lower leg. The referral letter states that Mr Salmon developed the ulcer 30 years ago, having fallen on the bus and developed a large haematoma. The GP was unaware of this situation until 1 month ago when he was asked to visit Mr Salmon by the district nurse attending his wife. During the 30 years since its development, Mr Salmon has been treating his own ulcer using antiseptic creams and dressings.

You are immediately struck by Mr Salmon's over-cheerful, euphoric behaviour. He greets you jovially and fidgets with his hands. You explain that he will be undergoing non-invasive investigations to try to determine the cause of his ulcer.

His investigations reveal a good arterial circulation. His resting pressure on both legs is normal and his Duplex ultrasound scan reveals that all vessels are patent. Duplex scan of his venous system reveals normal veins and no evident reflux in deep, perforating or superficial systems. Blood tests are within normal parameters with the exception of slight anaemia (haemoglobin 10.0 g/dl), and X-ray examination shows no underlying osteomyelitis. Wound biopsy reveals inflammatory changes only. His blood pressure is 140/90 mm/Hg, height 1.8 m and weight 76.2 kg. Examination of the wound reveals a deep ulcer extending through the fascia with little evidence of healthy granulation and rolled edges. The surrounding skin is normal (see Plate 7, between pp. 102 and 103).

Mr Salmon commences treatment at the hospital ulcer clinic. He attends regularly but makes little improvement. His bandage is always neatly in place and you begin to suspect that he is tampering with his dressings. He denies removing the bandage. Areas of new granulation disappear on future visits and the surrounding skin shows evidence of scratch marks. You discuss the situation with the consultant in charge of his case and decide that Mr Salmon may be causing deliberate damage to his ulcer. The consultant decides to apply a plaster of Paris cast to prevent him tampering with the wound and asks you to explain to him why this is necessary. He becomes very tearful when you do so.

Self-assessment   10 MINUTES

What factors indicate that Mr Salmon has an ulcer of traumatic origin?

FEEDBACK

You could have said that:

- it was the direct consequence of an injury that resulted in a haematoma
- it is not likely that the ulceration is related to arterial or venous disease as all investigations are normal

- blood tests show that he is not a diabetic and that he does not have autoimmune disease
- there is no evidence of changes to the surrounding skin which would indicate venous disease.

Self-inflicted (factitional) ulceration

Activity   15 MINUTES

What triggers in the scenario raise your suspicions that Mr Salmon has been deliberately tampering with and causing damage to his wound?

FEEDBACK

There are four indicators which might have triggered your suspicions.

1. Mr Salmon has had his ulcer for 30 years but has not sought professional help.
2. The bandage always seems to be neatly in place suggesting that it has been reapplied recently.
3. Scratch marks are evident on the surrounding skin.
4. There is loss of granulation tissue between appointments.

It is very important not to jump to conclusions about whether or not patients have deliberately interfered with their wounds with the intention of delaying healing. There is anecdotal evidence that this phenomenon may occur but no conclusive empirical evidence. There may be legitimate reasons for any of the indicators listed above. If, for instance, the surrounding skin has become irritated as the result of a bandage and dressing Mr Salmon may have an irresistible urge to scratch. This would account for the scratch marks, the loss of granulation tissue and disturbance of the bandage requiring him to tidy or reapply it before his appointment. His unwillingness to seek help for so long may be due to an irrational fear of hospitals and health care professionals. He may also have inadvertently damaged the wound by self-administering proprietary products.

Activity   5 MINUTES

Given the alternative explanations offered above, were your assumptions about Mr Salmon justified?

FEEDBACK

If Mr Salmon had identified the alternatives himself, your suspicions would not have been raised. The fact that he denies removing the bandage, when it is clear to you (because it has been applied differently) that it has been tampered with, is justification for your concern.

You may ask yourself why anyone would delay the healing of his or her own ulcer. The concept of the 'social ulcer' is discussed in Section 5. This case study shows the complexity involved in exploring this phenomenon.

Case study outcome

Mr Salmon did not have a plaster of Paris cylinder applied as it was thought that the level of exudate would cause severe maceration. His leg was dressed with a four-layer bandage but 3 months after treatment had commenced he had still failed to progress. Further investigations, including a bone scan, revealed osteomyelitis which was not evident on the first X-ray. Despite aggressive treatment it was decided to perform a below-knee amputation. Mr Salmon is now fully recovered and managing well with his prosthesis. It was never discovered whether or not Mr Salmon had been deliberately damaging his ulcer. Although frightened at the prospect of losing a limb, he adjusted very well and was clearly relieved. During his stay there was no evidence of non-compliance with treatment. He eventually revealed that he had sought professional help earlier, but never revealed why he did not continue with treatment.

CASE STUDY 9: LILY FRASER
—RHEUMATOID ARTHRITIS VASCULITIC ULCERATION

Scenario

This scenario places you in the role of a district nurse. Lily Fraser is a 57-year-old lady with circumferential, bilateral ulceration due to vasculitis, secondary to rheumatoid arthritis. Her deteriorating condition requires a complete nursing reassessment.

Mrs Fraser lives in a tiny first floor flat which is cluttered with furniture. Owing to her extreme immobility, she lives in one room which contains a bed, large armchair and commode. The room is heated by a gas fire and is swelteringly hot. As you

enter the flat you are aware of a strong odour, which you recognise is from the exudate from her legs.

You introduce yourself and ask Mrs Fraser about herself. You note that she is thin, pale and looks very tired. Her hands and fingers are grossly deformed and she seems to have little mobility in her arms or shoulders.

She explains that she has had severe rheumatoid arthritis for 30 years. During this time she has undergone knee replacements and has suffered several spontaneous fractures. Recently her arthritis had been less troublesome but 3 months ago she had an exacerbation, with severe pain and swelling in many joints. When this occurred she developed rapidly spreading ulceration on both legs.

Examination reveals large shallow granulating ulcers on both legs (see Plate 4, between pp. 102 and 103). The dressings you remove are sodden with exudate. During removal of her dressings Mrs Fraser is in extreme pain, begging you to stop on a number of occasions. The edges of the ulceration appear purple and both her feet are oedematous. Exposure of the ulcer increases the pain.

Examination of the nursing notes shows that many different dressings have been tried with little relief. Her current dressing regime involves twice-daily dressings, using a paraffin tulle dressing and absorbent dressing pads secured by a light bandage. The exudate on the dressing pads is fluorescent green. You note that she has received two courses of systemic antibiotics, although you are unable to find the results of the swabs taken. On both occasions, Mrs Fraser was given a 5-day course of flucloxacillin.

Mrs Fraser's medical history reveals that she has had bouts of chronic bronchitis and a cholecystectomy. Her current medication is methylprednisolone, 10 mg daily, and naproxen, 250 mg 6-hourly.

On questioning you find that Mrs Fraser has a poor diet and little appetite. She has refused meals on wheels and will not eat fresh vegetables or fruit. You note a fresh supplement drink on her table. You ask her to tell you what support she receives from family and friends. She tells you that her sister visits her three times a week and a niece every few weeks. The district nurses visit twice daily to re-dress her legs and this takes over an hour. The district nursing night service visit to put her to bed. She tells you that her GP is very supportive, visiting regularly when required. Home carers also provide daily support.

The home carer arrives during your visit and tells you that she feels the situation is becoming impossible.

During your nursing assessment, you note that Mrs Fraser has slight urinary incontinence and the skin on both groins and buttocks is erythematous despite the fact that she is sitting on an appropriate pressure-relief cushion.

What four factors in the scenario suggest that Mrs Fraser has a vasculitic ulcer?

FEEDBACK

You should have said the following.

1. She has rheumatoid arthritis with obvious gross deformity of her hands, feet and shoulders.
2. The ulceration coincided with the exacerbation of the rheumatoid arthritis.
3. The edges of her ulcer are purple and her feet are oedematous.
4. She has severe pain.

Patients, such as Mrs Fraser, who suffer from rheumatoid arthritis are prone to ulceration. It is often difficult to know the underlying aetiology in these patients which can be complex. Pun et al (1990) found that 10% of patients with the condition would suffer with an ulcer at some point. The same study found that in 18.2% of cases the cause was vasculitic, i.e. inflammation of the blood vessels.

Treatment of pseudomonas infection

What is the significance of the fluorescent green dressing pad?

FEEDBACK

The green fluorescence indicates the presence of *Pseudomonas aeruginosa* in the wound. *Pseudomonas aeruginosa* is an aerobic organism commonly found in soil and water. It frequently attacks areas of tissue damage and is capable of surviving with few nutrients.

There is considerable debate concerning the treatment of pseudomonas in wounds. The signs of cellulitis associated with clinical infection may be masked in this patient because she is on steroid therapy (methylprednisolone). Pseudomonas in wounds is sometimes treated with ciprofloxacin;

however, in Mrs Fraser's case this would need to be used with great care because one of the known side effects of this drug is the development of vasculitis.

Was the use of flucloxacillin appropriate? Give reasons for your answer.

FEEDBACK

You should have said that the use of flucloxacillin was probably not appropriate because:

1. flucloxacillin is normally prescribed in patients with staphylococcal infection
2. it is unclear whether she has true clinical infection
3. the courses of antibiotics she has been given are too short for effective treatment.

Structured assessment

The scenario highlights that Mrs Fraser has many problems. Using the four 'adaptive modes' described by Roy & Andrews (1991) 'physiological, role, interdependence and self-concept' illustrated earlier in the assessment undertaken in Case Study 2 (Box 6.1), undertake an assessment of her which identifies the factors to be addressed in planning her care both from a nursing perspective and a medical perspective.

FEEDBACK

Physiological factors

The physiological factors include the following.

- She is totally immobile and needs help to get into bed. Carers think this situation is becoming 'impossible'.
- She is tired and fatigued.
- She has deformities in her feet, hands and shoulders.
- Her appetite is poor and she is underweight.
- She is slightly incontinent.
- She has skin excoriations on her buttocks and groin and is at risk of developing pressure sores.

- She has large, possibly infected ulcers on both legs.
- She has heavy exudate from her ulcers with likely protein loss.
- She is in pain firstly from her ulcers and secondly from her joints.
- She is anaemic.
- She has suffered recent exacerbation of her rheumatoid arthritis.
- She has repeated bouts of chronic bronchitis.
- She has oedematous feet.
- She has suffered several spontaneous fractures.

Role factors

The scenario tells us little about her role function except that she is largely dependent on others, her primary role being that of patient.

Interdependence factors

- She has a sister who visits three times each week and a niece who visits less frequently.
- She is visited twice daily by district nurses and once a day by the 'night service'.
- She has daily support from home carers.
- She has regular visits from her GP.

Self-concept factors

Again the scenario tells us very little.

We are given considerable insight into the physiological dimension of Mrs Fraser's case but little regarding the psychosocial problems, i.e. the impact of her illness on her in terms of purpose and self-fulfilment, how she feels about herself and her relationship with others.

Activity   10 MINUTES

Take a good look at the physiological evidence you have so far and decide how you could make it more objective. For example, is describing a wound as 'large' comprehensive enough in an assessment? Describe what extra information you require and any problems you might encounter.

FEEDBACK

1. We know that she is underweight but just how heavy is she? Given her immobility and cluttered surroundings it may be very difficult to weigh her.

2. It is not enough to say that she is not eating. A food diary would give a better insight into her dietary status. In view of the number of carers involved, careful coordination of the process would be required.
3. Detailed information about her 'slight incontinence' is desirable.
4. The risk of developing pressure sores should be quantified using an appropriate assessment tool.
5. The size and position of her 'large ulcers' should be documented in detail including: exact size and precise location of each ulcer, the level of exudate, any odour, condition of surrounding skin, and details of any pain, etc. Morison & Moffatt (1994) give an example of a suitable assessment chart designed for this purpose.
6. A wound swab should be taken to determine the flora within the ulcer.
7. It is unlikely that you would be able to measure her resting pressure index in the home because of the extent of her ulceration and the associated pain.
8. Routine investigations of blood pressure, pulse and temperature should be taken.
9. Additional medical investigations include: blood tests to give more information on loss of protein and anaemia, and to help confirm the diagnosis; erythrocyte sedimentation rate and rheumatoid factor; biopsy of ulcer; and vascular status because of increased risk of arterial disease. She is clearly in pain from both the ulcer and her arthritis which is inadequately controlled by naproxen. This should be fully discussed with her GP. Patients with this type of ulceration frequently require opiates.

Activity   20 MINUTES

Now, think about the remaining three adaptive modes: role, interdependence and self-concept. Put yourself in the 'patient's shoes' and make notes on what you would be feeling, and what you would want changed.

Give one example for each mode, i.e. how does she feel about her role in life, her relationship with others and her own self esteem?

FEEDBACK

You should have picked some of the following points.

Role

Owing to her severe immobility and high dependency on others her ability to develop a meaningful role is severely compromised. She obviously cannot work, but her arthritis probably will prevent her even undertaking a hobby.

Interdependence

She is well supported by both professionals and family and as such has regular contact with other people. Her physical condition and the environment she lives in, however, are not conducive to developing relationships with others.

Self-concept

Given her medical history and current poor condition it is likely that she is severely depressed and has a poor opinion of herself. She may also feel anger and frustration at times.

● ●

Choosing an appropriate dressing

Activity   20 MINUTES

Look at the photograph of Mrs Fraser's ulcer in Plate 4 (between pp. 102 and 103), read the scenario again and perhaps review what we have said about dressings in Section 5.

1. What dressings could be used to dress her ulcer?
2. Which one would you try first and why?

● ●

FEEDBACK

There are no easy answers to these questions. The scenario tells you that many different dressings have been used before but the factors you should have taken into account when deciding how to dress her wounds were:

- her severe pain at dressing changes
- copious exudate
- the ulcer is large but shallow.

As you will see from the scenario outcome, the most appropriate primary dressing for Mrs Fraser proved to be a completely non-adherent dressing which could be left in place over several dressing changes.

● ●

Case study outcome

The situation with Mrs Fraser did not improve. She was finally admitted to a medical ward for reassessment of her situation. During her stay she was given a blood transfusion to correct her anaemia and skin grafts were applied to both legs. These grafts did not take well, and this is not unusual in patients with rheumatoid arthritis, particularly if the disease is active.

It was decided that Mrs Fraser would not be able to return to her flat. She agreed with this decision and appreciated the continuous care available to her in hospital.

Her ulceration continued to be difficult to manage. Changing her dressings was painful for her and this was controlled by the regular use of morphine and Entonox during the procedure itself. A number of dressings were tried, the most beneficial proving to be a completely non-adherent dressing that could be left in place over successive changes. This also helped relieve pain and prevented trauma to the wound bed. Exudate was contained by using orthopaedic wool, and a gentle elastic bandage (pressure 17 mmHg) was applied to reduce the oedema. The dressings were renewed on a daily basis.

During her admission her rheumatoid arthritis was reassessed and she began a programme of physiotherapy to prevent her becoming even more immobilised.

Mrs Fraser finally went to live in a nursing home as she required 24-hour care. This took nearly 9 months to arrange. However, by this time she had been discharged from the hospital, she had gained some weight and her pain was well controlled. It is unlikely that her ulcer will ever completely heal and she will need ongoing palliative care to prevent any deterioration

CASE STUDY 10: ROBIN POWERS
—CANCEROUS ULCERATION

Scenario

This scenario places you in the role of community staff nurse and leg ulcer clinic coordinator. Mr Powers presents with a small lesion on his left leg (see Plate 6, between pp. 102 and 103).

Mr Powers is a 40-year-old gentleman who self-refers to a community clinic. He has recently moved into the area and is not registered with a GP. He noted a small lesion on his left shin 4 months ago, which scabbed over but never healed. When the scab fell off the wound bled profusely.

Mr Powers is otherwise in excellent health and all investigations are normal. You explain to him that he must register with a local doctor. At this request he becomes abusive and demands to know why this is required. You explain the situation to him but he remains unconvinced. Your examination of the lesion leads you to suspect that it is malignant and you are anxious that he is referred to the local dermatology clinic for further investigation. He remains reluctant but you nevertheless write a letter to the GP you are attached to. You give Mr Powers the address and telephone number of the GP, dress his ulcer with a non-adherent dressing and light support bandage and try to stress, without frightening him, that it is important that he make an appointment as soon as possible.

Self-assessment   10 MINUTES

What five factors in this case study would lead you to suspect that Mr Powers possibly has a malignant ulcer?

FEEDBACK

You should have been able to pick out the following indicators.

- The ulcer forms a scab, bleeds easily and fails to heal.
- He is otherwise in excellent health.
- The condition of his skin is normal.
- The site of the ulcer is atypical.
- All other investigations, including pulse, blood pressure and resting pressure index are normal.

Making difficult decisions

Activity   60 MINUTES

Is there anything else you could have done about Mr Powers' reluctance to register with a GP? Are you under any obligation to check with the GP to see whether he has made contact?

If possible, ask three of your colleagues what they would do in this situation and compare their answers to your own.

FEEDBACK

The ethical principle of beneficence obliges you to act in a way which ensures the maximum benefit to Mr Powers as well as the minimum of harm. Unfortunately we cannot always agree on what is best for individual patients. This may be due to differences in professional emphasis. Nursing theory today is based largely on an individualised holistic

approach to care whereas rigid policies applied indiscriminately may stem from a more collective approach which is driven by economic and resource distribution factors. This conflict illustrates two further ethical principles: autonomy and justice. Autonomy involves acceptance of the individuality of people in terms of the opinions, values and feelings they hold and the right to act upon them. Problems arise with regard to autonomy when individuals differ in their perception of morality, i.e. what is right and what is wrong. Justice is concerned with fairness and what is owed to an individual. The aspect of justice which commonly relates to nursing practice is called 'distributive justice' and is concerned with the way in which health care resources are allocated.

Ethical principles

Gibson (1993) discusses these ethical principles and lists five kinds of controversial issues in nursing:

1. quality versus sanctity of life
2. freedom versus control and prevention of harm
3. truth telling versus deception or lying
4. desire for knowledge in opposition to religious, political, economic and ideological interests
5. issues of conventional, scientifically based therapy versus alternative, non-scientific therapies.

Activity   10 MINUTES

Which of the above list of 'controversial issues' relates to Mr Powers?

FEEDBACK

Two of these issues relate to Mr Powers. Firstly, 'freedom versus control and prevention of harm' is relevant in the sense that you may have to insist, cajole, persuade Mr Powers, against his will, to register with the GP. Secondly, 'truth telling versus deception or lying' applies because you have to decide whether or not to tell Mr Powers of your suspicions regarding the possible cause of his ulcer.

Ethical decision making

Gibson (1993) provides a framework for ethical decision making and describes three 'essential stages':

- information collection and problem identification
- consideration of alternative strategies
- selection of a course of action for implementation.

Activity 10 MINUTES

Should you tell Mr Powers of your suspicions? List your reasons for whatever decision you make.

FEEDBACK

- Your initial assessment has enabled you to identify the problem which is whether you tell Mr Powers that you think his ulcer might be malignant. You should now ask yourself if you have all the information you require. Is there anything that you might have missed? Should you get a second opinion? Why is he so reluctant to register? Does he perhaps have the same suspicions as you?
- What are the alternatives open to you? In simple terms the alternative is not to tell him and exercise the principle of autonomy in that you have given your professional advice and it is now up to Mr Powers to decide for himself. You may consider passing the responsibility over to another professional as an alternative but this does not get rid of the problem; the decision still has to be made by somebody. Of course, telling Mr Powers about your suspicions might be a very effective way of making him comply with the registration process and any treatment regime but this alternative has to be judged in terms of beneficence, i.e. balancing harm against benefit. If you decide on the latter option, how do you go about it with the minimum of harm?
- What course of action have you chosen? How sure are you of your diagnosis? Are you willing to take responsibility for your actions—especially if you are wrong? It would perhaps be unwise to say anything to Mr Powers without some histological evidence, but this takes time to obtain.

Self-assessment 5 MINUTES

Which of the principles of ethical decision making (beneficence, justice or autonomy) is most relevant in Mr Powers' case?

FEEDBACK

If you look at these three ethical principles you can see that they interrelate. The primary principle for nursing must be that no harm comes to Mr Powers (beneficence) but, while Mr Powers has the right to expect treatment (justice), he also has to make the decision to conform to the registration process (autonomy).

Case study outcome

Mr Powers responded well to the advice he was given. He registered with the GP who agreed to refer him for a dermatological opinion. He returned to the community clinic to thank the staff for their help.

When he was seen in hospital the leg ulcer clinic coordinator (the role you took in the scenario) made herself available, realising that he was very anxious. The dermatologist performed an excision biopsy which revealed, as suspected, that the lesion was a basal cell carcinoma. No further treatment was required (the lesion having been excised) and the wound healed uneventfully after 3 weeks. Mr Powers has not had any recurrence of his carcinoma and his prognosis is excellent.

This case again demonstrates that a multidisciplinary approach to care is essential. The close working relationship between the nursing team and the dermatologists proved very useful in managing Mr Powers' anxiety. It also shows that the nurse must develop good assessment skills if he or she is to identify the unusual ulcer and have the confidence to involve other members of the multidisciplinary team when necessary.

REFERENCES

Blair S D, Backhouse C M, Wright D D I, Riddle E, McCollum C M 1988 Do dressings influence the healing of chronic venous ulcers? Phlebology 3: 129–134

Boulton A J M, Connor H, Cavanagh P R (eds) 1994 The foot in diabetes, 2nd edn. Wiley, Chichester

Bridel J 1994 Risk assessment. Journal of Tissue Viability 4(3): 84–85

Cameron J 1995 The importance of contact dermatitis in the management of leg ulcers. Journal of Tissue Viability 5(2): 52–55

Cameron J, Powell S 1992 Contact dermatitis: its importance in leg ulcer patients. Wound Management 2(3): 12–13

Department of Health 1989 Working for patients. HMSO, London

Gibson C H 1993 Underpinnings of ethical reasoning in nursing. Journal of Advanced Nursing 18: 2003–2007

Hannuksela M, Salo H 1986 The repeated open application test (ROAT). Contact Dermatitis 14: 221–227

Morison M, Moffatt C J 1994 A colour guide to the assessment and management of leg ulcers, 2nd edn. Mosby, London

Powell S, Cameron J, Cherry G, Ryan T 1994 The safety of a new medicated paste bandage in patients with a history of sensitivity to other paste bandages. Abstract from the 4th European Wound Conference, Copenhagen

Pun Y L W, Barraclough D R E, Muirden K D 1990 Leg ulcers in rheumatoid arthritis. Medical Journal of Australia 153(10): 585–587

Roy C, Andrews H A 1991 The Roy Adaption Model: the definitive statement. Appleton & Lange, Norwalk

Shakespeare P 1994 Scoring the risk scores. Journal of Tissue Viability 4(1): 21–22

Wilson J 1995 Infection control in clinical practice. Baillière Tindall, London

Conclusion

Having completed this pack you should now have a good overview of the management of patients with a variety of leg ulcers. Research in recent years has begun to answer some of the complex problems facing practitioners who care for people with leg ulceration but there are many more important aspects still to be clarified such as the use of antiseptics in the cleansing of wounds, the use of dressings, understanding more about our patients' quality of life, and the issues of patient compliance with treatment.

We have progressed dramatically in our understanding of many aspects of venous ulceration in particular and given hope of healing to many who thought they would never heal. Other less common aetiologies, however, represent a considerable challenge to the multidisciplinary team as does the whole issue of why chronic wounds in general are so difficult to heal.

We hope that this introduction will inspire you to become actively involved in the pursuit of new knowledge and understanding in relation to leg ulceration in order that all our patients may benefit from even more effective professional intervention into what remains an extremely debilitating condition.

There have been many success stories in the field of leg ulceration with new services being developed all over the UK and elsewhere around the world. Health care providers and politicians are waking up to the idea that an efficient, comprehensive, collaborative and research-based approach can be very cost effective for the taxpayer and at the same time form the basis for a quality service to the patient.

Reader

Chronic ulceration of the leg: extent of the problem and provision of care

M J CALLAM,   C V RUCKLEY,   D R HARPER,   J J DALE

(Reproduced with kind permission from the BMJ Publishing Group.)

Abstract

A postal survey in two health board areas in Scotland, encompassing a population of about one million, identified 1477 patients with chronic ulcers of the leg. Women outnumbered men by a ratio of 2·8:1. The median age of the women was 74 and of the men 67. Seventy two (5%) were hospital inpatients, 174 (12%) were managed jointly by the primary care team and outpatient departments, and 1201 (83%) were managed entirely in the community.

Efforts to improve the management of chronic ulcers of the leg should focus on primary health care.

Introduction

Chronic ulceration of the leg appears to have perplexed physicians since medical records began. Although there are many reports on its management, little information is available on the overall size and extent of the problem or its clinical course.

Two European surveys into venous disease have been made, providing data on the prevalence of leg ulceration. The first was a study, based on a questionnaire, of the adult population of Klatov in Bohemia in 1961 by Bobek et al.[1] Those people who indicated that they had evidence of venous disease were subsequently examined. This survey showed that the prevalence of leg ulceration, either open or healed, was 1%. The second and more recent study, of factory workers in Basle, Switzerland, showed a similar proportion.[2]

Information concerning the United Kingdom is almost non-existent. In 1929 Dickson-Wright suggested a prevalence of 0.5% but admitted that this figure was an estimate.[3] In 1951 Boyd et al arrived at a similar figure based on the returns of patients registered as off work due to leg ulceration,[4] but this figure was probably an underestimate. In a study supplementary to that reported here and based on patients in a group practice in Edinburgh we recently estimated that 1% of adults suffer from chronic leg ulcers.[5]

Much of the information in reports on leg ulcers is based on small, selected populations, usually patients attending outpatient departments. An understandable conclusion that might be drawn from such reports is that all leg ulcers are managed by dermatologists, surgeons, or physiotherapists. A preliminary survey by our own group, however, showed that most patients were cared for in the community by district nurses and represented a formidable problem for the primary care services not only in terms of numbers but also in various aspects of management. We concluded that the first step towards improving care was to obtain better information on the scale of the problem, the clinical course of the condition, and how care was being provided.

The Lothian and Forth Valley leg ulcer study was therefore set up in 1981. This paper reports the first phase, the main aims of which were to establish a point prevalence of leg ulcers and to find out who was providing the care.

Methods

The survey was carried out in 1981–2 in the neighbouring health board areas of Lothian and Forth Valley, which have a mixed urban and rural population of about one million. The objective was to identify all patients receiving treatment for chronic leg ulceration from any branch of the National Health Service at the time of the survey.

To identify all patients receiving treatment in the community, recording forms were sent to all general practitioners, district and occupational nurses, and wardens of old people's homes. To identify patients receiving either outpatient or inpatient care at a hospital, forms were sent to outpatient departments, physiotherapy departments, and inpatient wards of general hospitals and all acute and long stay hospitals. In each case the correspondent was asked to identify all the patients currently undergoing treatment for active chronic leg ulceration or who had received treatment within three months. Efforts were made to obtain replies from non-responders by means of follow-up letters and telephone calls.

The resulting returns were cross checked to ensure that patients reported from more than one source were included only once in the final total.

Results

Of the 572 general practitioners approached, only 37 refused to cooperate with the study. Complete returns were obtained from all other correspondent groups. Notifications of 2128 patients were received, of which 651 were reported from more than one source, giving a total of 1477 patients (1765 83%) were reported by general practitioners, district nurses, occupational health services, and old people's homes; and 104 (5%) by physiotherapy departments, 148 (7%) by outpatient departments, and 111 (5%) by hospital inpatient departments). When patients were reported from more than one source, preference was given to those reported by general practitioners and district nurses as the primary providers of care. By these criteria 1282 (87%) were reported from the community and 195 (13%) from the hospitals.

From these figures the point prevalence of active leg ulceration known to health care workers in this area was established as 1·48/1000 total population. A considerable variation between geographical areas was evident, the range being 1·35–2.09/1000 population.

The patients were mostly women. Out of the total of 1477 patients who were identified by the survey, only 388 were men and 1089 women (ratio 1: 2·8). The table shows the distribution by age and sex of the 1311 patients on whom information on age was available. The median age of the men was 67 (range 22-96) and of the women 74 (range 26-100).

Leith Hospital, Edinburgh
M J CALLAM, MB, FRCSED, senior surgical registrar

Vascular Surgical Unit, Royal Infirmary, Edinburgh
C V RUCKLEY, MB, FRCSED, consultant surgeon

Surgical Unit, Royal Infirmary, Falkirk
D R HARPER, MD, FRCSED, consultant surgeon

Department of Nursing, Lothian Health Board, Edinburgh
J J DALE, SRN, MSC, senior nursing officer

Correspondence to: Mrs J J Dale, Lothian and Forth Valley Leg Ulcer Study, 40 Colinton Road, Edinburgh

Distribution of age and sex of patients (n = 1311) with chronic leg ulcers

	Men		Women	
Age* (years)	No (%)	Prevalence†	No (%)	Prevalence†
<25	1 (<1)	1: 191 846		
25–34	9 (2)	1: 7306	3 (<1)	1: 24 596
35–44	17 (5)	1: 2976	14 (2)	1: 3678
45–54	52 (15)	1: 922	57 (6)	1: 897
55–64	77 (22)	1: 576	153 (16)	1: 327
65–74	112 (32)	1: 290	288 (30)	1: 158
75–84	66 (19)	1: 195	315 (33)	1: 86
>85	13 (<4)	1: 139	134 (13)	1: 53
Total	347		964	

• In 166 patients information on age was not available.
† Prevalences specific to age and sex were calculated using Registrar General's census statistics for 1981 for area covered by the survey and corrected for 166 patients whose ages were not available.

Discussion

In seeking to quantify the great demand that the care of leg ulcers places on the health service we have highlighted the difficulties experienced in obtaining accurate and comprehensive information.

The first obstacle was that care is provided for this disease by many different specialties and in almost every part of the health service. Patients seen periodically in outpatient departments were often cared for by the district nurse between appointments. Patients also moved from one source of care to another during the survey. For this reason, although the totals attributed to each source of care are too high, the proportional distribution between primary and hospital care of roughly 5:1 is a fair reflection of what is happening in practice. Only 6% of general practitioners refused to collaborate, but we were nevertheless able to make up much of this deficit from information provided by other respondents in hospitals and the community, from whom total collaboration was obtained.

The clinical course of chronic leg ulceration is one of episodes of recurrence followed by periods when the ulcer is healed. Our survey, which looked at the point prevalence, identified only those patients who had had active ulceration within three months before the time of the survey and could not identify most patients who were 'between ulcers'. We chose to refer to point rather than period prevalence because, although we asked respondents to report ulcers that had occurred within the previous three months, virtually all ulcers were either open or had healed within one or two weeks of the inquiry. Thus the prevalence of active leg ulceration of 1.5/1000 population that we established represents only a proportion of the population of patients with chronic leg ulcers. The figures for the overall prevalence of the condition from our supplementary survey[5] and the work of Bobek et al[1] and Widmer[2] suggest that at any one time only 20-25% of ulcers are open. As one ulcer opens, however, another heals, and so the figure of 1·5/1000 represents the actual workload at any one time in terms of active ulceration.

A further obstacle to obtaining a complete survey is that we do not know what proportion of patients fail to report their ulcers to their doctors. In some instances that is because they think that they are able to dress the lesion themselves. Others may conceal the ulcer for various reasons such as fear of amputation. The size of this group is unknown, but we believe it to be small. It is in one sense irrelevant as we were concerned here with the scale of the problem as it impinged on health care resources.

Almost three times as many women as men were identified in the study. The table shows the distributions of age and sex among the 1311 patients whose ages were known, together with prevalences calculated from the Registrar General's census statistics for 1981 for the same geographical area. Our findings contrast noticeably with the figures found in the Basle study, in which the ratio was 1:1.[2] That study, however, was only of workers in factories, most of whom were men. All were of working age. Thus elderly women with leg ulcers would not have been detected. The survey by Bobek et al[1] comprised the entire adult population and showed a preponderance of women with a ratio of 1:1.5 (men: women). Anning, who reviewed a large series of referrals to hospitals in the 1950s, also showed a preponderance of women with a ratio of 1: 2·5.[6] It appears, therefore, that this condition is more common in women.

In considering the distribution of age and sex among our patients it is important to note that the ages given are those at the time of the survey and not at onset of the first episode of ulceration. In most cases the condition had been present for many years. In effect, this caused an accumulation of patients in the older age groups, particularly the women, who have a greater life expectancy. Two points can be noted from the table. Firstly, even though the age at the time of survey instead of the age at onset of ulceration was used, just under half of the men and a quarter of the women, were below the age of retirement. Thus leg ulceration is not only a problem for the elderly but also affects younger people, often resulting in substantial loss of working time. Secondly, as people's life span increases the size of the problem of leg ulcers will probably increase.

Identification of the sources of these patients was based on current or recent treatment and therefore broadly equates with the current provision of all or part of the care. Clearly, most patients with ulcers (87%) are managed by the primary care team, while a fairly small proportion are wholly under hospital care (13%).

If the figures from this study were extrapolated to the whole of the United Kingdom they would suggest that there are roughly 100 000 patients with active leg ulceration at any one time, drawn from a population with leg ulcers of 400 000. Much the largest share of the workload falls on district nurses. Any attempt to improve overall results must therefore include improvement of care in the community. Improvement in hospital care alone would make little impact.

Having ascertained the scale of the problem and learnt where care is being provided and by whom, our next objective was to study the clinical course of leg ulceration. We have assessed 600 of these patients in greater detail and shall report the findings later.

We thank our medical, nursing, and physiotherapy colleagues for their help. This study was made possible by a grant from the Health Service Research Committee of the Scottish Home and Health Department.

References

1 Bobek K, Cajzl L, Cepelák V, Slaisova V, Opatzny K, Barcal R. Étude de la frequence des maladies phlebologiques et de l'influence de quelques facteurs etiologiques. *Phlebologie* 1966; **19**: 217-30.
2 Widmer LK. *Peripheral venous disorders: prevalence and sociomedical importance.* Bern: Hans Huber, 1978.
3 Dickson-Wright A. The treatment of indolent ulcer of the leg. *Lancet* 1931; i: 457-60.
4 Boyd AM, Jepson RP, Ratcliffe AH, Rose SS. The logical management of chronic ulcers of the leg. *Angiology* 1952; **3**: 207-15.
5 Dale JJ, Callam MJ, Ruckley CV, Harper DR, Berrey PN. Chronic ulcers of the leg: a study of prevalence in a Scottish community. *Health Bull (Edinb)* 1983; **41**: 310-4.
6 Anning ST. *Leg ulcers: their causes and treatment.* London: J & A Churchill Ltd, 1954.

The physiology of wound healing

Colin Torrance

Colin Torrance is currently a postgraduate student in physiology at the University Medical School, Edinburgh. He trained at Queen Margaret College, Edinburgh, obtaining his RSCN and Diploma in Life Sciences qualifications. He then trained in general nursing at Fife College of Nursing, and subsequently held several staff nurse posts. Her completed his BSc in physiology at King's College, London. His interests include pressure sores, wound healing and reproductive physiology.

Wound healing is essentially an inflammatory reaction: the end result is repair by scar tissue formation (see *NURSING 3rd series 6*). The healing process is characterized by a sequential change in the types of cells infiltrating the wound. Each cell type has distinct requirements, and wound healing is a compromise between these competing demands. As with most compromises the final result is less than perfect, and scar tissue never regains the functional flexibility of the original tissue.

When considering wound healing it is natural to focus on events occurring at the site of injury. However, it cannot be overemphasized that wounds do not occur in isolation, they are only one aspect of a patient's condition. Nutritional factors, intercurrent illness and the patient's psychological state can all have a major impact on the rate and quality of wound healing. Circadian patterns can influence healing. When an individual is awake, catabolism (tissue degradation) is enhanced, while sleep favours anabolism (renewal). Thus, adequate sleep is as necessary for healing as adequate nutrition. The importance of nutrition in wound healing has been emphasized on pages 174–6. The cells involved in wound healing create heavy metabolic demands which require a good level of general nutrition and an adequate vascular supply to the injured area. Optimal healing occurs in the well-nourished individual, who has competent immune responses and well perfused tissues. Problem or chronic wounds often occur because some factor in the patient's general condition is impeding the healing process.

The sequence of events in wound healing can be conveniently described in four stages:
• the acute inflammatory reaction (0-3 days)
• the destructive phase, involving the removal of injured tissue (1-6 days)
• the proliferative phase, featuring angiogenesis and fibroplasia (3-24 days)
• the maturational phase of tissue remodelling (24 days to 1 year).
Two additional processes, epithelialization and wound contraction are also important.

The acute inflammatory phase

The primary goal of the immediate response to trauma is the control of haemorrhage. The body's initial response is vasoconstriction of the small blood vessels at the site of injury. Trauma disrupts the endothelial lining of the vessels and platelets stick to the exposed subendothelium. Interaction with subendothelial components, particularly collagen, stimulates the platelets to release serotonin and ADP (adenosine diphosphate), promoting further platelet aggregation. Activated platelets also mediate the conversion of fibrinogen to fibrin, stabilizing the clot. Other blood cells become incorporated into the clot, which then seals off the injured vessel (Figure 1). There is an initial release of histamine and other inflammatory mediators by the injured tissues, which causes a local vasoconstriction that may aid haemostasis.

The inflammatory mediators also cause vasodilation, with increased capillary permeability allowing fluid and plasma proteins to leak into the tissues. This is followed by the movement of white blood cells into the tissues. Vasodilation and increased capillary permeability result in the classical signs of inflammation: redness, warmth, swelling (oedema) and pain. The inflammatory response is not only beneficial, it is also essential if healing is to proceed. The first 24 hours of the acute inflammatory phase are characterized by the appearance of polymorphonuclear leucocytes and blood monocytes in the wound. Platelets may have a more extended role than simple haemostasis. When activated they release many substances, including growth factors, and it has been suggested that these may have a role in initiating the healing process.

Blood and exudate lost into the wound are rich in fibrin and form a clot, providing a limited degree of protection against bacterial or foreign body contamination. The fibrin forms a network holding the clot in place. As the clot dries out a scab is formed. This provides inferior protection against dehydration of the wound surface.

Although a degree of inflammation is essential, in very extensive trauma or where infection or foreign material contaminate a wound, inflammation may be prolonged and prove destructive. Prolonged inflammation will delay healing and may result in excessive granulation at a later stage. The presence of blood clots, dead or devitalized tissue and bacteria can all accentuate the inflammatory response. Foreign materials, including sutures, may have a similar effect. At this stage gentle handling, good asepsis and rigorous haemostasis are essential.

The destructive phase (Figure 2)

The main feature of this phase is removal of dead tissue and bacteria to make way for new growth. The presence of an extensive haematoma or necrotic tissue can delay healing by creating more dead space, encouraging bacterial proliferation and prolonging inflammation. This may inhibit both fibroplasia and epithelialization.

Neutrophilic, polymorphonuclear leucocytes are the first white cells to appear in the wound. These are short-lived cells which are soon replaced by macrophages. Neutrophils are active against bacteria, but are not essential for wound repair. In an experiment in which animals were treated with an antineutrophil serum to eliminate circulating neutrophils, no disruption of healing was noted (Simpson and Ross, 1972).

Macrophages are the central cells in this stage. They are responsible for the clearance of nectrotic tissue and are also active against bacteria. Neutrophils and macrophages contain several mechanisms for destroying ingested material. Microbial killing mechanisms include an acidic intracellular environment, and production of oxygen radicals and lysosomal enzymes. Neutrophils also contain an iron-binding protein, lactoferrin, which has bacteriostatic properties. Lysosomes contain enzymes capable of digesting proteins, peptides, carbohydrates and lipids. Administration of antimacrophage serum inhibits phagocytosis and markedly delays fibroblast migration, fibroplasia and collagen production. Macrophages are essential for healing; they play a role in attracting fibroblasts and also influence the growth of new blood vessels into the wound.

The proliferative phase (Figure 3)

This phase is characterized by intense proliferation of endothelial cells and fibroblasts. Endothelial buds grow into the space cleared by the macrophages. This ingrowth into areas of low oxygen tension occurs only after macrophage invasion. The endothelial buds carry fibroblasts with them, and these move into the wound, proliferate and begin to synthesize ground substance and collagen. Much of the hexosamine (a component of ground substance) manufactured at this stage seems to be derived from serum glycoproteins which have leaked into the tissues during the inflammatory phase. Collagen synthesis begins after 4 days. Initially the collagen is randomly organized, but as healing progresses its organization becomes more regular. During active fibroplasia the tensile strength of the wound increases roughly in parallel with the increase in collagen content. Fibroplasia is de-

Figure 1. Inflammatory phase

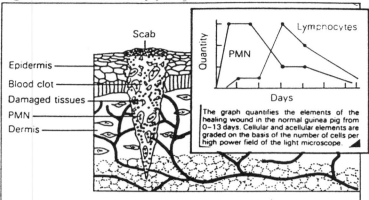

The graph quantifies the elements of the healing wound in the normal guinea pig from 0–13 days. Cellular and acellular elements are graded on the basis of the number of cells per high power field of the light microscope.

Figure 2. Destructive phase

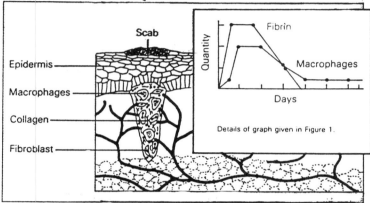

Details of graph given in Figure 1.

Figure 3. Proliferative phase

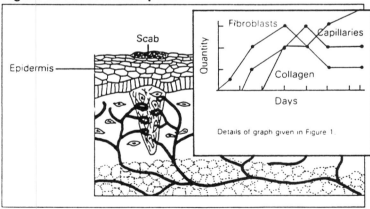

Details of graph given in Figure 1.

Graphs in Figures 1–3 adapted from Ross R, *Biol Rev* 1968; **43**: 51–96

pendent on the ingrowth of new blood vessels and an adequate supply of nutrients. Vitamin C is an essential stimulator of collagen synthesis, and a slightly acid pH also stimulates synthesis.

Granulation tissue consists of the new capillary loops, supporting collagen and ground surface matrix. Infection or the presence of foreign bodies prolongs inflammation and can result in excessive granulation and later hypertrophic scarring. Granulation tissue is highly vascular, but the new vessels are delicate and easily damaged. Granulation usually fills the defect but does not extend above the level of the normal epithelium. As the proliferative phase progresses the numbers of capillaries and fibroblasts begin to decline towards normal levels.

The maturational phase

The proliferative phase sees the most rapid increase in wound tensile strength. However, the wound still has only about 50% of the tensile strength of normal. During the maturational stage the collagen content continues to increase and collagen fibres increase in size and become reorientated, usually along the lines of tension in the wound (Figure 4). As remodelling progresses the wound loses its angry, red appearance and assumes the characteristic paleness of the scar. The scar softens and becomes flatter. Remodelling can be extensive, but scar tissue never regains the structure of the original tissue, and scar collagen is different from normal collagen. Even 100 days after injury wound collagen has a different microstructure from normal collagen. A scar remains weaker and usually has a thinner epithelial covering than surrounding tissues. Scar formation makes wound healing as much a pathological as a physiological process. There is some evidence that pharmacological agents which delay cross-linking of collagen fibres, allowing more remodelling during healing, may produce a more physiological scar. Drugs such as beta-aminoproprionite (BAPN) or penicillamine have been shown in animal models and clinical trials to improve the quality of scar tissue. The delay in cross-linking produced by these drugs may result in the collagen being more susceptible to remodelling by enzymes (collagenases). Pharmalogical control of

Figure 4. Maturational phase

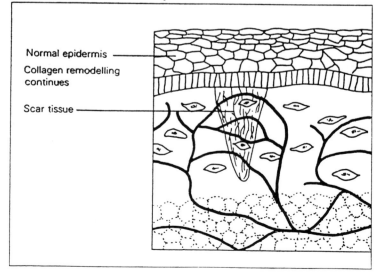

Normal epidermis
Collagen remodelling continues
Scar tissue

scar formation is in its infancy. Cohen (1985) provides a brief review of this area. Further information is also given by Hunt (1980).

Wound contraction

Initially, the edges of a full-thickness skin wound retract, increasing the wound area by 10-15%. After 3-4 days the edges of the wound begin to move inwards, and this contraction involves both the dermis and the epidermis. The mechanism of wound contraction is not fully understood, but a specialized form of contractile fibroblast, the myofibroblast, appears to be important. In uncomplicated wounds contraction can achieve excellent functional healing with minimal scarring. In areas where skin is less mobile contraction will not significantly contribute to healing.

Epithelialization

Following injury epithelial cells at the edges of the wound (and of hair follicle remnants) proliferate and migrate over the wound surface. They can only migrate over viable tissue and have to migrate under eschar. Migrating epithelial cells differentiate and lose their ability to divide. Optimal epithelialization occurs in a moist wound environment. The advantages of a moist environment can be illustrated by considering the effects of dehydration on skin wounds.

Normal scab formation results in an appreciable degree of wound dehydration with an increased loss of dermal tissue. Treatments such as blowing air or oxygen over the wound encourage even deeper scab formation with greater loss of tissue. The sources of new cells, hair follicles and other epidermal remnants are destroyed by dehydration and in deeper skin wounds the dermal papillary rate, a source of connective tissue growth, are also destroyed. An occlusive dressing, by preventing dehydration and keeping the wound moist, allows epithelialization to proceed directly across the wound surface (Winter, 1976). Epithelialization is about three times faster under an occlusive dressing than under normal eschar. However, infection may be a problem if the wound is heavily contaminated before the application of an occlusive dressing or where the patient's immunological defences are impaired.

Factors influencing wound repair

Both local and systemic factors can influence wound repair. Local factors include local blood supply, wound oxygen tension, temperature, infection and the effects of dressing or topical applications. Systemic factors include age, nutritional state and the presence of disease, particularly vascular disease, systemic infections or immunological incompetence. The influence of nutrition has been discussed on pages 174–6.

Oxygen and blood supply: trauma disrupts the vascular supply to the damaged tissues, and transport of oxygen and other essential nutrients to the wound edges can be precarious. Large areas of a wound are ischaemic. Wounds which are completely ischaemic do not heal. Pressure sores are an example of a wound caused primarily by disruption of the blood supply to a tissue. Vascular disease, shock or anaemia decrease the quantity or quality of the blood perfusing peripheral tissues impairing healing.

The new capillaries in a healing wound are very sensitive to changes in systemic circulation. Hypovolaemia causes capillaries to close leaving the growing edge of the wound unperfused. Conversely administration of fluids with low osmotic pressure to correct hypovolaemia can result in oedema in the growing tissues.

The growing edge of a wound is an area of high metabolic activity which utilizes most of the oxygen and other nutrients reaching the wound, leaving more central areas hypoxic. Mitotic activity occurring in a wound is likely to be confined to the oxygenated margins. Hypoxia can affect many aspects of wound healing: cell division, collagen synthesis and cross-linking, neovascularization and leucocyte activity. Macrophages can effectively remove debris in either aerobic or anaerobic conditions, but their ability to destroy ingested bacteria is reduced by hypoxia because the more effective mechanisms for bacterial killing (in both macrophages and leucocytes) are oxygen dependent.

Oxygen gradients have a complex influence on stimulating the growth of blood vessels into the wound. When hypoxic macrophages produce an angiogenic factor stimulating neovascularization, anoxic or well oxygenated macrophages do not secrete the angiogenic factor. Oxygen gradients create a gradient of angiogenic factor, and both are essential for healing to progress.

Fibroblasts require oxygen for collagen synthesis and for proliferation. A moderate increase in oxygen tension stimulates fibroblasts, but further increases may reduce their activity. This may not be due to a direct effect on the fibroblast, but may be associated with a reduction in blood supply, limiting the availability of some other substrate. Epithelialization is enhanced by an increased oxygen tension.

The influence of wound oxygen tension on healing is very complex. Oxygen is necessary for rapid, effective healing, but the presence of excessive oxygen may inhibit connective tissue healing. The pattern of oxygen gradients in the wound seem to be as important as the overall amount of oxygen available.

Temperature: a fall in wound temperature retards healing, partly due to vasoconstriction. Metabolic activity is reduced as the temperature falls and leucocytes in particular are sensitive to a drop in temperature; a fall of only 2°C is sufficient to reduce leucocyte activity to zero.

Movement: healing tissues are very fragile. In the early stages of epithelialization the migrating tongues of epithelium are only loosely attached to the dermis. Movement at the wound edges easily separates them from underlying tissues.

Infection: all wounds, including surgical incisions, are subject to bacterial contamination (see *NURSING 3rd series,* **3,** 92). Progression to a clinical infection depends on the balance between the numbers (and virulence) of the contaminating organisms and the competence of the host local and systemic resistance to infection. At the local level, bacteria can considerably alter the wound environment. Proliferating aerobic bacteria consume high levels of oxygen, causing a large fall in the wound's oxygen tension. They also compete for other nutrients in short supply. The increased activity of inflammatory cells combating the infection will further reduce the available oxygen.

Infection, by prolonging the inflammatory phase can alter the quality of subsequent healing. Foreign bodies increase the risk of bacterial colonization progressing into a wound infection. The anoxic wound centre is ideal for anaerobic bacteria. Macrophages will surround foreign bodies and reduce oxygen levels in the area, thus leading to proliferation of anaerobic bacteria. The presence of a blood clot or devitalized tissues also increases the risk of infection. Systemic factors reducing resistance to infection include age, poor nutrition and intercurrent illness (e.g. diabetes mellitus, anaemia). The management of infected wounds is discussed on page 178.

Drugs: at present no substance has been shown to be effective in accelerating the process of repair. However, certain drugs are known to have adverse effects. Three classes of drugs need to be used with caution: steroids, anti-inflammatory drugs and cytotoxic drugs. Cytotoxic drugs interfere with cell proliferation or produce immunosuppression, both actions which will retard wound repair. Radiotherapy has similar effects. High doses of steroids and anti-inflammatory drugs may suppress inflammation, modifying the progress of repair. When used in the normal therapeutic range, however, they are unlikely to have any significant effect on healing, particularly if their use is delayed until after the acute inflammatory phase.

The effects of wound dressings: a vast number of dressings and topical applications

● Practice point
Infection, by prolonging the inflammatory phase can alter the quality of subsequent healing.

have been used (the history of wound dressings is reviewed on pages 169–73). In the past there was limited understanding of the complexity of healing and the effects a dressing has on the wound environment. The dressings available today are more tailored to meet the individual requirements of each wound, and eventually we may reach the point when the needs of a particular patient and wound can be detailed and a suitable dressing prescribed. No single dressing will be suitable for all wounds, indeed as healing is a sequential process a wound must be continually reassessed. As conditions within a wound change different types of dressing may be needed.

Dressings, like hospitals, should do the patient no harm. Dressings which allow a wound to dry out, or adhere to the wound surface delay, rather than aid, healing. Fragments from gauze and paraffin gauze dressing can become incorporated into a healing wound. As with any foreign body this can prolong inflammation and encourage infection. Gauze does provide thermal insulation and is useful as an absorbent cover over a non-adhesive dressing, but it is not a barrier to infection. Removal of adherent dressings can damage the fragile new tissue.

A balance is necessary between keeping a wound moist and removing excess exudate, which can contain bacteria, cell debris and toxins. If these are retained on the wound surface tissue sloughing may occur. Occlusive dressings are suitable for clean, relatively uninfected wounds. Debridement or treatment of infection may be more important than maintaining a moist environment for some wounds.

Gaseous exchange is another important feature of a dressing. Generally it is assumed that a dressing should be oxygen permeable. Another important role is the prevention of bacterial contamination. An ideal dressing should cause minimum disruption of the wound environment, but avoid dehydration, prevent bacterial contamination and allow gaseous exchange.

Age: the ability to heal, as with many physiological functions, declines with age. The elderly ill often suffer from multiple pathology: poor nutrition, impaired blood supply and lowered resistance to infection, all of which contribute to slower healing.

Systemic disease: many diseases can adversely affect wound repair. Diseases affecting the integrity of the vascular system are of obvious importance. Shock in particular seriously impedes healing, and simple restoration of circulation volume may not be enough to re-perfuse the wound. Diseases which decrease resistance to infection, for example immune disorders or diabetes mellitus (diabetes also impairs healing due to its vascular effects), allow infection to become established. Conditions associated with poor nutrition, such as malignancy or liver diseases, tend to depress healing. Many diseases influence healing through more than one mechanism. The healing of chronic wounds can often be effected by treating a systemic factor, such as anaemia or chronic infection. Patients not just wounds must be treated.

Implications for nursing care

An understanding of the physiology of wound healing is essential for nurses involved in wound care. Nurses are in the best position to monitor the progress of healing and respond to the changing conditions within the wound. We see the wound on a daily basis and can relate improvements or deterioration in the wound to changes in the patient's general condition. It is important to remember that healing is a dynamic process; the needs of the wound alter as healing progresses. Healing is reliant on a good blood supply and an adequate level of nutrition. Healing tissues are very fragile and require extremely gentle handling. Devitalized tissues, foreign bodies and gross infection will seriously impede healing. Aseptic technique is essential at all stages. **N**

REFERENCES

Cohen IK. Can collagen metabolism be controlled: Theoretical considerations. *J Trauma* 1985; **25**(5): 410-12.

Hunt TK. *Wound healing and wound infection: Theory and surgical practice.* New York: Appleton-Century-Crofts, 1980: Ch 10.

Simpson D, Ross R. The neutrophilic leukocyte in wound repair: A study with anti-neutrophil serum. *J Clin Invest* 1972; **51**: 2009.

Winter G. Some factors affecting skin and wound healing. In *Bed-sore biomechanics.* (Kenedi RM *et al.*, eds) London: Macmillan, 1976: 47-54.

FURTHER READING

Henaker L. *Biological basis of wound healing.* Hagerston: Harper & Row, 1975.

Torrance C. Principles of moist wound healing. *Community View* 1973; September Supplement: 8-9.

Westaby S. *Wound care.* London: Heinemann Medical Books, 1985.

The physiology of wound healing

An examination of the processes involved in wound healing,
from reactions to injury through to scarring

Repair or replacement of damaged, obsolete and non-functional elements is a fundamental property of living things and occurs at the molecular and sub-cellular levels as well as at genetic, cellular and tissue levels. Tissue is exposed to injury not only from outside agents such as physical trauma, environmental poisons, infections and radiation, but also, somewhat surprisingly, from the products of its own metabolism.

For instance, the main system for production of energy, oxidative phosphorylation, produces as a side-effect highly reactive oxygen and hydroxyl radicals that are potentially harmful to cells. These radicals are normally destroyed by specific enzymes but are cunningly used by phagocytes for the destruction of infective agents such as bacteria or parasites. When internal protection against these radicals fails, most cells have mechanisms for repairing the damage they have caused themselves. Paradoxically, it is the period of renewed blood flow after a hypoxic/ischaemic episode when there is the greatest danger of oxygen radical damage[1,2], which may even be more severe than the original injury caused by the trauma or ischaemia.

It is worth considering this in relation to the treatment of pressure sores, where excess radical production when pressure is relieved suddenly may cause significant cell damage and contribute to irreversible injury. On a more global scale, as far as the body is concerned, it has been suggested that our lifespan may be determined by the accumulation of radical-induced injuries in vital tissues, which have not been properly repaired.

Normal 'remodelling' or 'tissue turnover' involves the removal of ageing cells, cell constituents and/or extracellular products and their replacement. Thus healing and replacement occur constantly, if

I.A. Silver, MA, FRCVS, is emeritus professor of pathology, University of Bristol, Bristol

Physiology

unobtrusively, even in the absence of trauma and provide the basic mechanism for healing on a larger scale when there is clinical injury.

Types of tissues
Tissues can be roughly classified into three types: labile, stable and permanent.

Labile tissues
Labile tissues have a naturally high cell turnover rate and are usually found either in sites where they are constantly exposed to destructive forces or are producers of something that is rapidly used in a natural biological process. The epidermis of the skin and the mucosa of the gut and vagina come into the first category and the lining of the seminiferous tubules of the testes fall into the second. Whatever the function, the effect is to provide a constantly renewed population of cells on the surface of the organ. Thus any damage to that surface is healed immediately by the normal renewal mechanism and, provided the injury does not extend significantly beyond the epithelial layer, no detectable evidence is left behind to show that an injury had occurred. This is healing by regeneration as opposed to repair and produces no scar tissue.

A slight variation on this process is seen in the liver, which is a labile organ, but one where the normal turnover of cells is relatively slow. However, after damage, the cells start to multiply extremely fast, following a latent period of about 12 hours. It is because of this behaviour that very large amounts of liver can be removed surgically in the expectation that the organ will rapidly regenerate itself.

Part of tissue remodelling is brought about by the loss of obsolescent cells through the process of apoptosis[3]. This involves loss of organelles, concentration of nuclear material, cell shrinkage and finally death. It is a physiological process and differs from death due to a pathological cause called necrosis and occurs to a greater or lesser extent in all wounds.

Stable tissues
Stable tissues, as compared with labile, have a low cell turnover and, when injured, heal by repair rather than by regeneration. The major element in repair is not the replacement of the damaged cells by similar ones, but the proliferation of the basic connective tissue cells, the fibroblasts. These live relatively quiet lives until stimulated by an injury in their neighbourhood when they divide, grow and produce fibres and a gelatinous space-occupying ground substance that fills the gaps between cells and structural elements.

The new fibres undergo maturation over months and sometimes years, to form tough, avascular scar tissue, which fills the space created by the injury but is different in texture, physical characteristics and function from the original tissue. It can therefore be likened to a dam in a piece of cloth that restores the continuity of the fabric but not the original appearance, texture and strength.

The essential difference between labile and stable tissue repair is that healing in the latter has to be actively 'switched on' rather than being part of normal cell replacement. In addition, it has to be 'switched off' when the tissue integrity has been restored. This control may not be effective: failure of the 'on' stimulus results in non-healing or slow healing while failure of the 'off' command allows formation of excessive granulation tissue or, later, hypertrophic scars or even keloids. Burn wounds are often slow to heal and subsequently engender proliferative scarring[4].

Permanent tissues

Permanent tissues are those such as the neurones of the central nervous system, which, in the adult, have virtually no power of regeneration or repair. Cells in these organs divide actively during the fetal and neonatal stage of growth, but are genetically programmed to cease dividing at a young age.

There is every reason to suppose that we will eventually learn the secret of gene manipulation to the extent we will be able to inhibit the suppressor genes that prevent nerve cells repairing themselves during the post-neonatal stage and adulthood. Such information will mean that traumatic injuries to the brain and spinal cord, which are currently permanent, may become reversible.

Steps in the process of healing

Although we all recognise a wound when we see one, are familiar with the progression from haemorrhage and clotting to epithelialisation, knitting together and final attainment of adequate strength, the apparently simple and well-ordered process is actually an extremely complex interaction of physical, chemical and cellular events. The most surprising thing is that the vast majority of wounds heal without difficulty unless there are specific complicating factors such as diabetes, malignancy, malnutrition or infection[5].

One of the simplest examples of healing is that of an uncomplicated incised skin wound where there is minimal loss of tissue and little surrounding trauma. The sequence of events is:
■ Destruction of cells, collagen fibres, ground substance and blood vessels in a narrow swathe
■ Depending on the tensions in the skin and direction of the wound, the latter may gape or the edges remain apposed
■ Haemorrhage occurs from the severed blood vessels
■ The blood flow slows and stops partly because of the blockage of larger vessels by platelet thrombi and partly because of blood clotting within the tissue and wound cavity.

Blockage of vessels and blood clotting are the first steps towards healing. Platelets are activated by contact with the structural

protein collagen, especially collagen Type IV, in the walls of the damaged blood vessels. The platelets stick to the collagen and release both clotting agents and a growth factor that stimulates fibroblast cells in their vicinity. The process of clotting not only precipitates the formation of the fibrous protein fibrin from fibrinogen (its soluble precursor in blood), but also activates a cascade of changes in a series of compounds in the complement system.

Fibrin forms a network of fibres joining the sides of the wound together, especially through the cut ends of the damaged blood vessels. This acts as a rather feeble glue in holding the edges of the wound together but, more importantly at this stage, provides a three-dimensional network that traps blood cells and forms a clot that seals the open surface of the wound against further external contamination. Later, the fibrin contracts as the fluid in the blood clot evaporates and pulls the wound edges together. The dried surface of the clot forms a scab over the wound during the next few hours, drying out and sticking tightly to the surrounding skin.

The inflammatory response

Following this biological emergency response there is a latent stage of about 12 hours before any obvious healing begins. This period is, however, one of intense activity in many cells and of radical adjustment in the metabolism of the tissue in the immediate vicinity of the wound. The major event is the development of an inflammatory response which is in itself a highly complex, multi-stage phenomenon initiated partly by the mechanical damage of wounding, but mostly by immunological and consequent chemical events. Inflammation has profound effects on tissue metabolism and increases demand for nutrients at a time when blood supply is likely to be compromised.

With regard to healing perhaps the most significant factors in the inflammatory response are:
■ The generation of various biologically active 'fragments' from complement
■ The effects of two families of inflammatory mediators, the kinins and the prostaglandins
■ The attraction and activation of phagocytic cells from the blood.

Complement fragments have many roles to play but the ones that are most important here are the chemotaxins which attract neutrophil leucocytes and

macrophages. The former are essential in combating bacterial infection and the latter in removal of tissue debris and orchestrating the healing process.

Both types of phagocyte arrive on the scene of the wound in a naïve and relatively quiescent state and require 'activating' before they realise their full biological potential. This process may be brought about in several ways, but when achieved makes the phagocytes better hunters and destroyers of foreign cells or identifiers and removers of damaged native tissue. In the case of the macrophages, activation causes them to produce growth factors which either start, accelerate or modify the healing process. It also causes them to produce and release simple chemicals (cytokines) that act as messengers between macrophages and other cells.

Macrophages are pivotal in bringing about the first stages of healing, and then controlling and directing it and finally stopping it when the repair is complete. These cells enter the wound from blood vessels as monocytes, which are formed in bone marrow. Once in the tissues and under the influence of various stimulatory factors, they divide and grow to form macrophages which then attack the debris left by tissue injury and bleeding. They erode the blood clot, become activated and start to release growth factors of various types.

Among the most important of these are angiogenic factors, which stimulate endothelium to divide and direct growth of new blood vessels; fibroblast growth factor(s), which causes fibroblasts to divide and later to form collagen fibres and ground substances (glycosaminoglycans); macrophage colony factor, which makes macrophages themselves divide and so increase their population rapidly, and possibly an epithelial stimulating factor.

These stimulatory factors, together with the platelet factor mentioned above, start the local cell populations dividing and moving into the wound space. Growth factors are usually small peptide molecules consisting of relatively few amino acids. They attach to cells by specific receptors on the cell surface and therefore affect only those cells carrying the appropriate receptor.

After attachment some may themselves become 'internalised' and switch a growth-promoting or inhibiting gene on or off, or they may cause the release of a 'second messenger' within the cell that brings about a change in cell behaviour.

Epithelial healing

While the macrophages have been increasing in numbers in the depth of a wound, having been brought there by the inflammatory response, the epithelial cells on the skin surface have been even more active. About 12 hours after an injury the cells in the basal layer(s) of the epidermis start to divide and, shortly afterwards, to migrate towards the gap in the skin caused by the wound. The precise route the migration takes depends on physical factors such as degree of hydration of tissue, the oxygen concentrations in or on the tissue, the presence or absence of bacterial toxins in the wound fluid and so forth.

Migration normally follows converging paths from every part of the wound edge and, because the cells are all guided by or are moving towards a physico-chemical 'ideal' environment, they inevitably meet, like well-organised tunnel construction crews, at the same level within the clot. The moving cells have many primitive characteristics and look rather similar to malignant epithelial tumour cells except in one very important respect. While they migrate from an original fixed position, they never lose contact with cells that have remained attached to the basement membrane that separates epithelium from connective tissue. When they have 'stretched' as far as they can without losing contact with a fixed cell they stop and form a new basement membrane. Thus the next cell can migrate over them to a point further into the wound space. The more moist the surface of the wound the nearer to that surface the migration occurs. If the surface of the clot is dried to form a scab, the cells burrow down into the clot until they find wet conditions that enable them to turn across the wound cavity within the clot.

When the migrating cells meet each other they stop moving because of a surface recognition process called contact inhibition, but they continue to divide and thus restore the thickness of the multicellular epidermis. In regions such as the mouth, where the environment is constantly moist, there are not many layers of cells in the epithelium and there is a growth factor in the saliva, healing is remarkably rapid. Partial simulation of this environment may be achieved by the application of occlusive dressings[6], but these have disadvantages as well as benefits associated with their use[7].

The stimulus to proliferation of epithelium appears to be in part caused by the suppression of inhibition of mitosis from loss of ageing products (chalones) in the dead upper layers of the epidermis and partly release and enhanced synthesis of growth factors by basal cells in the damaged area. The latter may be stimulated by interaction between activated macrophages and basal cells. The best characterised of these factors is epidermal growth factor (EGF) but there are probably many different factors involved in control of epithelial growth[8]. For instance, epidermal-derived growth factor not only stimulates epithelial but also hair growth. In addition, it inhibits

A wound in tissue and the effects and response to it may be likened to a civil or military disaster

connective tissue proliferation and primary wound contraction and is responsible, at least in part, for the cessation of granulation tissue growth in wounds that have been covered by epithelium[9].

Epithelial healing is by regeneration but the final result is not necessarily indistinguishable from the original appearance of the skin because the healing of damaged underlying connective tissue may lead to scar formation. Scars are relatively avascular and this restricts nutrition of the overlying epidermis, which therefore tends to become atrophic, thin and easily damaged by abrasion from clothing, and so on, as the scar matures.

Connective tissue repair

The healing of the dermis and most other non-epithelial tissues depends on the macrophage-induced formation of new blood vessels from the remains of damaged capillaries at the edges of the wound. As macrophages migrate into a wound cavity they encounter a hostile environment that is hypoxic and often lacking in nutrients because of failure of the damaged blood supply. This causes the macrophages to release angiogenic factors that diffuse towards the remains of the capillaries and induce division of the endothelial cells that line all blood vessels.

Because the concentrations of angiogenic factors are highest around the macrophages that are producing them, the endothelial cells nearest the macrophages divide fastest and therefore these new blood vessel-forming cells grow into the wound cavity. After a few divisions they form loops (capillary arcades) from which new sprouts form and continue to grow towards the rear of the advancing macrophages. The loops at first consist of solid cords of cells but then re-organise themselves to form tubes (new capillaries) which conduct blood flow. As soon as this happens the area becomes more oxygenated and better supplied by nutrients.

This change in the environment switches off production of angiogenic factors in any macrophages that have been left behind in the new tissue. However, those macrophages that are still advancing into the depths of the wound and are removing clot and debris, remain semi-starved of oxygen and continue to produce angiogenic factors until they have stimulated new blood vessel formation throughout the original wound space. As soon as the wound cavity is filled with functional capillaries the environment becomes oxygenated and this inhibits the production of angiogenic factors by the macrophages, so growth of new blood vessels ceases. This is an excellent example of a negative feedback mechanism.

While the formation of new connective tissue (granulation tissue) is critically dependent on the formation of new blood vessels it also involves another type of cell — the fibroblast. These are normal residents which act in a 'care and maintenance' role in normal tissue, keeping the collagen fibres in good condition and replacing or modifying the intercellular ground substance, the glycosaminoglycans. In their quiescent state they are extremely resistant to adverse conditions and survive well in excised tissue for many hours or even days. However, under the influence of macrophage and platelet-derived growth factors they become activated, enlarge and start to migrate and divide. They accompany the new blood vessels, producing a collagen network which surrounds the thin-walled capillaries and prevents them being ruptured by the blood pressure. They also secrete new fibres into the spaces between cells and build up tissue in the wake of the advancing macrophages and blood vessels.

In addition, they fill the tissue space with proteoglycans which coat the fibres, bind them together and give them greater flexibility. These somewhat glue-like substances were originally thought of as simple fillers, but it is becoming clear that they interact with and modify cell behaviour as well as confer particular properties on tissues[10]. For instance, in a long tendon the types of proteoglycans differ from one part to another depending on whether the region is subject only to a pulling force or also to compression, where the tendon runs in a groove over bone for example[11].

Fibroblasts are not confined to growth and secretion. All are capable of movement and some, the myofibroblasts, are specialised for contraction and behave somewhat like smooth muscle. In normal tissue they are inconspicuous but in open wounds where there is either tissue loss or gaping because of tension, they contract under the influence of inflammatory mediators, especially kinins, and produce the phenomenon of primary wound contraction. This is a mechanism by which the surface area of an open wound is reduced before cellular proliferation takes place. Thus there is less open wound surface to cover with new epithelium and less connective tissue required to fill the diminished wound cavity. Clearly this is a biological advantage in a wild animal, but there is a penalty to pay for it. Primary wound contraction is accompanied by a modification of the wounded area and the cosmetic effect in the long term is often unsightly.

In the more controlled conditions of a clinical environment, such contraction has no biological advantage. The application of skin grafts to open wounds greatly reduces the activity of myofibroblasts as does the factor called epidermal-derived growth factor[9]. Primary wound contraction is a good example of the functional compromises that appear in the evolution of a defence mechanism. The important thing for a wounded individual in the wild is to survive the immediate danger even if the longer-term effects may not be entirely positive.

Once a cavity has filled with new granulation tissue and the epithelium has grown across its surface, the proliferative phase of healing stops and maturation and remodelling take place. The control of this limitation and remodelling is crucial to the satisfactory outcome of the healing. Cessation of growth is partly brought about by elimination of the physical conditions that cause macrophages to become activated and to produce growth factors, and partly by the appearance of growth-inhibiting substances — inhibitory growth factors.

Although the complex interactions of such cellular and chemical elements are recognised, they are not properly understood. When they are, the knowledge will be a powerful tool in the hands of those who have to cope with difficult non-healing wounds such as leg ulcers or pressure sores. Equally, the clinical problems posed by excessive granulation tissue formation or hypertrophic scars and keloids will be more easily resolved when we have unravelled the complexities of growth control. Similarly, wound healing in fetuses is particularly rapid and takes place with minimal or no scar formation but the reason for this is obscure. Clarification of this phenomenon is likely to be achieved relatively soon and may well provide a basis for treatment of difficult, non-healing wounds in adults.

Scars

The final stage in most wound healing is the maturation of the scar. This is a prolonged stage that takes at least months and at most years. Once the wound cavity is filled with granulation tissue and growth stops, there is a gradual closure of the majority of the nutrient blood vessels and a reorganisation of the collagen into bundles that re-align partially along the direction of maximum stress. The effectiveness of this alignment is crucial in weight-bearing tendons and ligaments but less vital in skin wounds. Its failure in load-bearing structures accounts for the persistent weakness of joints after severe sprains. As well as re-alignment, the bundles of collagen are removed and resynthesised in such a way that the effect is to shorten them, thus pulling the edges of the original wound closer together. This is secondary wound contraction or cicatrisation, a slow but very powerful process, which, following wounds with extensive tissue loss, may cause distortion, disfigurement and functional disability. The control of this mechanism is not understood.

Nutrition

The role of nutrition in tissue repair is now beginning to be recognised, as are the ways in which fluid overload and oedema or underperfusión and shock in the very early stages of healing may damage new fibroblasts and delay healing.

A wound in tissue and the effects and response to it may be likened to a civil or military disaster such as an earthquake or Bosnia/Somalia-type civil war.

First there is physical damage and failure of the transport system, leading to loss of food supply just at a time when a new population of refugees and helpers (inflammatory cells) arrives on the scene. At this time of increased needs vulnerable members of the population die (in tissue these may be young, growing fibroblasts and cells cut off from blood supply). This is followed by site clearance by bulldozers (macrophages), the repair and opening of roads (blood vessels), re-establishment of supply routes and start of a rebuilding programme. Some of this is 'make do and mend' work, the equivalent of tissue 'repair' and some replacement equating with regeneration. Cooperation and communication is established between the local population and external helpers and emergency teams — the equivalent of cytokines and cell–cell communication and interaction. With the restoration of normality there is disappearance of the rescue crews and builders. Normal life is resumed but some scars still show that the disaster took place.

Conclusion

A great deal is now understood about the way in which healing is initiated and controlled, but equally there are vast areas of ignorance. It is, however, safe to say that healing requires a high level of nutrition to provide energy, carbohydrates and amino acids for synthesis of new tissue. Thus the old adage remains true — anything which compromises blood flow tends to reduce the capacity of a tissue to heal. ∎

REFERENCES
[1] Im, M.J., Hoopes, J.E. Effects of electrical stimulation on ischemia reperfusion injury in rat skin. In: Brighton, C.T., Pollack, S.R. (eds). *Electromagnetics in Medicine and Biology.* San Francisco: San Francisco Press, 1991.
[2] Schiller, H.J., Reilly, P.M., Bulkley, G.B. Antioxidant therapy for ischemia reperfusion, trauma and burn injury: an overview. In: Davies, K.J.A. (ed). *Oxidative Damage and Repair.* Oxford: Pergamon Press, 1991.
[3] Lackie, J.M., Dow, J.A.T. (eds). *Dictionary of Cell Biology.* London: Academic Press, 1989.
[4] Hunt, T.K. Burns. In: Hunt, T.K., Dunphy, J.E. (eds). *Fundamentals of Wound Management.* New York: Appleton-Century-Crofts, 1979.
[5] Pollock, A. *Surgical Infections.* London: Edward Arnold, 1987.
[6] Winter, G.A. Formation of the scab and rate of epithelialisation in the skin of the young domestic pig. *Nature* 1962; **193:** 293–295.
[7] Leek, M.D., Barlow, Y.M. Tissue reactions induced by hydrocolloid wound dressings. *J Anatomy* 1992; **180:** 545–551.
[8] Deuel, T.F. Polypeptide growth factors: roles in normal and abnormal cell growth. *Ann Rev of Cell Biol* 1987; **3:** 443–464.
[9] Eisinger, M., Sadan, S., Silver, I.A., Flick, R.B. Growth regulation of skin cells by epidermal, cell-derived factors: implications for healing. *Proceed Nat Acad Sci USA* 1988; **85:** 137–141.
[10] Clark, R.A.F., Henson, P.M. *The Molecular and Cellular Biology of Wound Repair.* New York: Plenum Press, 1988.
[11] Jones, A.J., Bee, J.A. Age- and position-related heterogeneity of equine tendon extracellular matrix composition. *Res Vet Sci* 1990; **48:** 357–364.

Leg ulcers: a chronology of related events

1975 BC

Majno described the washing of wounds in Mesopotamia and the eastern Mediterranean with water or milk and dressings of honey, conifer resin, myrrh and frankincense. Owing to the amount of references to it, honey was possibly the most important. Bandages were wool or linen.

1500 BC

The 'Ebers Papyrus' refers to 'serpentine windings'; this is possibly the first reference to varicose veins. The ancient Egyptian physicians, whenever possible, let wounds heal by themselves even though both medical and magical remedies were available. Wounds were sometimes covered with papyrus linen.

479–300 BC

Heang Ti Nei Ching Su Wen wrote about the treatment of ulcers in the 'Yellow Emperor's Classic of Internal Medicine' though it is not certain that he made a connection between abnormalities of the veins and ulceration. The ancient Chinese used bread mould to treat small wounds, occlusive bandages and sometimes elephant skin.

Circa 400 BC

A stone tablet, found at the Acropolis in Athens, shows what is possibly the oldest illustration of a varicose vein.

460–377 BC

Hippocrates makes many references to the venous system and ulceration including what is perhaps the first description of compression which was used to drive out 'evil humours'. He stressed the importance of careful assessment and cleanliness, recommending wound irrigation, preferably with boiled river water. He believed rest better than bandages or splints and preferred a dry wound rather than the use of ointments.

335 BC

Praxagoras of Cox was one of the first to distinguish arteries from veins. It was thought that the arteries contained air and the veins blood.

270 BC

Herophilos and Erasistratos, in Egypt, were the first to ligate blood vessels thus paving the way for modern surgery.

200 BC

The 'Sushruta Samhita', an Indian textbook of surgery, described both the debridement of ulcers with maggots and the use of inelastic cloth bandages. Leaves were used as dressings and skin grafting was undertaken.

14–37 AD

Aurelius Cornelius Celsus, the Roman physician, described the treatment of ulcers with plasters and linen bandages, the ligation of veins and the treatment of varicose veins through avulsion and cautery. He also described the four principal signs of inflammation and used antiseptics on wounds.

130–200 AD
Claudius Galen described the use of silk ligatures and the treatment of varicose veins through venesection and avulsion.

900 AD
Avicenna continued to promote the view of Hippocrates that ulcers should not be allowed to heal in case the 'evil humours' be prevented from escaping.

13th century
Saint Peregrinus, an impoverished monk, lived in northern Italy during the 13th century. Legend says that he avoided sitting or lying down which led to varicose veins and ulceration and an amputation was planned. On the night before his operation he prayed intensively, an angel appeared and, miraculously, his ulcer was healed by the following morning. He was canonised in the Servitenkirche in Vienna where there is a picture of him and where leg ulcer sufferers pray for healing.

1300–1370
Guy de Chauliac wrote extensively on wounds, discussing foreign bodies, bandages, suturing and compression. He proposed five principles regarding the treatment of wounds:

1. removal of foreign bodies
2. reapproximation of separated parts
3. maintaining this position
4. conservation of tissue
5. treatment of complications.

1306
Maitre Henri de Mondeville again describes the use of bandages to drive out evil humours. In so doing he realised that the compression promoted healing of the ulcer.

1346
At the Battle of Crécy all soldiers carried a box of spider's web to cover wounds when injured. It was recognised that the spider's web acted as a haemostat.

1452
Leonardo da Vinci produced highly detailed anatomical drawings of the venous system.

1493–1541
Paracelsus compared the unoccluded wound to a broken egg or apple in which the content rots.

1510–1590
Ambrose Paré described local compression bandaging extending from the foot to the knee and the ligation of varicose veins. He insisted on gentleness in handling tissues and deplored the practice of pouring boiling oil into battle wounds to cauterise them and the concept of 'laudable pus' which had been popular for hundreds of years and involved encouraging a wound to suppurate.

1547–1580
Fallopius made the first reference to venous valves. It is not clear whether the discovery was made by Amatus Lusitanus or Canano.

1514–1564
Versalius made the first complete description of the venous system.

1555
Sanctus of Barletta thought that varicose veins were the result of childbearing and too much standing before kings!

1585
Saloman Alberti published what is thought to be the first drawing of a venous valve.

1593–1603
Hieronymus Fabricius of Aquapendente gave the first full description of the venous valves.

1620
Fallopius made a connection between ulcers and varicose veins.

1628
William Harvey provided a revolutionary description of the circulatory system including the observation that valves are present to ensure the flow of blood in one direction only.

1669
Richard Lower made the first reference to 'venous tone' and the calf muscle pump.

1676
Richard Wiseman invented a lace-up stocking which is thought to be the precursor to the modern elastic stocking.

1688
Etmuller believed that menstrual blood collected in the leg during pregnancy causing varicose veins and ulceration.

1728–1793
John Hunter described healing by primary and secondary intention. He also noted that leg ulcers occurred most commonly in the poor and that they would heal readily if the patient was lying down.

1733
The Reverend Stephen Hale measured arterial and venous pressure in animals.

Mid-1700s
From this time onwards classification of ulcers began to appear in surgical texts.

1753
James Lind described scurvy and dealt at length with ulceration. A close link between scurvy and ulceration was suggested.

1758
Sharp noted the association between the effect of gravity and the development of gravitational oedema leading to ulceration.

1777

Benjamin Ben advised that healing of an ulcer would be safer if a wound on the other leg was created. He believed varicose veins were caused by ulcers.

1797

Home identified the relationship between patient height and weight and increased venous pressure leading to ulceration.

1795

As scurvy was effectively treated it was noted that leg ulceration in the Navy diminished.

1799

Charles Brown, a surgeon in London, made the following observation with regard to leg ulcers: 'It is a very melancholy fact that among the lower classes in the community, nearly in the proportion of one out of five, labour, and have many years, under this severe affliction'.

1799

Baynton developed the original paste bandage.

Circa 1800

Devon and Exeter Hospital—people with leg ulcers represented 16–23% of inpatients; only 3% were treated as outpatients. The average ulcer history was between 3 and 6 months but 30% had ulcers for longer than 10 years. The mean length of stay in 1816 was 14.8 weeks.

During the 1800s many patients were turned away from hospitals, many of which had a policy against the readmission of those patients with recurrent conditions. Leeches to treat oedema and haematoma were still popular, as they had been for many years. During the 19th century 40 million leeches were imported into France alone for wound care.

1880

The Bristol Royal Infirmary—19% of surgical inpatient admissions and 42% of outpatients had leg ulcers.

1825

Classification systems of this time included simple ulcers, fungous ulcers, gangrenous ulcers, and scorbutic ulcers.

1835

Spender was one of the first people to believe that ulcers were caused by varicose veins.

1854

Unna developed the 'Unna Boot' a form of plaster dressing for the treatment of ulcers.

Mid-1800s

Up until this time it was thought that if 'humours' were denied an exit, they would ascend and cause 'pulmonic inflammation' which might be fatal. From this attitude came the phrase 'ulcers improper to be healed'. The emphasis was on the alleviation of suffering.

1829

Stafford filled deep ulcers with wax.

1834
Pigeaux wrote that the drying of an ulcer was the cause of a cook having several abortions.

1855
Verneuil recognises the relationship between valve incompetence in the deep vein system and the development of superficial vein incompetence.

1818–1865
Philip Ignaz Semmelweis recognised that streptococcal infection in puerperal fever was higher when physicians did not wash their hands. This idea was met with derision at the time.

1809–1894
Oliver Wendell Holmes in the United States had similar ideas to those proposed by Semmelweis but found a much more receptive audience.

1821–1902
Karl Thiersch revived the ancient art found in Indian culture of skin grafting.

1859
Rudolph Virchow noted the association between deep vein thrombosis and the development of a pulmonary embolism. He developed an understanding of microscopic and cellular pathology during wound healing.

1863
Hilton observes that the medial malleolus of the foot is a common site for ulceration and that rest and elevation promote healing.

1866
John Gay, through detailed observations at autopsy, consolidated the view that varicose veins and ulcers are closely linked but also that ulcers occur in the absence of varicose veins. He noted that patients who had both were more difficult to treat.

1868
Spender identified that ulceration can occur in patients who do not have varicose veins, as a result of thrombotic damage to the deep vein system. As a result both Spender and Gay began to use the term venous rather than varicose ulceration.

1827–1912
Joseph Lister accepted Pasteur's theory of infection. His observation of effluent from a chemical factory in Glasgow led him to discover that it contained phenol. Together with the discovery that gypsies had used a phenol-containing tar on small wounds for centuries, this led him to develop his antiseptic policies which included spraying carbolic acid to kill microorganisms in the operating theatre thus paving the way for modern surgery.

1911
Hooker identified a relationship between exercise and venous pressure in the lower leg.

1928
Franklin produced a major historical survey of valves and stimulated much discussion.

1930
Dickson Wright introduced the concept of the gravitational ulcer and used adhesive bandage and local dressings to treat ulceration.

1936
Beecher et al were the first to measure the pressure in the dorsal veins of the foot using a saline manometer.

1960
Satomura and Kameko introduce the Doppler shift velocity manometer.

Sources

Browse N I, Burnand K G, Thomas M L 1988 Diseases of the veins: pathology, diagnosis and treatment. Edward Arnold, London

Dodd H, Cocket F B (eds) 1976 The pathology and surgery of the veins of the lower limb, 2nd edn. Churchill Livingstone, Edinburgh

Forrest R D 1982 Early history of wound treatment. Journal of the Royal Society of Medicine 75(March): 198–205

Kelman Cohen I, Diegelmann R F, Lindblad W J 1992 Wound healing—biochemical and clinical aspects. W B Saunders, Philadelphia

Lindholm C 1993 Leg ulcer patients clinical studies, from prevalence to prevention in a nurse's perspective. Department of Dermatology and Surgery, Malmö General Hospital, University of Lund, Malmö, Sweden

Loudon S L 1981 History of medicine, leg ulcers in the eighteenth and early nineteenth centuries. Journal of the Royal College of General Practitioners (May): 263–272

Negus D 1991 Leg ulcers: a practical approach to management. Butterworth Heinemann, Oxford

A prerequisite underlining the treatment programme
Risk factors associated with venous disease

CHRISTINE J. MOFFATT
RGN, NDN
*Director, Centre for Research and
Implementation in Clinical Practice,
Riverside Community Health Care NHS
Trust*

PETER J. FRANKS
PhD
*Director of Research, Centre for Research
and Implementation in Clinical Practice,
Riverside Community Health Care NHS
Trust*

Although venous disease affects about a quarter of the UK population, little is known about its epidemiology. An understanding of the associated risk factors, however, can help mitigate the progression, severity and outcome of the disease process.

An understanding of the risk factors associated with venous disease is required for an effective primary prevention programme to take place. This article offers a review of the risk factors associated with venous disease cited in the literature.

Historical view

During the long history of venous disease, many factors have been considered to cause or influence the disease process. The Egyptians were probably the first to provide written evidence of varicose veins (Dodd and Cockett, 1974), while Hippocrates was the first to describe the relationship between leg ulceration and enlarged veins (Scott, 1992). During the Dark Ages, strange theories emerged concerning venous disease: the release of body humours was thought to be essential to wellbeing, while binding or healing a leg ulcer was thought to lead to madness, as it prevented the escape of humours, and horrendous practices were used to ensure the ulcer remained open. Haly Abbas (994) recognised that varicose veins occurred in people who stood for long periods of time and believed the varicosities were full of black bile.

Ambrose Pare (1510-1590) attributed varicose veins to men of melancholy temper and to pregnancy in women. In 1555, Sanctus of Barletta thought they were the result of childbearing and too much standing before kings. The lack of understanding was such that it was thought the disease process was related to the female reproductive system, and Pigeaux (1834) wrote that drying an ulcer was responsible for a cook having several abortions. Etmuller (1688) considered that menstrual blood collected in the legs during pregnancy, causing varicose veins and ulceration. These theories held sway throughout the eighteenth and part of the nineteenth centuries, and were widely held throughout Europe.

By the nineteenth century, the importance of varicose veins was recognised as a cause of leg ulceration, while Gay and Spender (1868) both described venous thrombosis as a major cause of ulceration. Gay was also the first to use the term venous ulceration, but little was known of the relationship between the outcome of leg ulceration and venous thrombosis.

Key points
Moffatt, C. and Franks, P. (1994) A prerequisite underlining the treatment programme: risk factors associated with venous disease. *Professional Nurse*, **9**, 9, 637-42.

1. Venous disease affects about one quarter of the adult population.

2. Risk factors for venous disease include pregnancy, chronic standing and height.

3. Risk factors for venous ulceration have not been determined, though prolonged ulceration is associated with more severe venous disease, restricted mobility and limb movement.

4. Before a system of prevention can be initiated, these risk factors must be identified.

Venous disease today

Venous disease is known to affect approximately a quarter of the adult population in the UK (Franks *et al*, 1992). Despite this, and unlike other forms of vascular disease, it has received relatively little attention from epidemiologists interested in the identification of risk factors for disease. As well as predisposing a patient to a higher risk of developing a disease, a risk factor may also be implicated in the progression, severity and outcome of the disease process.

Although venous disease is rarely life-threatening, it is a considerable burden on health resources, and the identification of risk factors is essential. It is impossible to initiate primary prevention without first identifying which factors are important in the development of the disease.

Varicose veins

One of the major problems with investigations of varicose veins is the difficulty in assessing when a vein becomes varicosed, as there are few definitions in the literature. The most commonly used definition was given by Arnoldi (1957) as the presence of "any dilated, elongated or tortuous vessel".

References
Abramson, J.H. *et al* (1981) The epidemiology of varicose veins: a survey in western Jerusalem. *J. Epid. Comm. Health.* **35**, 213-17.

Alexander, C.J. (1972) Chair-sitting and varicose veins. *Lancet*, **i**, 822-23.

Allen, A.J. *et al* (1988) Impaired postural vasoconstriction: a contributory cause of oedema in patients with chronic venous insufficiency. *Phlebology*, **3**, 163-68.

Andreasen, C. and Krieger-Lassen, H. (1965) Fatal pulmonary embolism in a surgical department during a period of 15 years. *Acta. Chir. Scand. (Suppl)*, **343**, 42.

Arnoldi, C.C. (1957) Aetiology of primary varicose veins. *Dan. Med. Bull.*, **4**, 102-07.

Beaglehole, R. *et al* (1975) Varicose veins in the South Pacific. *Int. J. Epidem.*, **4**, 295.

Bersqvist, D. (1983) Postoperative Thrombo-embolism. Springer, Berlin.

Brand, F.N. *et al* (1988) The epidemiology of varicose veins: the Framingham study. *Am. J. Prev. Med.*, **4**, 96-101.

British Medical Journal (1979) Thrombo-embolism in pregnancy. *BMJ*, **1**, 1661.

Browse, N.L. (1962) Effect of bedrest on resting calf bloodflow of healthy adult males. *BMJ*, **1**, 1721.

Browse, N.L. *et al* (1988) Diseases of the veins: pathology, diagnosis and treatment. Edward Arnold, London.

Burkitt, D.P. (1972) Varicose veins, deep vein thrombosis, and haemorrhoids: epidemiology and aetiology. *BMJ*, **ii**, 556-61.

Callam, M.J. *et al* (1988) Chronic leg ulceration: socio-economic aspects. *Scot. Med. J.*, **33**, 358-60.

Colditz, G.A. *et al* (1986) Rates of venous thrombosis after general surgery: combined results of randomised clinical trials. *Lancet*, **2**, 143.

Coles, R.W. (1974) Varicose veins in tropical Africa. *Lancet*, **ii**, 474-75.

Cornwall, J.V. *et al* (1986) Leg ulcers: epidemiology and aetiology. *B. J. Surg.*, **73**, 693-96.

Dalrymple, J. and Crofts, T. (1975) Varicose veins in developing countries. *Lancet*, **i**, 808-09.

Dodd, H. and Cockett, F.B. (Eds) (1976) The Pathology and Surgery of the Veins of the Lower Limb (2nd Edn). Churchill Livingstone, Edinburgh.

Drury, M. (1965) Varicose veins in pregnancy. *BMJ*, **ii**, 304.

Ducimetiere, P. *et al* (1981) Varicose veins: a risk factor for atherosclerotic disease in middle-aged men? *Int. J. Epidem.*, **10**, 329-35.

Eberth-Willerhausen, W. and Marshall, M. (1984) Prevalenz riskofaktoren und kompkationen peripher venenorkrank-ûngen in der Munchner bevolkerung. *Hautarzt*, **35**, 68-77.

Fischer, H. (Hrsg) (1981) Venenleiden-Eine Reprasentative Untersuchung in der Bundesrepublik Deutschland. Urban and Schwarzenberg, Munchen.
continued

Age and sex A number of studies have demonstrated an increase in prevalence with age and significant differences between the sexes. In a study in Jerusalem, prevalence of varicose veins in women was nearly three times that of men, at 29 per cent and 10 per cent respectively, with a strong age gradient (Abramson *et al*, 1981). The only recorded study of incidence (proportion of patients who developed varicose veins over a period of time) was from the Framingham study (Brand *et al*, 1988), which found that the incidence did not change with age, suggesting the risk was similar for all age groups and not related to the ageing process.

Race It has long been considered that race may be important, with non-whites generally suffering to a lesser extent. During the 1970s a series of reports were published from developing countries, claiming that varicose veins were either rare or non-existent in them (Coles, 1974; Dalrymple and Crofts, 1975; Worsfold, 1974; Williams, 1974). These findings, however, must be treated with caution, since major differences in lifestyle may confound the results. Evidence that environmental factors play a significant role in the development of venous disease is seen in the Maori race; a significant difference in prevalence was detected in Maoris living on the New Zealand mainland (33 per cent of men and 44 per cent of women), compared with 3 per cent of men and 1 per cent of women living on the Tokelau Island (Beaglehole *et al*, 1975). These two groups were genetically identical, indicating that extrinsic factors play an important role in the development of the disease.

Social factors and venous disease It is often reported anecdotally that venous disease is a disease of the lower social classes. There have been inconsistent findings in the literature with regard to social class; some studies have indicated a gradient of higher risk in lower social classes, whereas others have failed to show a difference between classes (Abramson *et al*, 1981; Fischer, 1981; Ducimetierre *et al*, 1981).

Body shape Increased body weight has been consistently associated with the development of varicose veins (eg, Abramson *et al*, 1981; Fischer, 1981), but these studies have failed to adjust for height – in the Jerusalem study, patients with venous disease were on average 1.4cm taller than patients without disease (Abramson *et al*, 1981). When weight was adjusted for height, the association with weight disappeared, implying that height is the more important of the two factors. Obesity is, however, often accompanied by other factors, such as immobility, which may alter the patient profile considerably.

Pregnancy, menarche and menopause It has long been recognised that varicose veins are associated with pregnancy (Arnoldi, 1957). The Tubingen study demonstrated a doubling of risk in women who had two or more pregnancies; other studies report similar associations (eg, Fischer, 1981; Maffeii *et al*, 1986), although others have failed to demonstrate this association (Abramson *et al*, 1981; Drury, 1965; Weddell, 1969).

Increasing age at menarche has also been associated with an increased risk of varicose veins (Arnoldi, 1957) together with age at menopause (Arnoldi, 1957; Brand *et al*, 1988), although this observation has not been shown elsewhere (Abramson *et al*, 1981).

Related diseases and lifestyle

The coincidence of venous disease with other diseases has been examined. There appears to be an association between varicose veins and peripheral arterial disease (Ducimetiere *et al*, 1981), but no consistent finding for either hypertension (Abramson *et al*, 1981; Brand *et al*, 1988; Ducimetiere *et al*, 1981) or coronary artery disease (Abramson *et al*, 1981; Brand *et al*, 1988). Other disorders which may be linked are chronic constipation, haemorrhoids and inguinal hernia (Abramson *et al*, 1981). All these diseases are related to the development of high abdominal pressures, which may be a consequence of a low fibre diet (Burkitt, 1972). This may also explain why corset wearing has been identified as a positive risk factor (Abramson *et al*, 1981). Smoking may also be important, although the evidence for this is not strong (Abramson *et al*, 1981; Brand *et al*, 1988).

Reduced physical activity has long been associated with venous disease. Functional changes occur in immobile patients due to reduced calf muscle pump function and a rise in venous pressure which is exacerbated on dependency (Brand *et al*, 1988; Eberth-Willerhausen and Marshall, 1984). Some studies suggest a sedentary lifestyle increases the risk of developing venous disease (eg, Brand *et al*, 1988; Eberth-Willerhausen and Marchall, 1984). Physical activity and work posture may be important, but these results are inconclusive (Abramson *et al*, 1981; Alexander, 1972).

Deep vein thrombosis

Deep vein thrombosis (DVT) is important in the development of varicose veins and venous ulceration, but the true prevalence is difficult to estimate due to difficulties in diagnosis. The risk of DVT appears to increase with age, with an even distribution between the sexes (Harvey-Kemble, 1971). Some studies suggest that geographical and climatic factors influence the rate of DVT (Lawrence *et al*, 1977) but, as with varicose veins, it is difficult to distinguish these factors from race-related and other environmental factors. Other studies using more objective measurement of DVT have failed to confirm these findings (Andreasen and Krieger-Lassen, 1965).

It is well recognised that prolonged periods of bed rest (Browse, 1962) are associated with increased rates of DVT, while the type and length of operation also affect the outcome. Bersqvist (1983) summarised the published data and found a DVT incidence of 29 per cent in 1,081 patients undergoing general surgery. This figure has been confirmed in further prospective studies of patients undergoing surgery without prophylaxis (Colditz *et al*, 1986; Ruckley, 1976). Obesity appears to increase the risk of DVT (Havig, 1977) and is an additional risk factor in patients taking the contraceptive pill (Vessey and Doll, 1968). The true incidence of thrombosis in pregnancy is unknown, but studies suggest the risk of DVT may increase as much as fivefold (BMJ, 1979). General medical illnesses (Ochsner *et al*, 1951), heart failure (Short, 1952), myocardial infarction (Handley, 1972) and carcinoma have all been reported to increase the risk of DVT (Roberts, 1974). As with venous ulceration, patients with a history of DVT or pulmonary embolism are at greater risk of developing a further DVT (Kakkar *et al*, 1970).

Venous ulceration

Despite the large number of investigations into risk factors for varicose veins, little is known of the factors associated with venous ulceration, and it is likely that many risk factors for varicose veins will be important in patients with venous ulceration. As has been shown, the prevalence of varicose veins is high, but relatively few sufferers go on to develop leg ulceration (Cornwall *et al*, 1986). The risk of ulcer development appears to be directly related to the pattern of venous insufficiency, with patients with superficial and perforator incompetence having a higher risk of ulcer development than those with superficial disease alone (Zbinden *et al*, 1980). Deep vein thrombosis is a recognised risk factor, with more widespread thromboses leading to increased risk of ulceration than with calf vein thrombosis alone (Partsch *et al*, 1980; Stacey *et al*, 1991). Within the Riverside study, history of DVT was not found to influence ulcer healing, but since this may occur undetected patients may not recall an episode of thrombosis.

Oedema and inadequate treatment of chronic venous insufficiency have also been suggested as possible risk factors for ulcer development (Allen *et al*, 1988), while local trauma may play a contributory role in the

References (continued)
Franks, P.J. *et al* (1992) Prevalence of venous disease: a community study in west London. *Eur. J. Surg.* **158**, 143-47.
Handley, A. (1972) Low-dose deparin after myocardial infarction. *Lancet*, **2**, 623.
Havig, O. (1977) Deep vein thrombosis and pulmonary embolism: an autopsy study with multiple regression analysis of possible risk factors. *Acta. Chir. Scand. (Suppl)*, **478**, 1-120.
Harvey-Kemble, J.V. (1971) Incidence of deep vein thrombosis. *B. J. Hosp. Med.*, **6**, 721.
Kakkar, V.V. *et al* (1970) Deep vein thrombosis of the leg: is there a high risk group? *Am. J. Surg*, **1**, 20, 527.
Lawrence, J.C. *et al* (1977) Seasonal variation in the incidence of deep vein thrombosis. *B. J. Surg.*, **64**, 777.
Maffeii, F.H.A. *et al* (1986) Varicose veins and chronic venous insufficiency in Brazil. *Int. J. Epidem.*, **15**, 210-17.

continued below

Factors influencing

References (continued)
Moffatt, C.J. *et al* (1992) Community clinics for leg ulcers and impact on healing. *BMJ*, **305**, 1289-92.
Ochsner, A. *et al* (1951) Venous thrombosis: analysis of 580 cases. *Surgery*, **29**, 24.
Prasad, A., Ali-Khan, A., Mortimer, P. (1990) Leg ulcers and oedema: a study exploring the prevalence, aetiology and possible significance of oedema in venous ulcers. *Phlebology*, **5**, 181-87.
Roberts, V.C. and Cotton, L.T. (1974) Prevention of postoperative deep vein thrombosis in patients with malignant disease. *BMJ*, **1**, 358.
Ruckley, C.V. (1976) A multi-unit controlled trial of heparin and dextran in the prevention of venous thromboembolic disease. In: Kakkar, V.V. and Thomas, D.P. (Eds) Heparin, Chemistry and Clinical Usage. Academic Press, London.
Scott, H.J. (1992) History of venous disease and early management. *Phlebology Suppl.* **1**, 2-5.
Short, D.S. (1952) A survey of pulmonary embolism in a general hospital. *BMJ*, **1**, 790.
Skene, A.I. *et al* (1993) Venous leg ulcers: a prognostic index to predict time to healing. *BMJ*, **305**, 1119-21.
Stacey, M.C. *et al* (1991) Influence of phlebographic abnormalities on the natural history of venous ulceration. *B. J. Surg.*, **78**, 868-77.
Vessey, M.P. and Doll, R. (1968) Investigation of relation between use of oral contraceptive and thromboembolic disease. *BMJ*, **2**, 199.
Weddell, J.M. (1969) Varicose veins pilot survey 1966. *B. J. Prev. Med.*, **23**, 179-86.
Widmer, L.K. and Kamber, V. (1978) Who actually has peripheral venous disease? In: Widmer, L.K. (Ed) Peripheral Venous Disorders. Hans Huber, Bern.
Williams, E.H. (1974) Varicose veins in tropical Africa. *Lancet*, **i**, 1291.
Worsfold, J.T. (1974) Varicose veins in tropical Africa. *Lancet*, **ii**, 1322-23.
Zbinden, O. *et al* (1990) Long-term evolution of varicose veins: 11 year follow-up. Fifth European American Symposium on Venous Diseases, Vienna.

development of ulceration (Browse *et al*, 1988). Closely allied to treatment failure is the presence of oedema, which was identified in 55 per cent of ulcer patients (Prasad *et al*, 1990) – 77 per cent of community patients had oedema, compared to only 22 per cent of hospital patients. This difference can probably be explained by hospital patients receiving more effective compression therapy than those treated in the community, while diuretic use appeared to be associated with improved healing in this chronic group (Prasad *et al*, 1990).

Lifestyle factors have not been investigated in the development of venous ulceration, but the distribution of social classes in ulcer patients in Riverside was similar to that of the general population. A similar result was found in the Lothian and Forth Valley study, though they also found that patients in social classes IV and V had longer duration ulceration compared with those in social classes I, II and III (Callam *et al*, 1988). This may be explained by patients in social classes IV and V being slower to seek treatment, or environmental factors affecting the progress of their treatment. This is an area which requires considerable study to understand the poorer outcomes in these patients.

The only other information on risk factors for venous ulceration is restricted to factors which influence healing. Two studies have been performed in the UK to identify these factors. Information from a clinical trial was analysed which identified old age, large ulcer area, and long duration of ulceration as predictors of poor healing in 200 patients (Skene *et al*, 1993). There appeared to be little evidence that bacterial contamination influenced ulcer healing, although changes in bacterial flora were noted from month to month. This supports the clinical view that aggressive eradication of pathogens with topical agents such as antiseptics does not aid healing. In the Riverside Venous Ulcer Project, six factors led to significantly poorer healing. As expected, the chronic (>6 months) larger (>10cm^2) ulcers healed more slowly. General mobility (chair/bed-bound), restriction of limb mobility, treatment at home and male gender were all factors which significantly prolonged healing in patients treated with the four layer bandage system (Moffatt *et al*, 1992). It was surprising to find a reduction in healing in patients treated at home, as they received identical assessment and treatment. This group of patients was particularly immobile and had a multiplicity of problems. When multivariate analysis was performed, treatment at home and male gender were no longer significant factors. Even so, patients treated at home remain the greatest challenge within any health authority.

It is difficult to assess the role ulceration plays in mobility. Over 45 per cent of patients in the Riverside study had restricted mobility; in the Lothian and Forth Valley leg ulcer study, 11 per cent had reduced mobility as a direct consequence of leg ulceration, although 42 per cent had interference with work or leisure activities to a moderate or severe degree (Callam *et al*, 1988) – reduced limb mobility is often a consequence of ulceration. Pain around the ulcer site may cause the patient to keep the limb as still as possible, resulting in complete ankle arthrodesis and loss of calf muscle function, which can be difficult to rectify. Foot deformities are common in leg ulcer patients and further reduce mobility.

Mobility could be altered by encouraging people to walk. Patients in the Riverside study who walked with a walking aid had similar healing to those who were able to walk unaided (Moffatt *et al*, 1992). Clearly, the most important predictors of healing were ulcer size and duration. Only through immediate and effective treatment can these ulcers be hoped to heal quickly.

There is an obvious need to identify risk factors for venous ulceration in the community so a programme of prevention and health education can be initiated. Only then can the burden of treating these patients be reduced, albeit with effective treatments. We are, however, a long way from understanding the impact of venous disease on the patients and all its implications.

Nutrition and wound healing

A guide to the steps in the wound-healing response and to the role of nutrients in this process

G. Pinchcofsky-Devin, RD, FACN
vice-president, enteral services
Stat Homecare, Elmhurst, Illinois, USA

Nutrition; Physiology

The wound-healing response is a complex process following injury. Optimally, the process ends with complete restitution of tissue structure and function. However, delays in wound healing result in weak, poor-quality scars or, indeed, in complete failure to heal. An excessive healing response may cause keloids, contractions and other cosmetic functional alterations.

The classically described steps in the healing response involve and are dependent on nutritional substrates:
■ Inflammation, with recruitment of polymorphonuclear leukocytes, macrophages and lymphocytes
■ Fibroblast proliferation and collagen production
■ Collagen remodelling and re-epithelialisation when appropriate.

The strength and integrity of tissue repair depend on collagen cross-linking and deposition. Alterations in nutritional status or intake preceding or during injury may clearly alter the normal wound-healing response. The rebuilding of the body's immunologic defence system and the replacement of tissue destroyed by disease, surgery and problem wounds call for nutritional support. The best surgical and nursing care available will not heal the wound if there is inadequate nutritional substrate to make new tissue.

Role of specific macronutrients
Wound healing is aided by adequate oxygenation, blood flow and nutrient supply. All of the steps involved in wound healing require numerous synthesis and other energy-consuming reactions. It is possible that impaired healing may be a consequence of specific nutrient deficiencies. Proteins are the basic cellular component of all living organisms. Protein deficiency contributes to poor wound healing by prolonging the inflammatory response and impairing fibroplasia. When protein deprivation is prolonged, oedema secondary to hypoalbuminaemia occurs.

Methionine, a precursor to cysteine, is associated with collagen synthesis. The exact role of cysteine is not completely defined, but it may be needed as a co-factor in enzyme systems responsible for collagen synthesis — or it may contribute to the proper alignment and attachment to peptide chains in the formation of tropocollagen through disulphide bonds[1]. A possible role for arginine as a promoting agent for wound healing has also been suggested[2].

Carbohydrates and fats
Carbohydrates and fats provide a source of cellular energy. The specific roles of carbohydrates and fats in wound healing are less well defined. When glucose is not available for cellular function, the body catabolises protein and, to a lesser degree, fat, to produce glucose to meet energy requirements. Fats or lipids are the primary source of stored energy in the body. Fat is an essential component of intracellular organelles, such as the mitochondria, and is an integral component of cell membranes.

Protein and wound healing
Protein is an essential nutrient for healing. Forty per cent of the albumin pool is intravascular and 60% is extravascular.

Increased capillary permeability secondary to injury results in localisation of some acute phase proteins around the injury site[3,4]. This increase in plasma protein availability probably facilitates wound healing[5]. Albumin is the major plasma protein.

Albumin catabolism increases as a result of injury to the skin as does other plasma protein catabolism[6].

Protein requirements
Normal daily protein requirements in unstressed individuals can be met with as little as 0.5–0.8g/kg of protein. This is usually insufficient for the acutely ill patient, for whom intake should increase to 1.5 to 2.5g/kg to avoid negative nitrogen balance, which would place the patient in a state of anabolism[7]. The resultant increase in blood urea nitrogen from a high-protein diet is not significant provided the patient has no pre-existing renal condition. Providing adequate fluid for the patient is essential when providing a high-protein diet.

There is a clear correlation between a patient's dietary intake of protein and the development of pressure sores[8]. When calories supplied are less than required, muscle and organ proteins break down to supply amino acids for gluconeogenesis. A high-calorie diet with 50–60% of calories as carbohydrates will help spare protein stores of vital tissue.

Vitamins and wound healing
Vitamins play an essential role in wound healing[9-12]. Where specific vitamin deficiencies are diagnosed, individual supplements of up to 10 to 20 times the recommended daily allowance may be needed. Higher vitamin levels may be indicated because of increased excretion or decreased absorption as well as drug nutrient interaction.

Ascorbic acid plays an important role in wound healing. Vitamin C functions as a co-factor in the hydroxylation of proline to hydroxyproline, an essential step in the synthesis of collagen. Hydroxyproline is needed to stabilise collagen. The role of ascorbic acid in epithelialisation is less well defined; however, ascorbate is one of the stimulants for fibroblast mitosis and subsequent collagen synthesis[13].

Ascorbic acid has also been shown to enhance the cellular and humoral responses to stress. In *vitro* studies suggest there is an increased utilisation of vitamin C during phagocytosis and ascorbic acid may increase the activation of leukocytes and macrophages to the

NUTRITION AND WOUND HEALING

Poor nutrition can contribute to the development of chronic wounds, such as pressure sores or surgical wounds, in several ways.

A diet deficient in many nutrients, particularly those involved in protein synthesis, jeopardises tissue integrity and contributes to skin breakdown. In addition, inadequate caloric intake causes weight loss and a reduction in subcutaneous tissue, allowing bony prominences to compress and restrict circulation to the skin. The resultant reduction of the nutrients supplied to that area also promotes tissue catabolism.

PROTEIN

Protein is an essential nutrient for healing. The normal serum albumin concentration is 35–50g/l in the serum of the adult. This level is the equilibrium point between the production, distribution and degradation of albumin. The skin represents 30–40% of the extravascular albumin stores.

Albumin catabolism increases as a result of injury to the skin as does other plasma protein catabolism. Albumin is made available to regeneration tissue in proportion to the extent of injury and inflammation. Changes in temperature and pH at the injury site denature the native albumin. Macrophages are then able to utilise the constituents of the albumin.

Serum albumin in the wounded patient falls. If severe such a decrease in serum albumin synthesis or increase in albumin utilisation at a major wound site may impair wound healing in the patient.

As metabolic stress increases with injury, infection or open wounds the body uses protein as a greater portion of the total energy expenditure. Intake should increase to 1.5 to 2.5g/kg daily to avoid negative nitrogen balance and place the patient in a state of anabolism. With pressure sores healing can be achieved only with a high-protein diet. Providing adequate fluid for the patient is essential.

There is a clear correlation between the patient's dietary intake of protein and the development of pressure sores.

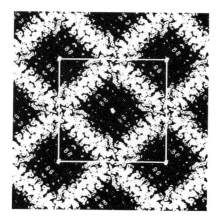

Albumin: computerised model

NUTRITIONAL ASSESSMENT

Early identification and monitoring of several nutrition risk factors may eliminate or reduce the complications associated with delayed wound healing. These nutrition risk factors include:
■ Decreased serum albumin level below 35g/l
■ Low serum transferrin level below 1800mg/l
■ Low total lymphocyte count below 1800 cells/mm³
■ Anemia; haemoglobin below 12mg/dl
■ Decreased oral intake.

The nutrition risk factors can be identified by performing a nutritional assessment.

The three major components of nutritional assessment are the visceral protein stores, the somatic protein stores and the vitamin and mineral status of the patient.

TRACE ELEMENTS

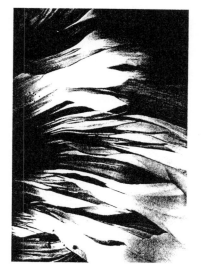

Zinc: polarised light micrograph

Zinc is needed for the transcription of RNA in the promotion of protein synthesis, cellular replication and collagen formation. Zinc deficiency has an adverse influence on wound healing through its effect on reducing rates of epithelialisation, decreasing of wound strength and collagen synthesis.

Iron is necessary for the hydroxylation of lysine and proline in the formation of collagen. Iron is necessary to transport oxygen in the body.

Copper is necessary for collagen cross-link formation. Together with iron, copper is essential to the production of erythrocytes.

The three steps in the healing response involve and are dependent on nutritional substrates: These steps are:

■ Inflammation with recruitment of poly-morphonuclear leukocytes, macrophages and lymphocytes

■ The proliferation of fibroblasts and the production of collagen

■ Collagen remodelling and re-epithelialisation when appropriate.

The strength and integrity of tissue repair will depend on collagen cross-linking and deposition.

CARBOHYDRATE AND FATS

Carbohydrates and fats provide a source of cellular energy. Glucose, the simplest form of carbohydrate, is the primary fuel for cellular metabolism of many tissues, including leukocytes, fibroblasts and macrophages. When glucose is not available for cellular function, the body catabolises protein and, to a lesser degree, fat, to produce glucose to meet energy requirements. Glucose is needed to meet the metabolic demand for wound healing and preserve the body's structural and functional protein.

Energy from fat metabolism is used in all normal cell functions, and fat metabolism results in the formation of prostaglandins and other regulators of the immune and inflammatory process.

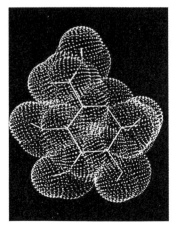

Glucose: computer graphic representation

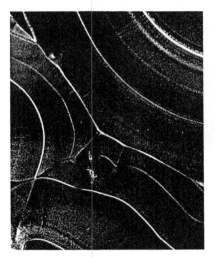

The natural process of wound healing requires numerous energy-consuming reactions and these all require increased amounts of vitamins. Where specific vitamin deficiencies are diagnosed, individual supplements of up to 10 to 20 times the recommended daily allowance may be needed. Supplementation is an extremely important component of the therapeutic nutrition care plan for the patient with a wound.

Vitamin C functions as a co-factor in the hydroxylation of proline to hydroxy-proline, an essential step in the synthesis of collagen. Vitamin C deficiency markedly delays the wound-healing process and causes capillary fragility. In vitamin C deficiency states, old wounds may re-open because of loss of tensile strength and degeneration of the extracellular matrix.

Ascorbic acid may increase the activation of leukocytes and macrophages to the injured site.

VITAMINS

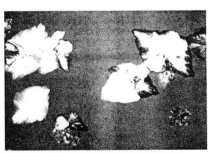

Vitamin A: dietary sources include butter, egg yolks and fish liver oils

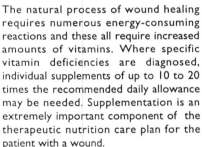

Vitamin C: water soluble, found in fresh fruit and vegetables

Vitamin A is important in maintaining the normal humoral defence mechanism and in limiting complications associated with wound infections either locally or systemically. Supplementation of retinoic acid has been shown to improve wound healing in patients receiving corti-costeroid treatment.

Vitamin A is required for an adequate inflammatory response, which is essential for the formation of mucopolysaccha-rides. These function as a protective sheath around collagen. The supplement-ation of vitamin A in steroid-dependent patients before surgery may promote a rapid healing response and reduce the incidence of wound dehiscence.

Vitamin E is essential for the stability of cell walls. Decreased levels of vitamin E are associated with shortened survival of red and white blood cells. Vitamin E also enhances the immune response. Vitamin K plays an essential role in coagulation, which is a prerequisite for healing.

injured site[14,15]. The reducing property of vitamin C may assist in preventing the oxidation of the membranes of chemotactic proteins, allowing for rapid response during inflammation[15].

Vitamin C deficiency markedly delays the wound-healing process and causes capillary fragility[16]. Reports of marginal vitamin C levels in institutionalised persons may substantiate the rationale for supplementation during hospitalisation, mainly where there is some evidence for its increased need during injury[17].

Vitamin A is important in maintaining the normal humoral defence mechanism and in limiting complications associated with wound infections either locally or systemically. Supplementation of retinoic acid has been shown to improve wound healing in patients receiving corticosteroid treatment[18]. Vitamin A counteracts the catabolic effect that glucorticosteroids exert on wound healing[18,19]. In vitro studies suggest vitamin A and retinoic acid enhance fibroplasia and collagen accumulation in wounds[20]. Vitamin A stimulates cellular differentiation in fibroblasts and collagen synthesis, thus hastening the healing process and enhancing tensile strength

Vitamin E, also known as tocopherol, is an antioxidant. It is essential for the stability of cell walls. Decreased levels of vitamin E are associated with shortened survival of red and white blood cells. Vitamin E also enhances the immune response.

Vitamin K plays an essential role in coagulation, which is a prerequisite for healing.

Trace elements and wound healing

Zinc acts as a co-factor in over 100 enzyme reactions. It is needed for the transcription of RNA in the promotion of protein synthesis, cellular replication and collagen formation. Zinc is required for synthesising and mobilising plasma proteins such as retinol-binding protein and albumin[21].

Iron is necessary for the hydroxylation of lysine and proline in the formation of collagen. It is also necessary to transport oxygen in the body.

Copper is a component of many enzyme systems including lysyl oxidase. It is also necessary for collagen cross-link formation. Together with iron, copper is essential to the production of erythrocytes.

Nutritional assessment: correlation of development and healing of wounds

Early identification and monitoring of several nutrition risk factors may eliminate or reduce the complications associated with delayed wound healing.

There are three major components of a nutritional assessment. They are the visceral protein stores (which include serum albumin, transferrin, total protein and total lymphocyte count), the somatic protein stores (which include creatinine, height index and anthropometric measurements) and the vitamin and mineral status of the patient.

Research suggests that the patient's serum albumin level is closely correlated with the development of pressure sores[22-24]. Further, the lower the serum albumin the more advanced the pressure sore stage.

A patient may be below standard body mass (thin) by subjective assessment and thus diagnosed as marasmic but have a normal albumin level. If mobile, this patient is less likely to develop pressure sores than if he or she were hypoalbuminaemic and obese. A patient found to be hypoalbuminaemic on nutritional assessment and thus diagnosed as having adult Kwashiorkor-like malnutrition may be obese but at greater risk of pressure sore development.

Another index of a standard nutritional assessment is a total lymphocyte count; a decreased total lymphocyte count positively correlates with the occurrence of pressure sores.

Healing wounds are intensely anabolic and malnutrition need not be severe to affect the healing process adversely. Additionally, overt symptoms or physical signs may not accompany specific nutritional or metabolic abnormalities.

Conclusion

Wound healing is a complex interaction of mechanical, physiological and biochemical events. An alteration in any facet of this intricate process will inevitably lead to prolonged or abnormal wound healing.

Early nutritional assessment and intervention will help meet the protein, energy, vitamin and mineral requirements necessary to optimise healing.

The prevention and treatment of wounds depends heavily on adequate nourishment and the correction of nutrient deficiencies. Without the correction of nutritional deficiencies, concomitant with the correction of external factors, the application of proper wound-care techniques alone cannot be expected to result in wound healing. Thus, nutrition assumes an equal footing with the other time-honoured pathogenic considerations in wound prevention and treatment. ∎

REFERENCES
1 Ruberg, R.L. Role of nutrition in wound healing. *Surg Clin N A* 1984; **64**: 705.
2 Barbul, A., Retture, G., Levenson, S. M. et al. Arginine: a thymotropic and wound-healing agent. *Surg Forum* 1977; **28**: 101.
3 Fischer, C.L., Gill, C., Forrester, M.C. et al. Quantitation of acute-phase proteins postoperatively. *Am J Clin Path* 1976; **66**: 840.
4 Agostoni, A., Binagh, B. C., Radies, F. et al. Acute phase proteins and healing of myocardial infarction. *J Molecular Cell Cardiol* 1972 **4**: 519.
5 Powanda, M.C., Moyer, E.D. Plasma proteins and wound healing. *Surg Gynecol Obstet* 1981; **153**: 857.
6 Owen, J.A. Effect of injury on plasma proteins. *Adv Clin Chem* 1967; **9**: 72.
7 Chernoff, R., Milton, K., Liphitz, D. The effect of a very high protein liquid formula (replete) on decubitus ulcer healing in long-term tube-fed institutionalised patients (abstract) *J Am Dietet Assoc* 1990; **90**: 9, A-130.
8 Bergstrom, N., Braden, B. A prospective study of pressure sore risk among institutionalised elderly. *J Am Geriatrics Soc* 1992; **40**: 8, 747–758.
9 Alvarez, O.M., Gilbreath, R. Thiamine influence on collagen during the granulation of skin wounds. *J Surg Res* 1982; **32**: 24–31.
10 Burr, R.G., Rajan, K.T. Leucocyte ascorbic acid and pressure sores in paraplegia. *Br J Nutrition* 1972; **28**: 2, 275–281.
11 Grenier, J., Aprahamian, M., Genot, R. et al Pantothenic acid (vitamin B5) efficiency on wound healing. *Acta Vitamina Logica* 1982; **4**: 1–2, 81–85.
12 Taylor, T.V., Rimmer, S., Day, B. et al. Ascorbic acid supplementation in the treatment of pressure sores. *Lancet* 1974; **2**: 7880, 544–546.
13 Orgil, D., Denling, R.H. Current approaches to wound healing. *Crit Care Med* 1988; **16**: 899–908.
14 Leibowitz, B., Seigel, B.V. Ascorbic acid neutrophel function and the immune response. *Int J Vit Nutr Res* 1978; **48**: 159–164.
15 Shilotry, P.G. Phagocytosis and leukocyte enzymes in ascorbic acid-deficient guinea pigs. *J Nutr* 1977; **107**: 1507–1512.
16 Irvin, T.T., Challopadhyay, D.K., Smythe, A. Ascorbic acid requirements in postoperative patients. *Am J Surg* 1978; **147**: 49.
17 Mason, M., Matyk, P.W., Doolan, S.A. Urinary ascorbic acid excretion in postoperative patients. *Am J Surg* 1978; **147**: 49.
18 Ehrlich, H.P., Hunt, T.K. Effect of cortisone and vitamin A on wound healing. *Ann Surg* 1968; **167**: 324–328.
19 Hunt, T.K., Ehrlich, H.P., Garcia, J.A. et al. Effect of vitamin A on reversing the inhibitor effect of cortisone on healing of wounds in animal and man. *Ann Surg* 1969; **170**: 633–641.
20 Demetriou, A.A., Levenson, S.M., Retture, G. et al. Vitamin A and retinoic acid-induced fibroblast differentiation *in vitro. Surg* 1985; **98**: 931–934.
21 Henken, R. Zinc and wound healing. *New Eng J Med* 1974; **292**: 13, 675–676.
22 Pinchcofsky-Devin, G.D., Kaminski, M.V. Correlation of pressure sores and nutritional status. *J Am Geriatrics Soc* 1986; **34**: 6, 435–440.
23 Ek, A.C., Unosson, M., Bjunlf, P. The modified Norton scale in nutritional state. *Scand J Caring Science* 1989; **3**: 4, 183–189.
24 Hanan, K., Scheele, L. Albumin vs weight as a predictor of nutritional status and pressure ulcer development. *Ostomy Wound Man* 1991; **33**: 2, 22–27.

Measuring wounds

A guide to the use of wound measurement techniques

P. Plassmann, Dipl-Ing. (FH), PhD, is a research fellow at the Medical Electronics and Imaging Group, Department of Electronics & Information Technology, University of Glamorgan, Wales

Wound measurement

Accurate measurement of the physical size of wounds is vital for assessing the progress of healing. Owing to the increasing range of interventions that may affect wounds at different stages of the healing process, the need for accurate and practical methods of measuring wound dimensions is growing in importance. Simple and straightforward approaches using rulers and transparency tracings have been followed by more sophisticated measurement methods involving cameras and computer vision technology.

Wounds have a three-dimensional, dynamic structure which is difficult to measure. All measurement techniques have to deal with three general problems which directly affect their accuracy:
■ *The definition of a wound's boundary.* This is determined by the subjective assessment of the human observer who performs the measurements and decides whether or not a particular part of the area in question belongs to the wound
■ *Wound flexibility in wounds that are undermined, large or deep.* Such wounds are capable of changing their appearance significantly, thus jeopardising the reproducibility of measurements
■ *The natural curvature of the human body.* Measurement devices that do not account for surface curvature will produce inaccurate results.

Despite these problems, various attempts have been made to measure the area and volume of wounds.

Area measurement
Area measurement techniques may be divided into three major groups: ruler-based assessment schemes, transparency tracings and photographic methods.

In 1985 Kundin[1] reported on a patented gauge which measures the length, breadth and depth of a wound in a single measurement. In 1989 two formulae were published[2] which allow the calculation of the approximate area

and volume from these three measurements. The area is calculated as follows:

$$Area = length \times breadth \times 0.785$$

In 1990, Thomas and Wysocki[3] found that area measurements made with the gauge correlated with those made using transparency tracings and photographs. The Kundin method, however, underestimated area by several orders of magnitude when wounds were of irregular contour. Compared with other methods, ruler-based schemes were found to be the least reliable, with the highest standard deviations.

The practice of tracing the outline of a wound through a transparent sheet appears to be the most popular and practicable method for area measurements. An improved version uses flexible two-layer transparencies with an imprinted metric grid. The tracing is made on the upper sheet, and the lower sheet, which is in contact with the wound, is disposed of after use.

The main source of error in this method is the ability of observers to define precisely the edge of a wound[4,5]. After the tracing is taken, a variety of methods can be used to obtain its area. A straightforward but time-consuming approach is to place the transparency on metric graph paper and count the number of $1mm^2$ squares[6]. Less tedious is the practice of cutting out the tracing and weighing it on a precision scale[5]. This method is faster, but the second transfer of wound shape reduces the accuracy of the measurement.

Wound tracings may be transferred onto a computer and the measurements can be taken using hand-held scanners[7]

or electronic cameras. The computer software automatically identifies the boundaries of the tracing and is faster and more accurate than other devices such as planimeters[5,6] and digitising tablets[3].

The accuracy of photographic measurements is reduced by the need to scale the photographs and by the curvature of the wound area. Palmer et al.[8] used a computer-linked electronic camera to evaluate the effect of camera angle on the measurement of the wound. They found that a camera angle of 20 degrees from the perpendicular resulted in a reduction of the measured area of approximately 10%. Instead of using a computer-linked camera, a viewing box may be used to project slides onto paper[9]. The projection may then be traced with a pen and calculated using one of the area measurement techniques mentioned above.

The practice of tracing wounds through transparencies remains the most effective method of measuring the area of a wound. The technique is rapid and inexpensive, requires minimal training and provides instant results (especially with computer-assisted calculation methods).

Volume measurement
Healing of deep wounds usually begins at the base rather than the edge of the wound. Area measurements do not reflect the early changes in wound shape; attempts have been made, therefore, to assess wound volume. Volume measurement is complicated by the problems of boundary definition, changing wound shape and body curvature. Some wounds are also extensively undermined and their volume may change with the patient's position.

Ultrasonic surface scanners are available for industrial applications and reports of attempts to use this technology in patients have been

AREA MEASUREMENT TECHNIQUES

Performance parameters of three area measurement techniques

	Ruler-based	Transparency tracings	Photography
Ease of use	Easy	Easy	Moderate
Time consumption	One minute	Several minutes	Several minutes
Cost	Very low	Low	Moderate
Availability	Good	Good	Good
Type of record	Figures	Tracing/figures	Image/figures
Wound contact	Yes	Yes	No
Training	Little	Some	Some

Fig 1. Precision of three area measurement techniques

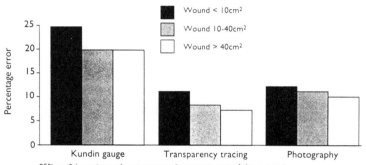

Wound < 10cm²
Wound 10-40cm²
Wound > 40cm²

Percentage error

Kundin gauge   Transparency tracing   Photography

95% confidence intervals are presented as percentages of the respective areas.
The 95% confidence interval is approximately two standard deviations wide (1.96)

Note that for all methods the precision increases with increasing wound size. Owing to the different circumstances in which measurements are taken using the various methods (different users, rules, definitions or environmental conditions), the percentages shown in Fig 1 are only indicators of their respective precision.

ALGINATE CAST TECHNIQUE

Wound volume may be measured using dental impression materials. The materials come as a powder which is mixed with water to form a paste that sets to an elastic cast in one-and-a-half to three minutes (depending on the temperature of the water). This method is easy to learn and to perform at the bedside[24]. The alginate does not stick to the wound or equipment and can be extracted without difficulty. The volume of the cast may be calculated by dividing its weight by the density of the material or by placing the cast in a graduated cylinder where the volume of displaced water indicates the volume of the cast[25].

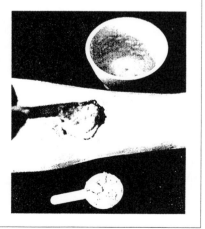

SALINE MEASUREMENT TECHNIQUE

Wound volume may be determined by covering the wound with a transparent adhesive film and then filling the lesion with sterile saline by injecting it through the film. The accuracy of the method is influenced by the clinician's ability to inject the exact amount of saline into the cavity that is necessary for the adhesive film to follow the former undestroyed surface of the skin. The tendency of wounds to absorb saline is also a limitation. Removing the adhesive film may be painful for the patient; in addition, possible spillage of the saline, which may be contaminated by wound exudate, makes this procedure less than ideal.

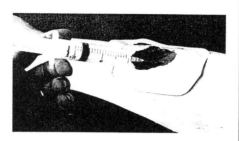

STRUCTURED LIGHT TECHNIQUE

Pictures from the patient are taken in a few seconds and digitised colour pictures of the wound may be stored on computer disk for later reference. The operator provides the system with information on the boundary of the wound which is then used to calculate its area, volume, circumference and depth. The measurement process takes less than five minutes for each wound.

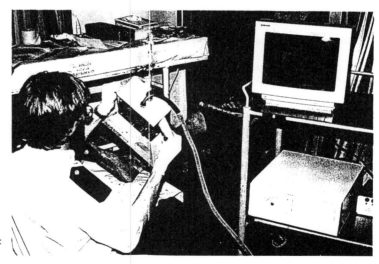

A wound measurement instrument based on the structured light technique

VOLUME MEASUREMENT TECHNIQUES

Performance parameters of six volumetric wound measurement methods

	Ultra-sound	Ruler-based	Casts	Saline	Stereo-photo-graphy	Struc-tured light
Ease of use	Difficult	Easy	Moderate	Moderate	Difficult	Moderate/ difficult
Time consumption	30 minutes	One minute	Several minutes	Several minutes	20-30 minutes	4-5 minutes
Cost	High	Very low	Low	Low	Very high	High
Availability	Research instrument	Good	Good	Good	Research instrument	Prototype available
Type of record	Three-dimensional printout	Figures	Cast/ figures	Figures	Three-dimensional image/figures	Images/ figures
Wound contact	Yes/no	Yes	Yes	Yes	No	No
Training	Several hours	Little	One hour	One hour	Several hours	Several hours

Fig 2. The precision range of the different volume measurement methods. The upper margin of each range represents the precision of measurement for large and shallow wounds, the lower margin represents the precision for relatively small, deep wounds.

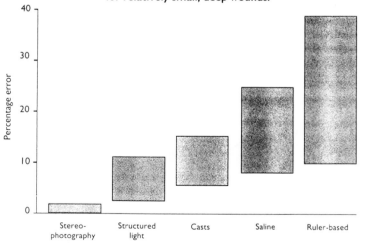

Precision range (one standard deviation as % of the respective volume)

The methods used for measuring wound volume are more accurate in the case of wounds which are small in area but have a significant volume. These wounds may be measured with much higher precision than those which are large and shallow. This is a result of the need to reconstruct the original healthy skin surface in order to determine the volume of a lesion. The larger the wound area, the greater the margin of error this reconstructing process produces.

made[10]. Compared with an optical camera, the resolution is always poor since it is difficult to focus the ultrasonic waves to a sufficiently narrow beam. Recent developments which use techniques adapted from microwave range finders (radar)[11] still have relatively poor resolution, but this may be improved by taking multiple pictures from different positions[12].

Ultrasonic depth scanners are useful for measuring small wounds and scars. Whiston et al.[13] used a 20MHz ultrasound B mode scanner to analyse the tissue patterns of healing wounds.

Using rulers, wound volume may be calculated as follows:

Volume = area x depth x 0.327

Provided that all measurements are taken with the rulers in exactly the same position, the progress of healing may be documented with some precision; however, experiments on wound models with known volumes have shown that standard deviations may reach up to 40% of the volume[14].

The volume of a wound may be measured with impression materials such as a high-viscosity vinyl poly-siloxane (for example, Reprosil)[15] but cheaper and faster measurements may be made using dental alginate hydrocolloid materials (for example, Jeltrate or Bluemix). It is suitable for many types of wounds with the exception of those being extensively undermined. Generally the cast can be extracted without difficulty from a lesion, but if the shape of a wound makes it impossible to verify that no material is left in the cavity, this method should not be used.

In 1990 Berg et al.[16] suggested that volume measurements could be made by covering the wound with a transparent adhesive film and filling the lesion with sterile saline by injecting it through the film. Experiments have shown that on wound models a precision of more than 10% is rarely achievable[14]. In some cases it is not possible to position the patient in a way which allows the wound to be filled with saline[15].

As well as avoiding all the problems which result from physical wound contact, optical measurement techniques can provide additional information. Boardman et al.[17] found that the colours within a healing wound can indicate its biological condition: infected wounds show distinct differences in hue compared with wounds which are healing normally. The major disadvantage of optical techniques is their inability to measure wound features which are not visible because of undermining or surface curvature.

An approach by Bulstrode et al.[18] and Erikson et al.[19,20] uses stereophoto-grammetry to obtain true three-dimensional measurements. Early models of this instrument were awkward to use, but it has been redesigned, and errors in accuracy and precision are in the order of 1%[21]. Time consumption is the main disadvantage of the method since photographs of the wound have to be developed before a trained operator can make measurements.

Another three-dimensional measurement system is based on the structured light technique[22,23]. The wound area is illuminated by a projector with a set of parallel strips of light. A camera is connected to an image-processing computer and from the known positions of camera and projector and the observed intersection points of the stripes of light with the wound's surface, a three-dimensional represen-tation of the observed area can be produced by triangulation.

Methods used for measuring wound volume are complex and not ideal. The advantages and disadvantages of each method have to be weighed. The most practical and appropriate technique, determined by the type of wound and the availability of equipment, should be used.

Conclusion

For everyday use on the ward or in the community, where suitable, alginate casts are probably the preferred method as they are easy to produce and inexpensive. For research purposes, however, greater accuracy becomes more important and the more expensive and complicated stereo-optical or structured light methods are preferable. The additional advantage of combining dimensional measurements with a colour analysis of the wound using structured light instruments may allow healing time to be predicted or give an early indication of complications in the healing process. ∎

REFERENCES
1. Kundin, J.I. Designing and developing a new measuring instrument. *Perioperative Nurs Quart* 1985; 1: 4, 40–45.
2. Kundin, J.I. A new way to size up wounds. *Amer J Nurs* 1989; **89**: 2, 206–207.
3. Thomas, A.C., Wysocki, A.B. The healing wound: a comparison of three clinically useful methods of measurement. *Decubitus* 1990; **3**: 1, 18–25.
4. Ramirez, A.T., Sorof, H.S., Schwartz, M.S., et al. Experimental wound healing in man. *Surg Gynecol Obstetr* 1969; **128**: 283–293.
5. Bohannon, R.W., Pfaller, B.A. Documentation of wound surface area from tracings of wound perimeters. *Physical Therapy* 1983; **63**: 10, 1622–1624.
6. Majeske, C. Reliability of wound surface area measurements. *Physical Therapy* 1992; **72**: 2, 138–141.
7. Ahroni, J.H., Boyko, E.J., Pecoraro, R.E. Reliability of computerized wound surface area determinations. *Wounds: A compendium of clinical research and practice* 1993; **4**: 4, 133–137.
8. Palmer, R.M., Ring, E.F.J., Ledgard, L. A digital video technique for radiographs and monitoring ulcers. *J Photog Sci* 1989; **37**: 65–67.
9. Katelaris, P., Fletcher, J.P., Little, J.M. A new means of assessing healing in chronic venous ulceration. *Austr N Z J Surg* 1986; **56**: 99–102.
10. Ide, M., Noboyoshi, M. Multiple section tomograms simultaneous display ultrasound diagnostic equipment. In: *Proceedings of the Ultrasonics International Conference, Brighton 1977*. Brighton: IPC Science and Technology Press, 1977.
11. Pavy H.G., Jr., Smith, S.W., von Ramm, O.T. An improved real time volumetric ultrasonic imaging system. In: Schneider, R.H. (ed). *Medical Imaging V: Image Physics 1991*; Proceedings 1443. Bellingham, Wa: SPIE, 1991.
12. Chen, Y.C., Yang, C.W., Hen C.F. An ultrasonic imaging system for 3-D object recognition. In: *Proceedings of the International Conference on Industrial Electronics, November, 1987* Volume 2. New York: IEEE, 1987.
13. Whiston, R.J., Melhuish, JM., Harding, K.G. High resolution ultrasound imaging in wound healing. *Wounds: A compendium of clinical research and practice* 1993; **5**: 3, 116–121.
14. Plassman, P., Melhuish, J.M., Harding, K.G. Methods of measuring wound size: a comparative study. *Wounds: A compendium of clinical research and practice* 1994; **6**: 2, 54–61.
15. Covington, J.S., Griffin, J.W., Mendius, R.K., et al. Measurement of pressure ulcer volume using dental impression materials: suggestions from the field. *Physical Ther* 1989; **69**: 8, 690–694.
16. Berg, W., Traneroth, C., Gunnarson, A., et al. A method for measuring pressure sores. *Lancet* 1990; **335**: 1445–1446.
17. Boardman, M., Melhuish, J.M., Palmer, K., et al. Hue, saturation and intensity in the healing wound. In: *Proceedings of the 3rd European Conference on Advances in Wound Management, Harrogate, UK., October 1993*. London: Macmillan Magazines, 1994.
18. Bulstrode, C.J.K., Goode, A.W., Scott P.J. Stereophotogrammetry for measuring rates of cutaneous healing: a comparison with conventional techniques. *Clin Sci* 1986; **71**: 437–443.
19. Erikson, G., Eklund, A.E., Torlegard, K., et al. Evaluation of leg ulcer treatment with stereophotogrammetry. *Brit J Dermatol* 1979; **101**: 123–131.
20. Erikson, G., Eklund, A.E., Liden, S., et al. Comparison of different treatments of venous leg ulcers. *Cur Therapeut Res* 1984; **35**: 678–684.
21. Walsh, M.S., Goode, A.W. A scientific approach to wound measurement: the role of stereophoto-grammetry. In: Janssen, H., Rodman, R., Robertson, J. (eds). *Wound Healing*. Wrightson Medical Publishing, 1991.
22. Plassmann, P., Jones, B.F. Measuring leg ulcers by colour-coded structured light. *J Wound Care* 1992; **1**: 3, 35–38.
23. Frantz, R.A., Johnson, D.A. Stereophotography and computerized image analysis: a three-dimensional method of measuring wound healing. *Wounds: A compendium of clinical research and practice* 1992; **4**: 58–64.
24. Resch, C.S., Kerner, E., Robson, M.C., et al. Pressure sore volume measurement. *J Amer Geriatr Soc* 1988; **36**: 444–446.
25. Pories, W.J., Schear, E.W., Jordan, D.R., et al. The measurement of human wound healing. *Surgery* 1966; **59**: 5, 821–824.

Hand-held Doppler assessment for peripheral arterial disease

An update on the use of continuous-wave Doppler ultrasound for the measurement of blood pressure and calculation of the ankle brachial pressure index in the assessment of patients with arterial disease

Patients presenting with vascular disease usually give a history of symptoms that points to an accurate diagnosis. This is not often the case when a patient presents with a leg ulcer. Here the question is whether the patient has occult sub-clinical arterial disease that may influence the choice of treatment.

The hazards of inappropriate compression bandaging are well recognised[1]. The information required to reach a diagnosis of arterial insufficiency can be gained from the history and examination of the patient and from simple non-invasive investigations.

History
Systematic inquiry may reveal underlying risk factors for arterial disease[2]. There may also be specific symptoms related to lower limb arterial disease. There may be sudden rapid deterioration in a previously asymptomatic leg or a history of chronic arterial insufficiency.

Acute arterial occlusion is said to present with the five Ps: pain, pallor, pulselessness, paraesthesia and paralysis. This, however, is not always the case, and the severity and number of symptoms will vary with the level of ischaemia[3].

Chronic arterial insufficiency of the lower extremity causes two classic symptoms – intermittent claudication and rest pain[3]. Claudication is usually described as a cramp-like tightening in the calf and occasionally in the foot, thigh or buttock, brought on by walking a certain distance and relieved by resting, often for several minutes[4].

Rest pain is a different and far more significant symptom. The pain is usually felt in the foot or the toe, often the great toe, and comes on soon after going to bed. It is usually relieved by hanging the foot out of the bed, and the patient is often forced to sleep in a chair[4].

K.R. Vowden, RGN, FETC, is a clinical nurse specialist; V. Goulding, BSc, is a vascular technician; P. Vowden, MD, FRCS, is a consultant vascular surgeon; all at Bradford Royal Infirmary

Peripheral arterial disease; Assessment; Doppler; ABPI; Leg ulcers

It is important to remember that other conditions can mimic the symptoms of rest pain and intermittent claudication[4]. These should be excluded by physical examination or simple investigations.

Examination of the lower limb
Detailed examination of the legs can give valuable information on the state of the peripheral circulation[4]. Ulceration and gangrene are indications of possible arterial disease. The site and appearance of an ulcer can give an indication of its type[5-7], but the diagnosis should never be based on the ulcer appearance alone.

Thickening of the nails and slow nail growth is characteristic of chronic arterial insufficiency[3,5], as is shiny, scaly skin. There may also be thickening of the skin with fissuring, particularly over the heel[5]. Oedema can indicate severe ischaemia, the patient having to keep the limb dependent to relieve rest pain[3,5].

Palpation and auscultation of the proximal lower limb pulses can give a good indication of the condition of the underlying vessels[3,4,8]. Once the state of the proximal vessels has been assessed and documented, attention should be directed to the ankle and foot pulses.

Doppler assessment
In 1842, Christian Doppler[9] stated that the frequency of sound emitted or reflected from a moving object varied with the velocity of the object. This so-called 'Doppler effect' explains the change in frequency of a wave when either the transmitter or the detector is moving relative to

the other. This effect can occur with any wave-form, not just ultrasound, and can be used to examine movement.

Unlike the Korotkoff sounds that are generated directly by blood flow in the blood vessel, the sound that is heard when using Doppler ultrasound is produced by amplification of the frequency shift that occurs in the ultrasound signal when it is reflected by a moving object. The movement of the red blood cell within the circulation as it reflects the sound transmitted by the Doppler probe produces the frequency shift. The extent of the shift depends on the speed of movement of the blood cell.

This principle was first applied in medicine in 1957 by Satomura to study the structure and function of the heart[10]. In 1960 Satomura and Kaneko described a study, based on this technique, of instantaneous changes in blood flow in the peripheral arteries[10].

Franklin produced an ultrasonic flowmeter based on the Doppler effect from which the portable continuous-wave Doppler was developed[11]. This technique was successfully applied in patients with peripheral arterial and venous disease, evaluating both the pulse wave-form and the systolic blood pressure[11].

Doppler pressure readings
Continuous-wave Doppler ultrasound is just one of several methods that can be used to derive blood pressure. A stethoscope is routinely used to measure the systolic and diastolic pressure in the arm, and has been used to measure ankle blood pressures[12]. However, the arteries at the ankle do not lend themselves to this technique[13] which relies on the detection of Korotkoff sounds to measure both systolic and diastolic pressures[12,13]. Continuous-wave Doppler can be used to measure only systolic pressure[13].

PHYSICAL EXAMINATION OF THE LOWER LIMB

Subtle colour differences between the feet, particular pallor of the skin on one foot, can be an indication of arterial disease (Fig 1).
Other signs are slow capillary return after blanching, or fluttering of the veins with slow refilling after elevations and Buerger's sign of pallor on elevation.
Rubor (redness) on dependency (Fig 2) indicates serious ischaemia[4].

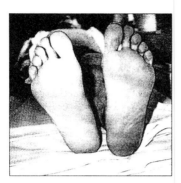

Fig 1. Pallor of the foot when the patient is lying flat, an indication of ischaemia

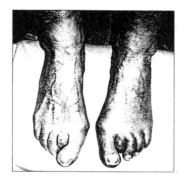

Fig 2. Sunset foot, Buerger's sign of rubor on lowering and ischaemic limb indicating severe ischaemia

ARTERIES IN THE LOWER LEG

The posterior tibial (PT) pulse is located in the hollow behind the medial malleolus, and the dorsalis pedis (DP) pulse is felt between the first and second metatarsals (Fig 3).

Although the PT pulse is almost always present[3], the DP pulse may be absent in almost 10% of the healthy population[1]. In these subjects the terminal branch of the peroneal artery is usually palpable at the ankle[3].

Three recent studies have concluded that palpation of the pedal pulses in patients with arterial disease is subject to significant observer error and should be used only in combination with objective measurements (such as Doppler pressure measurement) as a guide to clinical management[29-31].

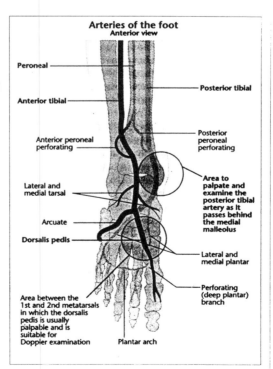

Fig 3. Location of the main arteries in the lower leg and foot

THE HAND-HELD DOPPLER

The modern hand-held Doppler probe consists of two crystals. One crystal oscillates, emitting ultrasound of a frequency in the range 2-10MHz (the exact frequency varies for each probe). Probes for arterial and venous flow detection are usually 5 or 8MHz while for obstetric work 2 or 3MHz is used[32].

The transmitted ultrasound beam is directed towards the blood vessel of interest. Ultrasound waves are reflected or 'echoed' back, and are detected by a second receiving crystal.

These waves consist of reflections from stationary objects such as fat and skin and from moving objects such as red blood cells. The latter signals will have undergone the 'Doppler effect' and will thus contain the resulting frequency shift (Fig 4).

The signal received by the Doppler probe therefore consists of a mixture of frequencies. This signal is filtered to leave only the frequency-shifted signal which is then amplified and fed to a loud speaker or converted to a graphic output.

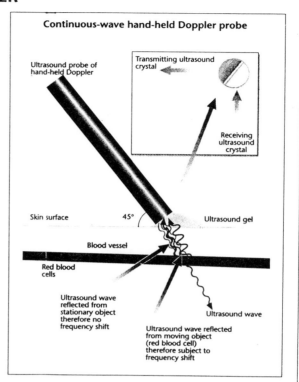

Fig 4. Diagram of continuous-wave hand-held Doppler probe demonstrating frequency shift

TYPICAL DOPPLER WAVEFORMS

As well as the audible signal output, the reflected wave-form from the Doppler probe can also be analysed graphically and data from this can be used to give further information on the arterial tree[17]. Typical zero-crossing output from the common femoral artery is shown in Fig 5.

In the absence of disease, the wave-form is triphasic. It becomes progressively more monophasic as arterial disease progresses. More complex analysis of the data can be used to obtain flow velocities and an estimate of the severity of any stenosis[15,17].

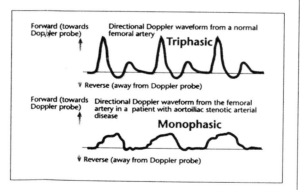

Fig 5. Typical Doppler wave-forms

ANKLE BRACHIAL PRESSURE INDEX

The basis of the ABPI is a comparison between the highest ankle pressure and the best estimate of central systolic blood pressure[4,18] (Fig 6). This later measurement is taken to be the higher of the two (left and right) brachial pressures[33].

It is important to realise that the brachial pressure can vary between the left and right arms even in subjects with a 'normal' circulation[34]. Differences above 15mmHg suggest underlying arch vessel disease[35].

Widespread arterial disease may involve the circulation to both arms and in such a situation the arm systolic blood pressure will not reflect true central systolic pressure. Any calculations based on this pressure will be inaccurate.

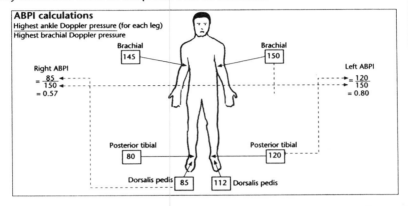

ABPI calculations
Highest ankle Doppler pressure (for each leg)
Highest brachial Doppler pressure

Brachial 145   Brachial 150

Right ABPI
$= \dfrac{85}{150}$
$= 0.57$

Left ABPI
$= \dfrac{120}{150}$
$= 0.80$

Posterior tibial 80   Posterior tibial 120

Dorsalis pedis 85   112 Dorsalis pedis

TABLE 1. HOW TO CALCULATE THE ABPI

Criteria	Action
Resting	10-20 minutes[12,28]
Position	Supine with no pressure on the proximal vessels
Anxiety	Explain the procedure and reassure the patient
Arms	Place an appropriately sized cuff around the upper arm
	Locate the brachial pulse by palpation and apply ultrasound contact gel
	Angle the Doppler probe at 45° and move to locate the best signal
	Inflate cuff till signal is abolished, then deflate slowly and record the pressure at which the signal returns. Take care not to move the probe from the line of the artery
	Record this pressure, then repeat the process for the other arm
	Use the highest of these two values to calculate the ABPI
Legs	Place an appropriately sized cuff around the ankle immediately above the malleoli (having first protected any ulcer that may be present)
	Locate the DP pulse by palpation or with the Doppler probe and apply ultrasound contact gel
	Continue as for the brachial pressure reading
	Record this pressure, then repeat the measurement for the PT pulse (and, if required, the peroneal pulse)
	Use the highest reading obtained to calculate the ABPI for that ankle
	Repeat for the other leg

Notes 1. Repeatedly inflating the cuff, or leaving the cuff inflated for prolonged periods, can cause the ankle pressure reading to fall by producing a hyperaemic response
2. If the pulse is irregular (as in atrial fibrillation) it may be difficult to measure the systolic pressure as it can vary markedly from beat to beat.

Strain-gauge plethysmography, isotope clearance, transcutaneous oximetry and photo-sensor techniques can all be used to measure peripheral blood pressure but none are as portable or as easy to use as the Doppler flow velocity detector[13,14].

As with all blood pressure readings it is important that an appropriately sized cuff is chosen to occlude the artery[13,15]. It is recommended that the width of the cuff be 40% of the circumference of the mid-point of the limb or 20% wider than the diameter. The length of the bladder should be twice its width[13]. The pressure recorded is not that at the site of the Doppler probe application but is the pressure required to occlude the artery at the level of the cuff[4].

For this reason, when measuring the ankle pressure, the cuff should be placed as close to the ankle as possible. The highest occlusion pressure for the three distal ankle pulses (the anterior tibial – AT, the posterior tibial – PT, and the peroneal) and the pedal pulse (the dorsalis pedis – DP) should be taken as the best estimate of the ankle systolic pressure. In practice, readings are usually limited to the PT and DP arteries. If an ulcer is present it should be protected before the cuff is applied[16].

If the ulcer site is too painful, and the cuff therefore has to be placed higher than the ankle, the pressure reading obtained is not the ankle systolic pressure and should not be used to calculate the ankle brachial pressure index (ABPI).

As the pressure measurement relates to the cuff position, it is possible, by placing an appropriately sized cuff at different sites along the leg and measuring the occlusion pressure in an artery immediately distal to the cuff, to obtain a series of segmental pressures[13,17,18]. This can be of value in localising arterial disease.

Provided a standard protocol is followed, ankle pressure measurements are remarkably free of error[18]. Absolute pressures rarely vary by >10mmHg. When the pressures are standardised by taking variations in central pressure into consideration, results are even more consistent[18]. A variation in the ABPI of >0.15 usually implies a significant pathological change[18].

The test is subject to inter- and intra-observer variations[19,20]. Calcification of the medial layer of the artery can make the underlying arteries resistant to compression and can therefore cause a falsely high reading. This can be a particular problem in people with diabetes[18,21]. If it is suspected that a falsely high pressure has been obtained the leg can be elevated and the height of the foot above the bed at which the Doppler signal disappears can be measured[18,22,23]; multiplying this height in centimetres by 0.735 will convert this height to a pressure in mmHg[18].

Ankle pressure measurements can be taken at rest or combined with a stress test such as exercise or hyperaemia[18,24]. Stress testing in this way can reveal occult arterial disease[25]. Even in mild peripheral arterial disease, the ankle pressure falls and then slowly recovers to the pre-exercise level. The extent of the fall in pressure and the time for recovery reflect the severity of the underlying arterial disease[25,26].

Ankle brachial pressure index
The ABPI is an important and easily repeated assessment of the severity of lower limb peripheral arterial disease[4,18]. The sensitivity and variability of Doppler pressure readings and of the ABPI itself are well recognised[18,27]. The ABPI has now taken on a far more demanding role in the management of patients with leg ulcers, determining who should receive compression bandaging[1,16,28].

As the ankle pressure normally exceeds the brachial pressure by 10-20mmHg[4,26], the resting ABPI should be >1[4,18]. An ABPI of <0.9 can be taken as indicating some arterial disease[28]. The majority of patients with claudication have an ABPI between 0.8 and 0.4, while patients with rest pain generally have an ABPI of <0.4[18]. In general, compression bandaging should not be used in patients with an ABPI of <0.8[16].

Conclusion
Continuous-wave Doppler assessment forms only part of the overall assessment of the patient who may have arterial disease. It is important that the whole patient is assessed so that treatment does not solely concentrate on the wound or leg ulcer but takes into account other factors that influence healing. Without a holistic approach, Doppler pressure measurement and the calculation of the ABPI taken in isolation are meaningless. ∎

REFERENCES
1. Callam, M.J., Ruckley, C.V., Dale, J.J. et al. Hazards of compression treatment of the leg: an estimate from the Scottish Surgeons. Br Med J 1987; 295: 1382.
2. Vowden, K., Vowden, P. Vascular surgery: Risk factors for arterial disease. J Wound Care 1996; 5: 2, 89-90.
3. Rutherford, R.B. The vascular consultation. In: Rutherford, R.B. (ed.). Vascular Surgery (3rd edn). Philadelphia, Pa: WB Saunders, 1989.
4. Marston, A. Clinical evaluation of the patient with atheroma. In: Bell, P.R.F., Jamieson, C.W., Ruckley, C.V. (eds). Surgical Management of Vascular Disease. London: WB Saunders, 1992.
5. Fairbairn, J.F. Clinical manifestations of peripheral arterial disease. In: Fairbairn, J.F., Juergens, J.L., Spittell, J.A. (eds). Peripheral Vascular Disease (4th edn). Philadelphia: WB Saunders, 1972.
6. Morison, M.J. A Colour Guide to the Nursing Management of Wounds. London: Wolfe, 1992.
7. Negus, D. Leg Ulcers: A practical approach to management. Oxford: Butterworth Heinemann, 1991.
8. Nicholson, M.L., Byrne, R.L., Steele, G.A., Callum, K.G. Predictive value of bruits and Doppler pressure measurements in detecting lower limb arterial stenosis. Eur J Vasc Surg 1993; 7: 59-62.
9. Doppler, C. Uber das Farbige Licht der Dopplesterne und Einiger Anderer Gestirne des Himmels. Prague: Abh K Bohm Ges Wiss 1842; 2: 465.
10. Yao, S.T. Experience with the Doppler ultrasound flow velocity meter in peripheral vascular disease. In: Gillespie, J.A. (ed.). Modern Trends in Vascular Surgery 1. London: Butterworth, 1970.
11. Franklin, D.L., Schlegel, W.A., Rushmer, R.F. Blood flow measured by Doppler frequency shift of back-scattered ultrasound. Science 1961; 134: 465.
12. Hocken, A.G. Measurement of blood-pressure in the leg. Lancet 1967; 1: 466-468.
13. Yao, S.T. Pressure measurement in the extremity. In: Bernstein, E.F. (ed.). Vascular Diagnosis (4th edn). St Louis, Mo: Mosby, 1993.
14. Beard, J.D., Scott, D.J.A. Investigation of chronic lower limb ischaemia. Hospital Update 1991; 17: 6, 496-509.
15. Standness, D.E. Doppler ultrasonic techniques in vascular disease. In: Bernstein, E.F. (ed.). Vascular Diagnosis (4th edn). St Louis, Mo: Mosby, 1993.
16. Cameron, J. Using Doppler to diagnose leg ulcers. Nurs Stand 1991; 5: 40, 25-27.
17. Sumner, D.S. Objective diagnostic techniques: role of the vascular laboratory. In: Rutherford, R.B. (ed.). Vascular Surgery (3rd edn). Philadelphia, Pa: WB Saunders, 1989.
18. Sumner, D.S. Non-invasive assessment of peripheral arterial occlusive disease. In: Rutherford, K.S. (ed.). Vascular Surgery (3rd edn). Philadelphia, Pa: WB Saunders, 1989.
19. Fowkes, F.G.R., Housley, E., Macintyre, C.C.A. et al. Variability of ankle and brachial systolic pressure in the measurement of atherosclerotic peripheral arterial disease. J Epidemiol & Comm Health 1988; 42: 128-133.
20. Ray, S.A., Srodon, P.D., Taylor, R.S., Dorinandy, J.A. Reliability of ankle brachial pressure index measurement by junior doctors. Br J Surg 1994; 81: 188-190.
21. Hobbs, J.T., Yao, S.T., Lewis, J.D., Needham, T.N. A limitation of the Doppler ultrasound method of measuring ankle systolic pressure. VASA 1974; 3: 160-162.
22. Goss, D.E., Stevens, M., Watkins, P.J., Baskerville, P.A. Falsely raised ankle/brachial pressure index: A method to determine tibial artery compressibility. Eur J Vasc Surg 1991; 5: 23-26.
23. Smith, F.C.T., Shearman, C.P., Simms, M.H., Gwynn, B.R. Falsely elevated ankle pressures in severe leg ischaemia: the pole test – an alternative approach. Eur J Vasc Surg 1994; 8: 408-412.
24. Nicholaides, A.N. Basic and practical aspects of peripheral arterial testing. In: Bernstein, E.F. (ed.). Vascular Diagnosis (4th edn). St Louis, Mo: Mosby, 1993.
25. Laing, S., Greenhalgh, R.M. The detection and progression of asymptomatic peripheral arterial disease. Br J Surg 1983; 70: 628-630.
26. Carter, S.A. Role of pressure measurements. In: Bernstein, E.F. (ed.). Vascular Diagnosis (4th edn). St Louis, Mo: Mosby, 1993.
27. Yao, S.T. Haemodynamic studies in peripheral arterial disease. Br J Surg 1970; 57: 10, 762-767.
28. Keachie, J. Making sense of Doppler ultrasound. Nurs Times 1992; 88: 10; 54-56.
29. Brearly, S., Shearman, C.P., Simms, M.H. Peripheral pulse palpation: an unreliable physical sign. Ann Royal Coll Surg Eng 1992; 74: 169-171.
30. Magee, T.R., Stanley, P.R.W., Mufti, R.A. et al. Should we palpate foot pulses? Ann Royal Coll Surg Eng 1992; 74: 166-168.
31. Moffatt, C., O'Hare, L. Ankle pulses are not sufficient to detect impaired arterial circulation in patients with leg ulcers. J Wound Care 1995; 4: 3, 134-138.
32. Williams, C. HNE diagnostic Doppler ultrasound machines. Br J Nurs 1995; 4: 22, 1340-1344.
33. Carter, S.A. Clinical measurement of systolic pressure in limbs with arterial occlusive disease. JAMA 1969; 207: 10, 1 869-1874.
34. Sutton, G.C. Examination of the cardiovascular system. In: Julian, D.G., Camm, A.J., Fox, K.M. et al (eds). Diseases of the Heart. London: Baillière Tindall, 1989.
35. Carter, S.A. Role of pressure measurements in vascular disease. In: Bernstein, E.F. (ed.). Non-invasive Diagnostic Techniques in Vascular Disease. St Louis, Mo: Mosby, 1985.

Ankle pulses are not sufficient to detect impaired arterial circulation in patients with leg ulcers

C. Moffatt, RGN, NDN, is director of education and clinical practice, and L. O'Hare, BA, RGN, is a lecturer/practitioner, Centre for Research and Implementation of Clinical Practice, London

Much debate has taken place on the use of Doppler ultrasound in the community setting. A sequential study of patients attending a community ulcer clinic was undertaken to identify community nurses' ability to detect arterial disease by palpation of pedal pulses and to compare these figures with the recording of a resting pressure index. A total of 462 patients (553 limbs) were studied; 167 (31%) had no detectable pulses at the ankle. Of the 93 limbs with a reduced resting pressure index (< 0.9), 37% had detectable pulses. Of the 440 with a normal resting index (≥0.9), 25% had no detectable ankle pulses. A number of risk factors were identified. Palpation of pedal pulses alone by community nurses is a poor prediction of arterial disease and should be accompanied by the recording of a resting pressure index

Discrepancies in current methods of nursing assessment for patients who present with leg ulcers have been highlighted[1]. One fundamental area of controversy is that which surrounds the use of Doppler ultrasound as part of the nursing assessment. The dilemma centres on the relevance, reliability and validity of Doppler ultrasound as a guide to detecting arterial disease in the lower limb, compared with manual palpation of pedal pulses, when these techniques are used by community nurses. Evidence supporting the reliability of palpating pedal pulses as a way of detecting arterial disease has come from studies carried out within a vascular unit by a

> Doppler ultrasound; Compression therapy; Leg ulcers

trained observer rather than during routine nursing assessment of patients with leg ulceration[2].

In considering the significance of the Doppler ultrasound in recording a resting pressure index (RPI), it is important to acknowledge that this tool does not constitute a diagnosis but, in conjunction with a comprehensive nursing and medical assessment, is an indicator of the underlying aetiology of the ulceration. Between 70% and 90% of leg ulcers are likely to be venous in origin. However, up to 20% of these patients may present with mixed pathology with the risk of concurrent arterial disease increasing with age[3]. The Doppler ultrasound used in this context

REFERENCES
[1] O'Hare, L.J. Implementing district-wide nurse-led venous leg ulcer clinics: a quality approach. *J Wound Care* 1994; 3: 8, 389–392.
[2] Callam, M.J., Harper, D.R., Dale, J.J., Ruckley, C.V. Arterial disease in chronic leg ulceration: an underestimated hazard? Lothian and Forth Valley Leg Ulcer Study. *Brit Med J Clin Res* 1987; 294: 6577, 929–31.
[3] Cornwall, J.V., Dore, C.J., Lewis, J.D. Leg ulcers: epidemiology and aetiology. *Brit J Surg* 1986; 73: 9, 693–696.

provides a screening procedure necessary to safeguard against the inappropriate use of high compression therapy in patients with significant arterial disease. The assumption that the recording of a resting pressure index by a nurse is diagnostic of venous ulceration by the elimination of arterial disease is fundamentally incorrect. More extensive tests are required to assess the presence and distribution of venous disease[4]. The formulation of a medical diagnosis remains the responsibility of the doctor. With the exception of nurses working in specialist centres, diagnostic testing is rarely part of the community nurse's role[5].

Alarmingly, in practice, the evidence suggests that many nurses take responsibility for diagnosis[6]. One study found that in 52% of cases, the diagnosis of ulcer aetiology was made by the nurse, with only 25% of cases diagnosed by the GP and 23% by the consultant (Stockport Health Authority, unpublished data). In the same study, it was reported that 51% of the respondents based their assessment solely on the appearance of the ulcer. More recently, a wound care audit showed that 38% of patients were recorded as having unclassified disease owing to the nurse's inability to denote the ulcer aetiology[7]. This result reflects the uncertainty among practitioners of their ability to provide a differential diagnosis, and may be a factor in studies which report a low incidence of venous ulceration and a high rate of mixed disease.

Furthermore, a study in South Lincolnshire and Leicestershire found that only 10% of nurses reported that their patients had been seen by their GPs and that, although 45% were seen on initial assessment, this was often only at the request of the district nurse (Shepperson, unpublished data). In addition, other studies demonstrate that at present as many as 80% of patients remain under the care of the primary care team and are not referred to hospital[5]; the Harrow and Wirral studies suggested that a large percentage of patients with chronic long-standing ulceration had never been referred[3]. Findings from Doppler studies form an integral part of the referral criteria in a number of areas and allow the rapid transfer of patients with arterial disease to a hospital unit for further investigations[8].

District nurses appear to be taking the primary responsibility for treatment choice once a diagnosis has been made. A questionnaire by the *Journal of District Nursing* in 1986 found that of the 474 nurses who responded, 98% had patients classified with venous ulcers on their caseload[9]. In further studies, Ertl found that the district nurse was responsible for treatment choice in 71% of cases (Ertl, unpublished data). Practice nurses are also playing in increasing role in the management of this patient population. A study by Mundy in Andover reported that practice nurses attended to 38% of the leg ulcers (Mundy, unpublished data), although within the Riverside study the figure was slightly lower at 15%[8].

Study aim

Increasing numbers of nurses have access to Doppler ultrasound yet receive little or no training in its use. Within the context of the primary health-care team, community nurses play a dominant role in providing care for patients with leg ulcers. This prompted us to consider the difficulties of nursing assessment and wound management, and, specifically, the role that the recording of a resting pressure index plays in clinical practice. It is imperative that the nursing assessment identifies patients for whom compression therapy is contraindicated. To achieve this, a resting pressure index should be taken in the context of a detailed patient history, a comprehensive physical assessment and an awareness of the importance of social and psychological factors in the wound healing process.

The recording of a resting pressure index is a well recognised and validated procedure for detecting peripheral arterial disease, first described by Yao[10]. Significant arterial disease causes a narrowing of the lumen of the affected vessel which results in blood flow disturbance. With the patient at rest and/or following exercise, the Doppler ultrasound probe is used to assess the function of specific blood vessels within segments of the limb. This procedure makes it possible to detect arterial disease, clinically identified as an abnormal drop in the systolic pressure.

The aim of this study was to incorporate all patients sequentially referred to community clinics with a leg ulcer of any type and to examine the use of Doppler ultrasound by nurses in the community setting.

Method

It is routine practice within Riverside Health Authority for all patients to have a resting pressure index recorded as part of their initial nursing assessment. During the study, all community nurses who treat leg ulcers attended an in-service training programme. During the assessment, nurses recorded

False classification of arterial status could lead to inappropriate treatment

[4] Browse, N.L., Burnand, K.G. *Diseases of the veins: Pathology, Diagnosis and Treatment.* London: Edward Arnold, 1988.
[5] Lewis, J.D., Cornwall, J.V. The assessment, management and prevention of leg ulcers. *Care of the Elderly* 1989; 1: 2, 83–85.
[6] Cullum, N. *The Nursing Management of Leg Ulcers in the Community* Liverpool: University of Liverpool, 1994.
[7] Moffatt, C.J., Lambourne, L. The South Bedfordshire wound care audit. *Nurs Standard* [In press].
[8] Moffatt, C.J., Oldroyd, M.J. A pioneering service to the community: The Riverside Community Leg Ulcer Project. *Professional Nurse* 1994: 9: 7, 486–497.
[9] Anon. *Your data on leg ulcers.* J Dist Nursing 1987; 5: 5, 4–6.
[10] Yao, S.T. Haemodynamic studies in peripheral disease. *Brit J Surg* 1970; 57: 761–766.

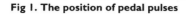

Fig 1. The position of pedal pulses

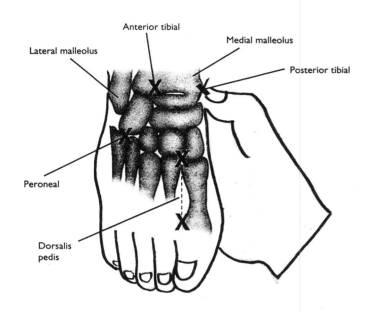

Anterior tibial

Medial malleolus

Lateral malleolus

Posterior tibial

Peroneal

Dorsalis pedis

Fig 2. The procedure for recording the resting pressure index

Stage 1   Ensure that the patient is lying flat and feels comfortable and relaxed.

Stage 2   Secure sphygmomanometer cuff around arm.

Apply ultrasound gel over brachial pulse.

Hold Doppler probe gently over brachial pulse until a good signal is obtained.

Inflate cuff until Doppler signal disappears then gradually lower pressure until the signal returns. This is the brachial systolic pressure record. (Diastolic pressure is not recordable with Doppler.)

Stage 3   Examine the foot for posterior tibial and dorsalis pedis pulse using fingers and/or Doppler probe.

Stage 4   Secure sphygmomanometer cuff just above ankle.

Locate posterior tibial and dorsalis pedis pulse using Doppler probe and gel.

Inflate cuff until signal disappears, then gradually reduce pressure until the signal returns. Repeat with second pulse.

This is the ankle systolic pressure. (Spuriously high readings may be obtained in elderly or diabetic patients as the cuff may not fully compress the calcified vessels.)

Stage 5   To calculate the resting pressure index, divide the higher ankle pressure by brachial pressure.
R.P.I. ≥ 0.8 suitable for compression
R.P.I. < 0.8 not suitable for full compression

whether they were able to detect manually palpable pulses at the dorsalis pedis, posterior tibial and peroneal sites (Fig 1). Any factors which contributed to difficulties in achieving palpation were recorded. The nurse then recorded a resting pressure index using a standard procedure, again concentrating on the dorsalis pedis and posterior tibial pulses (Fig 2). In addition, the patient's medical history was taken using a standardised assessment form, and information was compiled on concurrent arterial disease, current and previous history of ulceration and presenting signs and symptoms. The patient's attitude, level of co-operation with the procedure and any other factors influencing these were also noted.

It was integral to the validity of the study to determine the number of false positive and false negative diagnoses and to identify the factors which could lead to the false classification of arterial status and, potentially, to inappropriate treatment regimes with the risk of damaging consequences.

Results

During the study period, 462 patients presenting with 533 ulcerated limbs were assessed. The mean age of the patients was 74 years and 67% of the study population were female (Fig 3). Sensitivity and specificity were calculated to assess the value of pedal pulse palpation in the detection of arterial disease, using resting pressure index measurements as the 'gold standard'. The sensitivity for lack of pulses as a predictor of arterial disease was 63%, with a specifity of 75% and a positive predictive value of only 35%. This could lead to 37% of patients having inappropriate treatment. Of the limbs assessed, 167 (31%) had no detectable pulses at the ankle for a variety of reasons. Within the study population, 93 limbs had a resting pressure index of less than 0.9, which is generally agreed to signify the presence of arterial disease, yet 37% of these patients still had palpable pedal pulses.

Of the remaining 440 limbs with a normal resting pressure index, 25% had no detectable pulses despite the absence of significant arterial disease within the lower limb (Fig 4). Several independent risk factors have been associated with the lack of pulses in this patient group. These include a history of cardiac failure, a fixed ankle joint, the presence of diabetes mellitus, and no history of phlebitis (an unexplained anomaly). In this study, 9% of the patient population had a degree of heart failure for which they were receiving treatment and any oedema present, however mild, can make palpation of the pulses difficult.

Reduced mobility, which is common in this age group, can lead to a fixed ankle joint. It is often linked to chronic joint and bone disorders such as arthritis, and is compounded by the discomfort of an ulcer situated on the malleoli site, which further reduces the limb's range of movement. In this study, 57% of the patients had reduced mobility, with 45% suffering from osteoarthritis and 12% rheumatoid arthritis. Restricted mobility can have a dramatic effect on the function of the calf muscle pump, particularly when the Achilles tendon becomes shortened (Fig 5), and, as demonstrated by this study, also affects the ability to palpate pedal pulses.

Discussion

The results indicate that the recording of a resting pressure index by qualified and competent nurses is an essential part of the nursing assessment of all patients with circulatory disorders of the lower limb.

In the Lothian and Forth Valley study, 65% of limbs with a resting pressure index of 0.9 had palpable pulses, whereas 5% of the patients with normal healthy legs had impalpable pulses[2]. Barnhorst and Barner noted that the dorsalis pedis pulse is congenitally absent in 12% of individuals[11]. Cornwall found that the prevalence of arterial disease in the 85-year-old age group can reach 50%[5]. In the light of such evidence, and in conjunction with our findings, it can be demonstrated that this group of patients may have received inappropriate compression therapy if the Doppler ultrasound had not been used as an aid to accurate assessment.

The presence of diabetes also affects the manual palpation of pedal pulses. It is well recognised that the recording of an ankle pressure index for patients with diabetes mellitus can be misleading owing to calcification of the vessels. Since the vessels cannot be compressed, falsely elevated readings can result[12]. In this patient group, an understanding of changes within the wave signals is an important adjunct to the resting pressure index recording.

An additional consideration is that with these patients, arterial disease often occurs distally and patients may present with a normal resting index but gross distal disease. The situation may be further compounded by the presence of neuropathy which masks the symptoms of critical ischaemia. Denervation of the autonomic nervous system in these patients causes an alteration in blood flow so that the foot appears warm

Fig 3. Patient and limb characteristics of study population

Patient characteristics			Limb characteristics		
	Patients (n = 462)			Limbs (n = 553)	
Mean age (sd)	74.0	(12.2)	Median ulcer duration (months)	3	(0.25-756)
Body mass index (kg/m²)	26.4	(6.6)	Varicose veins (%)	133	(25)
Female (%)	311	(67)	Oedema (%)	106	(20)
Diabetes (%)	31	(7)	Eczema (%)	194	(36)
Hypertension (%)	96	(21)	Deep vein thrombosis	63	(12)
Rheumatoid arthritis	55	(12)	Phlebitis (%)	78	(15)
Osteoarthritis	206	(45)			
Congestive cardiac failure	43	(9)			

Fig 4. Results of pedal pulse palpation and resting pressure index recording of study population

RPI	<0.9	≥0.9	Total
Pulses			
Present	34	332	366
Absent	59	108	167
Number of ulcerated limbs	93	440	553

False positive values=34 at risk of damage
False negative values=108 at risk of suboptimal treatment

and red. Inexperienced practitioners may assume that the foot is well perfused. This may occur in 10% of patients with neuropathy and in this group of patients the Doppler ultrasound may give misleading results.

A variety of other clinical conditions have been reported to influence Doppler findings, including chronic renal failure and the presence of gross oedema[13]. Oedema, which can confound an accurate assessment, is a recognised complication of progressive venous disease and affected 20% of patients within our study.

For those patients who present with peripheral vascular disease (PVD) there also exist constraints and difficulties in achieving an accurate assessment. It is accepted as a normal occurrence that a patient with mild PVD may have a normal ankle pressure index which falls after exercise[14]. With this patient group, intermittent claudication may be difficult to identify since a generalised level of reduced mobility can prevent patients walking far enough to induce ischaemic pain. Often this only presents once rest pain has been established. When intermittent claudication occurs, it has been

11 Barnhorst, D.A., Barner, H.B. Prevalence of congenitally absent pedal pulses *N Engl J Med* 1968; **278**: 264–5.
12 Hobbs, J.T., Yao, S.T., Lewis, J.D., et al. A limitation of the Doppler ultrasound method of measuring ankle systolic pressure. *VASA* 1974; **3**: 2, 160–162.
13 Williams, I.M., Picton, A.J., McCollum, C.N. The use of Doppler ultrasound 1: Arterial disease. *Wound management* 1993; **4**: 1, 9–12.
14 Laing, S., Greenhalgh, R.M. The detection and progression of asymptomatic peripheral arterial disease. *Brit J Surg* 1983; **70**: 628–630.

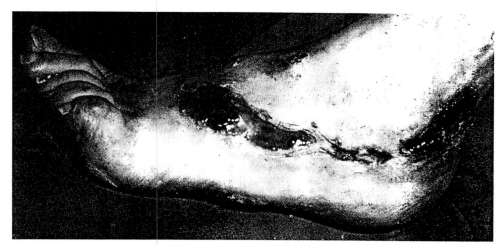

Fig 5. Fixed ankle joint

High-
compression
therapy carries
considerable
risk if used
inappropriately

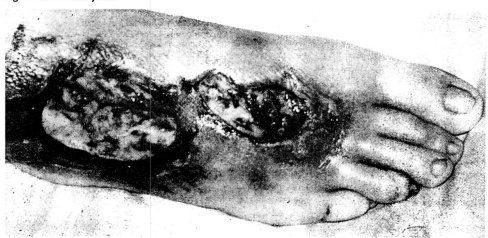

Fig 6. Result of inappropriate compression therapy

shown to be a sensitive indicator of arterial disease, with 70% of patients with claudication in the Harrow study demonstrating a reduced resting pressure index[5].

High-compression therapy remains the cornerstone of treatment for patients with known venous ulceration, yet it carries considerable risk if used inappropriately (Fig 6). An RPI of 0.9 is generally accepted as the point at which arterial disease is present, but an RPI of 0.8 is the point below which compression therapy is contraindicated. Studies have shown that skin perfusion is markedly reduced in patients who have limb ischaemia, and an exacerbation of the original ulceration becomes further compounded by the application of external compression[15]. Compression damage was documented in a study involving 154 consultants who practised general surgery in Scotland. Over a five-year period, 49 (32%) reported at least one case of compression-induced damage out of a total of 147 patients. More alarmingly,

seven of these patients required an amputation[16]. Although this is probably an underestimate of the real extent of the problem, it reminds all professionals involved in the management of leg ulceration of their accountability in the provision of safe and effective care.

Many areas within Britain are now establishing leg ulcer services. Accurate patient assessment is a fundamental consideration for all concerned. Education and training in wound care is a prerequisite to achieving quality in service delivery[17]. It is not only the practitioners' responsibility to provide the optimum treatment, but also the managers' duty to recognise that a skilled and knowledgeable workforce can facilitate effective outcomes. This study reinforces the message that nursing assessment, as well as treatment, must be based on valid research and that the use of the Doppler ultrasound plays a vitally important role. ∎

15 Pabst, T.S., Castronuevo, J.J., Jackson, J.D., et al. Evaluation of the ischaemic limb by pressure and flow measurement of the skin microcirculation as determined by laser Doppler velocimetry. *Curr Surg* 1985; **42:** 29–31.
16 Callam, M.J., Ruckley, C.V., Dale, J.J., et al. Hazards of compression treatment of the leg: an estimate from Scottish surgeons. *Brit Med J* 1987; **295:** 1382.
17 Moffatt, C.J., Karn, E.A. Answering the call for more education: Development of an ENB course in leg ulcer management. *Professional Nurse* 1994; 708–12.

The Use of Doppler Ultrasound 1: Arterial Disease

IM Williams, FRCS, *Research Registrar;* AJ Picton, BSc, *Vascular Technician; and* CN McCollum, MD, FRCS, *Professor of Surgery; Department of Vascular Surgery, University Hospital of South Manchester, Nell Lane, West Didsbury, Manchester M20 8LR.*

Simple Doppler ultrasound techniques may be used to confirm a clinical diagnosis or detect the severity of arterial insufficiency. Wider use of these techniques may improve patient care by reducing the incidence of misdiagnosis and ensuring early referral of arterial disease to a vascular consultant.

The adequacy of the vascular supply is perhaps the single most important factor determining the rate of healing in any wound or ulcer. Peripheral vascular disease causes considerable morbidity throughout the western world and may produce symptoms in the legs such as intermittent claudication, rest pain, ulceration and gangrene (FIGURE 1). Arterial disease with low ankle blood pressures

may also contribute to the development of pressure sores and ulceration in venous disease. The assessment must therefore include a thorough history and full clinical examination, including palpation of all relevant pulses.[1] Careful examination in this way can give the clinician a good idea of the anatomical location of significant atheromatous disease. Simple Doppler ultrasound techniques may then be used to confirm a clinical diagnosis or detect the severity of arterial insufficiency. As the palpation of pulses is subjective and prone to considerable error, for most health care professionals the measurement of arterial pressure by Doppler is a more reliable method of detecting arterial disease.

The Doppler principle

The frequency of sound from a constant source may be influenced by movement of the source. When the sound source moves away from or towards an observer there will be an apparent decrease or increase in the sound frequency heard. This phenomenon was first explained over a century ago by an Austrian physicist, Christian Doppler. The phenomenon can be illustrated by a racing car which sounds more strident and high pitched as it approaches and immediately drops in pitch as it passes and moves away.

Moving red blood cells do not emit sound: the vibration of a piezoelectric element in a

FIGURE 1: Gangrene of the great hallux due to severe arterial disease.

probe produces an external source of ultrasonic sound waves. This sound wave is directed at the moving blood flow and the reflected waves detected by the same probe (FIGURE 2). The received signal, which has been compressed by reflection from blood cells moving towards the probe or elongated by cells moving away, is then amplified into an audible signal or converted into a waveform on an oscilloscope. High frequency Doppler ultrasound probes in the range 6–10 MHz are used for the assessment of vessels close to the skin surface, whilst lower frequency probes with greater penetrating power (1–5 MHz) are used to assess the deeper vessels. The complex array of reflected frequencies produce a characteristic signal (audible or waveform) representative of blood flow through the artery or vein.

Significant disease of the arterial lumen produces blood flow disturbances resulting in deviation from the normal Doppler ultrasound signal. This allows identification of disease proximal to the site of insonation. If significant arterial disease is present in the lower limb vessels, the blood pressure distal to the diseased artery is reduced. Yao first used Doppler ultrasound to replace the conventional stethoscope for measuring systolic blood pressure and a simple method was devised to assess lower limb arterial disease by comparing the ankle and brachial systolic pressures. This is expressed as the ankle/brachial pressure index (ABPI).[2]

The ankle/brachial pressure index technique

The patient is rested supine for 10 minutes eliminating the effect of previous exercise on the blood pressure. A sphygmomanometer pressure cuff is placed around the upper arm, the brachial arterial pulse is identified by palpation and contact jelly then applied.

To achieve the best Doppler signal, there should be an angle of 45 to 60 degrees between the probe and the artery. As the underlying artery may not be parallel to the skin surface, the angle of the probe may require adjustment to achieve the highest quality signal. The cuff is inflated until the signal is lost as blood flow ceases when the brachial artery is occluded.

Care must be taken to ensure the optimum signal is maintained throughout cuff inflation by slight adjustment of the probe position. The brachial systolic blood pressure is recorded as the pressure at which the Doppler signal returns on slow cuff deflation.

To measure the ankle pressure a normal upper arm sphygmomanometer cuff is placed just above ankle. If there is an ulcer at this level,

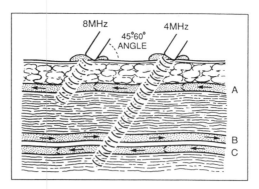

FIGURE 2: An 8 MHz probe assesses the superficial veins (A) with the 4 MHz probe isonating deeper arteries (B) and veins (C).

a non-adherent dressing may be used to protect the wound and prevent the cuffs from being soiled. In patients with painful ulcers the cuff can be placed above the ulcer around the calf but the pressure recorded will be the calf, not ankle pressure. If the posterior tibial artery (located just posterior to the medial malleolus) cannot be identified, then the dorsalis pedis can usually be found on the dorsum of the foot between the first and second metatarsals. A similar procedure to the measurement of the brachial systolic pressure is then performed and the ankle systolic pressure recorded (FIGURE 3).

If the ABPI is more than 0.8 (the lower limit of normal) but the clinical history suggests claudication, an exercise challenge can be performed. The patient walks on a treadmill inclined at 10 degrees at four kilometres per hour for one minute.[3] On completion of the exercise the patient immediately lies supine on the couch and the ankle pressure is measured within 45 seconds.

If the ABPI remains above 0.8, then the arterial supply to the limb will be essentially normal. Although a greater than 20 mmHg fall in ABPI following exercise would indicate

FIGURE 3: Posterior tibial artery systolic pressure being measured.

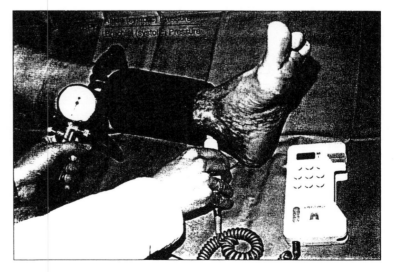

arterial disease, it is likely that wound healing will still be adequate when arterial pressures are above 80–100 mmHg and with an ABPI greater than 0.6.

An ABPI of less than 0.8 indicates significant arterial disease and patients may require more extensive arterial assessment. If the ABPI is less than 0.6, any ulceration may be due primarily to arterial insufficiency. Compression bandaging, recommended for venous ulceration, should not be attempted until further expert assessment has been carried out. Failure to identify arterial signals at the ankle, despite careful examination using Doppler ultrasound, requires a vascular specialist opinion as soon as possible.

In some patients, especially diabetics, the calf and ankle arteries may be incompressible due to calcification of the arterial wall. In these cases the ABPI ratio is unreliable. Experienced Doppler ultrasound users may be able to detect the audible difference between a relatively non-diseased biphasic Doppler waveform and a diseased monophasic waveform.

Another simple test to identify severe arterial disease is to locate a Doppler signal at the ankle with the patient lying supine and raise the foot and leg with the Doppler probe held in place over the artery. If the signal weakens and disappears on elevation, severe arterial disease is likely and further assessment or a vascular specialist's opinion will be required.

FIGURE 4: Spectral waveform analysis and segmental pressure ratios demonstrating left superficial femoral artery occlusion. Normal triphasic waveforms recorded down the right limb, with a monophasic waveform at the left popliteal artery.

Waveform analysis and segmental pressures

As indicated earlier, the frequency shifts caused by blood flow may be converted into a frequency waveform.[4] When this is combined with segmental pressure ratios, the vascular surgeon has the opportunity to investigate the extent and anatomical location of significant arterial disease in an entirely non-invasive way.[5]

Procedure

The common femoral and popliteal artery waveforms are obtained using a 4–5 MHz probe. Normally, all the waveforms should be triphasic: biphasic waveforms indicate mild disease proximal to the site of insonation and a monophasic waveform is indicative of more severe disease (FIGURES 4 and 5). Segmental pressures are done whenever arterial disease has been detected with an ABPI of 0.8 or less. A reduction in ratio of more than 0.2 between cuffs suggests a haemodynamically significant arterial stenosis. When symptoms suggest arterial insufficiency but the ABPI is more than 0.8, an exercise challenge is carried out.

Tests such as these have the advantage that they can be used repeatedly to follow disease progression without undue discomfort or risk of morbidity. This allows the vascular consultant to select the appropriate time for intervention with angiography delayed until immediately before possible reconstructive surgery (if performed at all).

Other applications for Doppler ultrasound

Doppler ultrasound may be used in the pre-operative mapping of veins for arterial bypass surgery. This invariably means detecting and marking the long saphenous vein. Post-surgery, all our lower limb bypass grafts are entered into a graft surveillance programme, where colour flow duplex ultrasound-Doppler is used to

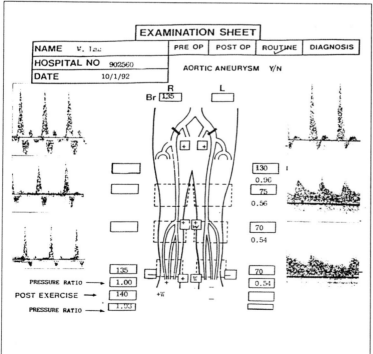

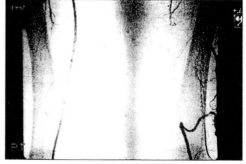

FIGURE 5: Pre-operative arteriography confirming non-invasive vascular findings: a left femoro-popliteal block.

detect haemodynamically significant graft stenoses before graft occlusion occurs.

Interest has recently developed in the screening of abdominal aortic aneurysms (AAA) both in the first degree relatives of patients with symptomatic or operated AAA and also randomly in the community. This has shown that up to six per cent of the male population over the age of 65 years has an AAA.[6] Screening programmes using portable ultrasound monitors are now being set up to reduce the number of patients suffering rupture of aortic aneurysms—normally a fatal event.

Ultrasound can also be used to assess the superficial and deep venous systems. Venous insufficiency in either or both of these systems can present with lower limb ulceration and, if the ABPI is above 0.8, chronic venous insufficiency must be excluded.

Simple Doppler techniques in community medicine

An assessment of the arterial supply to the lower limb can be achieved easily by simple Doppler ultrasound ABPI measurements. Following appropriate training this technique can be performed reliably by general practitioners or community nursing staff.

In addition to the diagnosis of arterial insufficiency as a cause of ulceration, the simple hand-held Doppler may be used for correct diagnosis of other arterial and venous problems. However, this test is only an indicator of the extent of any arterial disease and suspicious results, especially in patients with diabetes, should be referred to a vascular consultant.

Wider use of the Doppler ultrasound technique may improve patient care by reducing the incidence of misdiagnosis and ensuring early referral of arterial disease to a vascular consultant.

References

1. Bouchier-Hayes D, Broe PJ, Grace PA, Mehigan D. *Case presentations in arterial disease.* Oxford: Butterworth-Heinemann, 1991.
2. Yao ST, Hobbs J, Irvine NT. Pulse examination by an ultrasonic method. *Br Med J* 1968; 4: 555–557.
3. Laing SP, Greenhalgh RM. Standard exercise test to assess peripheral arterial disease. *Br Med J* 1980; 13: 1–7.
4. Evans DH, McDicken WN, Skidmore R, Woodcock JP. *Doppler ultrasound—physics, instrumentation and clinical applications.* Chichester: Wiley Medical Publications, 1989.
5. Zwiebel WJ. *Introduction to vascular ultrasonography.* 2nd edition. London: WB Saunders, 1986: 308–311.
6. Collin J, Wallen J, Araiyo L, Lindsell D. Oxford Screening Programme for Abdominal Aortic Aneurysm in men aged 65 to 74 years. *Lancet* 1988; 2: 613–615.

The Use of Doppler Ultrasound 2: Venous Disease

AJ Picton, BSc, *Vascular Technician;* IM Williams, FRCS, *Research Registrar; and* CN McCollum, MD, FRCS, *Professor of Surgery; Department of Vascular Surgery, University Hospital of South Manchester, Nell Lane, West Didsbury, Manchester M20 8LR.*

Simple hand-held Doppler probes can be used to assess both the deep and superficial venous systems.

The venous system returns blood from the tissues to the heart. In the lower leg, veins are categorised into (1) the superficial system and (2) the deep system, interconnected along the length of the leg by a series of perforators communicating the superficial with the deep system. Studies show that chronic venous insufficiency is the single most frequent cause of leg ulceration with over 90 per cent of patients suffering from significant venous incompetence[1] (FIGURE 1). However, arterial insufficiency may be the cause of ulceration in five to 10 per cent and arterial disease may contribute to ulceration in up to 15 per cent of all patients. It is vitally important to exclude arterial insufficiency in patients with leg ulcers and the ankle/brachial pressure index (ABPI) may be used to achieve this.[2] Compression bandaging is the treatment of choice for venous ulceration and may cause pressure necrosis where the arterial blood pressure is lower than the normal pressure.

FIGURE 1: Typical appearance of a large laterally situated venous ulcer.

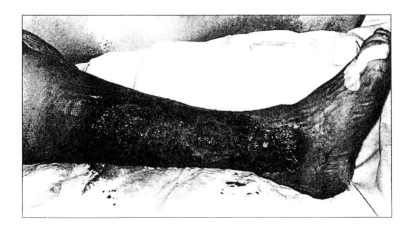

Venous incompetence and insufficiency

Blood is pumped back towards the heart from the legs by the action of the calf muscle pump. During walking the calf muscles contract with each step taken. This compresses the deep veins and forces blood proximally. Normal deep veins have within their lumen a series of valves preventing blood flowing retrogradely. Incompetent valves allow blood to 'leak' down the leg increasing the pressure distally.

Venous incompetence may be identified in the superficial system by examination alone but will only be reliably detected by Doppler ultrasound. Deep venous incompetence is less obvious but is still frequently found in patients with venous disorders. Valvular incompetence may be primary or secondary to venous thrombosis or trauma.

Symptoms of chronic venous insufficiency

Chronic venous insufficiency describes the features of chronic venous hypertension which may be due to incompetence, obstruction and immobility. The main symptoms include:

- Leg oedema.
- Low calf and ankle pigmentation.
- Eczema.
- Induration.
- Postural discomfort.
- Cramps.
- Leg ulceration.

Superficial venous incompetence may be detected in the vast majority of patients with leg ulcers and is often the major or only contributing factor. This highlights the need to assess all patients with severe venous insufficiency in order to select those who could benefit from very simple vein surgery that may even be conducted under local anaesthesia.

Venous Doppler ultrasound

Simple, hand-held Doppler probes can be used to assess both the deep and superficial venous systems. Most large veins have a characteristic audible Doppler ultrasound signature. The signal is usually spontaneous and continuous but is cyclic with respiration; inspiration results in an increased signal volume with a decrease on expiration. The venous signal may then be augmented by compressing the calf. During venous examination with a hand-held instrument, failure to obtain a venous signal may be an indication of venous thrombosis and this should be confirmed by venous duplex Doppler imaging.

Superficial venous Doppler ultrasound (8 MHz probe)

Doppler ultrasound may be used simply to distinguish between pure deep and pure superficial incompetence. This is achieved with the patient standing, with all their weight on the contra-lateral limb so ensuring that the calf muscle is relaxed (FIGURE 2).

The long saphenous vein can be located using

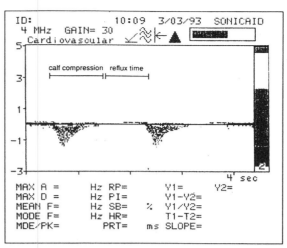

FIGURE 3: **Normal venous spectral waveform.**

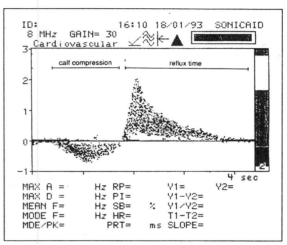

FIGURE 4: **Abnormal venous spectral waveform displaying two second reflux.**

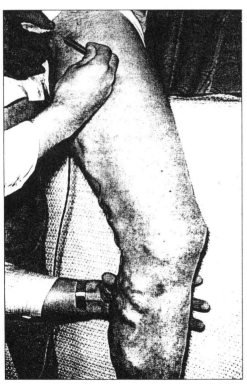

FIGURE 2: **Recommended stance of patient for venous assessment.**

an 8 MHz probe by finding the superficial femoral artery in the thigh which will appear muted due to its greater depth. Moving the probe medially and compressing the calf muscles causes a rush of blood through the femoral vein which will be heard as a muted signal. Moving the probe a little further medially to a spot 2–3 cm below and lateral to the pubic tubercle will reveal a much clearer signal from the long saphenous vein (FIGURE 3).

The venous signal can be distinguished from the arterial signal by its characteristic sound and direction of flow. On release of the calf there should be no reflux (return flow) which would indicate incompetence (FIGURE 4).

To ensure the long saphenous vein, rather than the superficial femoral vein (part of the deep venous system), is being assessed a narrow tourniquet around the lower thigh inflated to approximately 100 mmHg should reduce or prevent flow through the long saphenous but not the deep veins. The short saphenous can be located in the popliteal fossa usually just lateral to the popliteal artery signal and can be mapped down the postero-lateral aspect of the calf. Calf compression when assessing both the popliteal (deep system) and the short saphenous (superficial system) should be carried out low in the calf to prevent movement of skin interfering with the signal.

Competent perforators connect and allow flow from the superficial to the deep venous system. Incompetent perforators result in retrograde blood flow and a reduced efficiency of the deep muscle pump. This is detected by the characteristic high volume signal over the perforator and by failure of a tourniquet above the perforator to control retrograde flow in the relevant vein.

Deep venous Doppler (4 MHz probe)
The assessment is started in the groin region using a 4–5 MHz Doppler probe where the superficial femoral artery is identified. The superficial femoral vein is immediately adjacent and medial and may be followed as far as possible down the leg with intermittent calf compression to assess for reflux. Care should be taken to ensure that the arterial signal can be heard relatively close to the vein distinguishing it from the long saphenous vein. The popliteal vein may be examined in a similar manner and the probe moved radially around the deep vein to ensure that an overlying superficial vein is not the source of the signal.

Reflux time
The duration of reflux in seconds on release of calf compression is a simple and reproducible measure of the severity of venous reflux. The shorter the reflux time the more severe is the venous incompetence. Chronic venous insufficiency is associated with venous refilling times of less than four to five seconds. It may well be that this simple examination will be used in the future to screen for people likely to develop venous ulcers.

Treatment
The accepted method of treating venous ulceration is by four-layer compression bandaging which achieves healing rates of 74 per cent by 12 weeks[3] (FIGURE 5). This overcomes the gravitational effect, prevents blood pooling at the ankle and reduces oedema. Once the ulceration has healed, grade two compression stockings are issued for the same purpose of reducing ulcer recurrence. Recurrence remains a major problem

and occurs in 25 per cent of patients with recently healed venous ulcers each year.

Where the superficial veins are incompetent or where there are incompetent perforators early surgery may enhance healing and help reduce the chance of recurrence. Simple surgery of this type may be performed on Doppler ultrasound findings alone but it is wise to carry out functional investigations such as ambulatory venous pressure (AVP) measurements.[4] AVP allows the direct measurement of venous pressure in foot veins. (Narrow tourniquets to occlude the superficial veins may then be used to simulate the effects of venous surgery.) An incorrect diagnosis of superficial incompetence as the main contributor to venous hypertension in the presence of deep venous incompetence is a major cause of recurrence following either surgery or injection sclerotherapy.

Conclusions
Simple, portable Doppler ultrasound devices may be used to detect both arterial disease and venous incompetence and are becoming indispensable for clinicians and nurses treating leg ulcers. With the correct training most staff soon become adept at the technique and able to distinguish the more unusual causes of ulceration by the exclusion of both arterial and venous insufficiency.

Arterial and severe venous disease are indications for referral to a consultant vascular surgeon with a fully equipped vascular laboratory and experienced vascular technicians. Colourflow duplex-Doppler combines real time arterial and venous imaging by ultrasound with colour-Doppler blood flow to provide an accurate assessment of both vascular anatomy and function. As machine time is limited for these expensive instruments increased awareness of simple arterial and venous Doppler ultrasound techniques permits more efficient usage of vascular laboratory time.

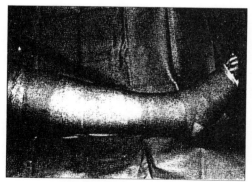

FIGURE 5: Patient with four-layer compression bandaging.

References

1. Cornwall JV, Lewis D. Leg ulcers: epidemiology and etiology. *Br J Surg* 1986; 73: 693.
2. Callam MJ, Ruckley CV, Dale JJ, Harper DR. Hazards of compression treatment of the leg: an estimate from Scottish surgeons. *Br Med J* 1987; 295: 1382.
3. Blair SD, Wright DDI, Backhouse CM, Riddle E. McCollum CN. Sustained compression and healing of chronic venous ulcers. *Br Med J* 1988; 297: 1159.
4. Hopkin NFG, Wolfe JHN. The Investigation of Deep Vein Thrombosis. In: Bell PRF, Jamieson CW, Ruckley CV (Eds). *Surgical management of vascular disease.* Cambridge: Saunders. University Press, 1992.

Wound cleansing – which solution?

MOYA J. MORISON, MSc, BA, RGN
Staff Nurse, Stirling Royal Infirmary

It is an instinctive reaction in both humans and animals to lick a wound. This is the most natural method of wound cleansing and is comforting, providing some temporary pain relief, perhaps by triggering the release of endorphins (opiate-like substances produced by the brain). A review of written records of wound care, dating back 4,000 years suggests, however, that man has used many other methods (Forrest, 1982). Hippocrates (400 BC) recommended that wounds be washed in tepid water, with or without vinegar. Wine and vinegar were probably the first antiseptics to be used systematically. Galen (AD 129-200), a surgeon to the gladiators, washed wounds in sea water which was relatively uncontaminated compared to the urban water supplies. Normal saline is a very useful cleansing agent today. Fortunately some other cleansing agents such as lizards' dung, pigeons' blood and boiling oil, which delayed healing and invariably resulted in suppuration, have gone out of fashion!

The purpose of wound cleansing

The aim of wound cleansing is to help to create the optimum local conditions for wound healing, prior to the application of a wound dressing which should maintain an optimum microenvironment. Wound cleansing therefore involves the removal of state exudate and debris:
- foreign materials (soil, grit, grease, splinters of wood, metal or glass, clothing, chemicals, etc);
- bacteria and other micro-organisms;
- devitalised (dead or ischaemic) soft tissue;
- slough;
- necrotic tissue.

Continued presence of debris might delay the wound's healing and act as foci for infection.

Approaches to cleansing in different wounds

Where tissue is heavily contaminated by dirt and bacteria or is devitalised, *surgical removal* is often the treatment of choice (Haury et al, 1980). Devitalised soft tissue acts as a culture medium, promoting bacterial growth, and the anaerobic environment created inhibits the ability of leucocytes to ingest bacteria and kill them. Unless radical excision of damaged tissue is performed it will not be possible to remove all bacterial contaminants. The difficulty is to decide when a wound is 'clean enough'. Van Rijswijk et al (1985) showed that colonisation of healthy granulating tissue by saprophytes and even low levels of pathogens had little effect on the success of wound healing under an occlusive dressing so it is not always necessary to maintain a *sterile* wound surface, especially if to do so would involve damage to healing tissues by powerful antiseptics.

Decontamination of all but the most minor traumatic wounds is usually done in the A&E department, where treatment methods will generally be decided upon by the casualty officer. In extreme cases, for example severe burns, debridement may need to be done under general anaesthetic, if the patient's condition permits.

Removal of more trivial foreign bodies, such as splinters, fish hooks and superficial grit and grease may be left to the nurse. David's (1986) book on wound management gives an excellent illustrated account of wound care in casualty. The aim is to remove gross contaminants with the minimum of pain to the patient and trauma to the tissues. Immersing the injured part in water or saline at body temperature eases the pain and often helps to loosen debris. *Asepsis is unnecessary until all gross contamination is removed.*

- A moderate to severe irritant response is usually seen within 4-5 days of commencement of use.
- They are toxic to fibroblasts in animal models.
- They can delay the production of collagen.
- They may impair epithelial migration.
- They may prolong the acute inflammatory response stage of healing.

EUSOL has the following additional disadvantage

- It can cause the release of endotoxins from coliforms leading to effects ranging from mild uraemic toxaemia to serious renal failure (the Schwartzmann reaction).

Table 1. The harmful effects of hypochlorites on healing tissues.

Which solution now?

- Kills a wide range of micro-organisms.
- Is effective over a wide range of dilutions.
- Is non-toxic to human tissues.
- Does not easily give rise to sensitivity reactions, either locally or systemically.
- Acts rapidly.
- Works efficiently even in the presence of organic material (eg pus, blood, soap).
- Is inexpensive.
- Has a long shelf life.

Table 2. Characteristics of the ideal antiseptic.

A different approach is needed when cleansing surgically made wounds, which are initially 'clean'. Here *strict asepsis* is needed from the beginning to prevent endogenous or exogenous wound infection, and the possibility of cross infection of other patients.

When cleansing chronic open wounds such as pressure sores or leg ulcers there is some controversy surrounding the need for strict asepsis, especially in the community. Some wound care specialists advise that a 'clean' procedure is sufficient but there is always the risk that the nurse might unwittingly act as a vector for cross infection which could have serious consequences if organisms such as ß-haemolytic streptococci or pseudomonads are involved. Methods for removing necrotic tissue in chronic wounds were discussed in detail by Morison (1987 a and b). Briefly, the main alternatives to surgical excision are:

- **enzymatic treatment,** eg Varidase – which is specific to necrotic tissue and is at a physiological pH;
- **hydrocolloid dressings,** eg Granuflex which rehydrate necrotic tissue and create conditions that encourage the body's natural debriding processes;
- **hypochlorite agents** – which are effective debriding agents but toxic to tissues with prolonged use (Table 1).

Assuming the nurse is dealing with a wound which is not covered with necrotic tissue, which solution should she use to remove loose debris and stale exudate?

For wounds which are not grossly contaminated sterile water or a 0.9 per cent saline solution are the cleansing agents of choice. These simple solutions, or an approximation of them, have been used quite effectively for the last 2,000 years. They are non-toxic and inexpensive. However, where there is a reasonable to high risk of wound infection, for instance in contaminated traumatic wounds and burns, in debilitated patients, or where wounds are so sited that they are likely to have become contaminated by urine or faecal material, an antiseptic solution may be indicated.

The advantages and disadvantages of a number of antiseptics were reviewed by Morison (1987a) and the characteristics of the ideal antiseptic are listed in Table 2. When choosing an antiseptic it is necessary to balance the antiseptic's effectiveness as a bactericidal or bacteristatic agent against the likely degree of damage to healthy human tissues. **Eusol and hypochlorites** are known to delay healing (Table 1) (Brennan et al, 1985; 1986). Although they are undoubtedly effective in debridement (Leaper and Simpson, 1986) it is inadvisable to use such toxic agents routinely.

Aqueous chlorhexidine solutions, however, have many of the characteristics of the ideal antiseptic. They have a low toxicity to living tissues in animal models (Brennan et al, 1985; 1986; Platt and Bucknall, 1984; Saatman et al, 1986) and are effective against a wide range of Gram-positive and Gram-negative organisms, but they are not effective against acid-fast bacilli, bacterial spores, fungi or viruses and their activity, too, is reduced by organic matter such as blood, pus and soap (Reynolds, 1982).

Some cleansing solutions combine the proven broad spectrum, antimicrobial properties of chlorhexidine with the detergent properties of **cetrimide** and are useful in cleansing grossly contaminated traumatic wounds and burns. Cetrimide alone has certain specific uses (Table 3), but precautions are required by pharmacy when making up the diluted solutions, to guard against bacterial contamination, especially by *Pseudomonas* spp.

Povidone-iodine is a potent antimicrobial agent used widely and effectively in pre- and postoperative skin disinfection and cleansing (Gilmore and Martin, 1974; Gray and Lee, 1981), and in outpatient open wound management (Helm, 1978). It has a special part to play in reducing wound sepsis in burns (Parks et al, 1978; Boswick, 1978; Zellner and Bugyi, 1985). In a burn injury there may be irreversible damage to the microcirculation so that neither the body's own immune system components nor parenterally administered antibiotics are able to penetrate rapidly to the site where they are most needed, and micro-organisms can proliferate in the nutrient medium provided by the dead tissue. Wound sepsis remains the commonest cause of death in such patients, and local treatment of infected burns with antiseptics is needed.

The value of antiseptics in the management of other open wounds is more difficult to assess and further studies of the interactions between antiseptics, bacteria and the immune system are needed *in humans* to determine the situations where their use is most beneficial (Leaper and Simpson, 1986). Antiseptics require *time* in contact with bacteria if they are to kill them or inhibit their division. Where an antiseptic is only used in passing, as a cleansing solution, and does not remain in contact with the wound after the wound toilet is completed, it may not have time to be effective. If bacteria are merely being removed by the physical action of cleaning, at a dressing stage, then normal saline should be as effective a cleansing agent as any, and has no unwanted side-effects.

Applying the cleansing solution

There are two basic methods for mechanically cleansing a wound: irrigation or direct 'scrubbing' with a cotton wool ball or gauze. The difficulty with irrigation is how to apply the cleansing solution under sufficient pressure to dislodge the debris, without damaging the underlying tissue (Westaby, 1985). It is also possible to damage wound tissue by rough handling with cotton wool balls or gauze swabs. Many different swabbing techniques are practised in Britain and America, but a study by Thomlinson (1987) found that, of the three methods she tested in discharging surgical wounds, no technique was significantly better than the others, and all techniques merely resulted in the redistribution of micro-organisms.

The meaning of pain

Dressing changes and wound cleansing can be painful procedures, especially at the first time of treatment. The procedure should be explained to the patient beforehand and any prescribed analgesia given. If the patient becomes distressed during the procedure, then Entonox may be indicated. However, if painful dressing changes become the normal experience for a particular patient then the nurse should question her own treatment methods:

- **Is a cleansing agent being used which is *known* to produce an irritant response with prolonged use, eg hypochlorites, eusol?** If so, discontinue use.
- **Is the dressing being changed too infrequently?** – even 'non-adherent' dressings may adhere if left in place too long, especially in a wound where the exudate strikes through the dressing and dries out. Delicate underlying tissues may then be traumatised when the dressing is removed, causing unnecessary pain and delayed healing.
- **Is the wound infected?** – the classical signs of infection may not be obvious at first but it may well be worth sending a wound swab off to the Bacteriology department for culture and sensitivity testing.
- **Does the patient feel the nurse is lacking in empathy?** Is the nurse minimising the psychological and social significance of the wound to the individual? It might be timely to discuss the meaning of the wound with the patient, as well as the treatment plan and likely prognosis, if this has not already been done.

Product directory

Table 3 summarises uses, advantages and disadvantages of individual products. This is useful for reference on the wards. In addition, two solutions are included which have been available for many years and which still have certain specialist uses: silver nitrate and potassium permanganate. Incorrectly used, however, these solutions can be very hazardous and special attention is drawn to the information on adverse effects included in the table.

Do we need to cleanse wounds at every dressing change?

If a wound is *grossly contaminated* by foreign material, bacteria, slough or necrotic tissue, wound cleansing is necessary at every dressing change to prevent delayed healing. If a wound is clean, there is little exudate, and it is healthily granulating, however, repeated cleaning may do more harm than good, by traumatising newly produced and delicate tissues, by reducing the surface temperature of the wound, and by removing exudate which itself may have bactericidal properties (Hohn et al, 1977).

Why nurses find it hard to choose

There are many reasons why nurses find it hard to choose the most appropriate cleansing agent in a particular situation. There is, for instance, a shortage of information on cleansing agents in most nursing textbooks. A glance at Table 3 shows that the problem is compounded by the number of products with similar active ingredients. It is hoped this article will help sort out some of the confusion.

References

Boswick, J.A. (1978) The use of Betadine antiseptics in treating burns and other wounds of the hand. The Proceedings of the World Congress on Antisepsis. New York, H P 160-162.

Brennan, S.S. and Leaper, D.J. (1985) The effect of antiseptics on the healing wound: a study using rabbit earchamber. *British Journal of Surgery*, **72**, 10, 780-782.

Brennan, S.S., Foster, M.E. and Leaper, D.J. (1986) Antiseptics toxicity in wounds healing by secondary intention. *Journal of Hospital Infection*, **8**, 3, 263-267.

David, J.A. (1986) Wound management: a comprehensive guide to dressing and healing. Dunitz, London.

Forrest, R.D. (1982) Early history of wound treatment. *Journal of the Royal Society of Medicine*, **75**, 198-205.

Gilmore, O.J.A. and Martin, T.D.M. (1974) Aetiology and prevention of wound infection in appendicectomy. *British Journal of Surgery*, **61**, 281-287.

Gray, J.G. and Lee, M.J.R. (1981) The effect of topical povidone-iodine on wound infection following abdominal surgery. *British Journal of Surgery*, **68**, 310-313.

Haury, B. et al (1980) Debridement: an essential component of traumatic wound care. In: Hunt, T.K. (ed) Wound Healing and Wound Infection: Theory and Surgical Practice. Appleton Century Crofts, New York.

Helm, P.A. (1978) Outpatient wound management with Betadine products (Povidone-iodine). The Proceedings of the World Congress on Antisepsis. New York H P 105-108.

Hohn, D.C. et al (1977) Antimicrobial systems of the surgical wound. *American Journal of Surgery*, **133**, 5, 597-600.

Leaper, D.J. and Simpson, R.A. (1986) The effect of antiseptics and topical antimicrobials on wound healing. *Journal of Antimicrobial Chemotherapy*, **17**, 2, 135-137.

Morison, M.J. (1987a) Preventing delayed wound healing. *The Professional Nurse*, **2**, 9, 298-300.

Morison, M.J. (1987b) Priorities in wound management: part I. *The Professional Nurse*, **2**, 11, 352-355.

Parks, D.M. et al (1978) Wound healing in burns. The Proceedings of the World Congress on Antisepsis, New York. H P 138-140.

Platt J. and Bucknall, R.A. (1984) An experimental evaluation of antiseptic wound irrigation. *Journal of Hospital Infection*, **5**, 181-188.

Reynolds, J.E.F. (ed) (1982) Martindale: The Extra Pharmacopoeia. The Pharmaceutica Press (28th edition), London.

Saatman, R. et al (1986) A wound healing study of Chlorhexidine digluconate in guinea pigs. *Fundamental and Applied Toxicology*, **6**, 1-6.

Thomlinson, D. (1987) To clean or not to clean? *Nursing Times*, **83**, 9, 71-75.

Van Rijswijk et al (1985) Multicentre clinical evaluation of a hydrocolloid dressing for leg ulcers. *Cutis*, **35**, 173-176.

Westaby, S. (ed) (1985) Wound Care. Heinemann Medical Books, London.

Zellner, P.R. and Bugyi, S. (1985) Povidone-iodine in the treatment of burn patients. *Journal of Hospital Infection*, **6**, (Supplement) 139-146.

CLEANSING AGENT	BRAND NAME	PHARMACEUTICAL COMPANY	COLOUR OF SOLUTION	USES	PRECAUTIONS/ CONTRAINDICATIONS/ ETC.
Purified water	Aquasol	S + P	Colourless	Topical irrigation of 'clean' wounds.	Warm to body temperature if irrigating a large area.
Sodium chloride (0.9% w/v)	Normasol Topiclens	S + P / S + N	Colourless	Topical irrigation and cleansing of wounds, burns and eyes.	As for sterile water.
Chlorhexidine gluconate (0.05%)	Hibidil Unisept Bacticlens	ICI / S + P / S + N	Pink	Cleansing of wounds and burns where an antiseptic solution is indicated.	Products containing **CHLORHEXIDINE** should *not* come into contact with (a) eyes (b) middle ear (c) brain or meninges.
Chlorhexidine acetate (0.05%)	Chlorasept 2000	T(B)			
Chlorhexidine gluconate (0.015%) & cetrimide (0.15%)	Savlodil Tisept Cetriclens	ICI / S + P / S + N	Yellow	Cleansing contaminated, traumatic and infected wounds and burns, surgical wounds, and swabbing in obstetrics.	Products containing **CETRIMIDE** can cause skin irritation and occasionally sensitisation.
Chlorhexidine acetate (0.015%) & cetrimide (0.15%)	Travasept 100	T(B)			
Chlorhexidine gluconate (0.015%) & cetrimide (0.5%)	Cetriclens Forte	S + N	Amber yellow	Initial cleansing of physically contaminated wounds eg, traumatic wounds and burns.	*Contraindications:* in patients who have previously shown a hypersensitivity reaction to chlorhexidine or cetrimide. Such reactions are extremely rare.
Chlorhexidine gluconate (0.05%) & cetrimide (0.5%)	Savloclens	ICI			
Chlorhexidine acetate (0.05%) & cetrimide (0.5%)	Travasept 30	T(B)			

CLEANSING AGENT	BRAND NAME	PHARMACEUTICAL COMPANY	COLOUR OF SOLUTION	USES	PRECAUTIONS/ CONTRAINDICATIONS/ ETC.
Cetrimide (40%) (aqueous stock solutions should contain at least 4% v/v isopropanol or 7% v/v ethanol as a precaution against bacterial contamination).	Cetavlon	ICI	Pale straw	*0.5-1% solution:* cleansing wounds contaminated by dirt or grease. *1-3% solution:* in skin diseases, cleansing skin of scabs, crusts and ointments.	**Contraindications:** previous hypersensitivity to cetrimide. *Precautions:* **DILUTE BEFORE USE:** concentrated solutions can cause severe burn-like reactions. Keep out of eyes, and avoid contact with brain meninges or middle ear. Avoid prolonged and repeated applications to skin as hyper-sensitivity may result.
Povidone-iodine (0.5%) (aerosol dry powder spray)	Disadine DP	Stuart	Golden Brown	Treatment and prevention of infection in wounds including burns, leg ulcers and pressure sores.	**Contraindications:** non-toxic goitre. **Warning:** Prolonged treatment with povidone-iodine of patients with *severe and extensive burns* may cause: metabolic acidosis, hypernatraemia, and renal impairment. Also avoid prolonged use in *pregnant or lactating women* as absorbed iodine can cross placental barrier and is secreted into breast milk. **Precautions:** Known iodine-sensitive patients – very rarely produces skin reactions. Avoid inhalation and contact with eyes.
Povidone-iodine (2.5%) (pressurised aerosol)	Betadine dry powder spray	Napp		Treatment and prevention of infection in ulcers, burns, incisions, minor injuries etc.	
Povidone-iodine (5%) (pressurised aerosol)	Betadine antiseptic spray	Napp			
Povidone-iodine (10%) (in alcoholic solution)	Betadine alcoholic solution	Napp		Pre- and postoperative skin disinfection.	
Povidone-iodine (10%) (in aqueous solution)	Betadine antiseptic	Napp			
Hydrogen peroxide (3%)	–	Hospital pharmacy	Colourless	Cleansing and deodorising wounds and ulcers.	Possible irritant response with prolonged use. Bleaches fabric.
Chlorinated lime (1.25%) and boric acid (1.25%) with at least 0.25% available chlorine	eusol	Hospital pharmacy	Colourless	Disadvantages greatly outweigh any advantages, therefore use is **NOT** recommended (see Table 1).	**SEE TEXT** Avoid contact with eyes. Protect surrounding intact skin with yellow soft paraffin or equivalent ointment. Discontinue use if severe or prolonged irritation occurs.
Surgical chlorinated soda solution: chlorinated lime, sodium carbonate and boric acid with 0.5-0.55% available chlorine	Dakin's solution				
Sodium hypochlorite with 0.3-0.4% available chlorine	Chlorasol	S + P Hospital pharmacy			
Silver nitrate (0.5% solution)	–	Hospital pharmacy	Colourless	Was used to reduce infection rate in burns but no longer first choice. Can be used in short term to seal suppurating lesions and to reduce hypergranulation.	Adverse effects can include: hypochloraemia and hyponatraemia with prolonged use in burns patients; argyria; methaemoglobinaemia. Stains skin black.
Potassium permanganate solution (1 in 8000 dilution)	–	Hospital pharmacy	Purple	Cleansing and deodorising suppurating eczematous wounds and acute dermatoses, especially useful prophylactically where there is risk of secondary infection.	Irritant to mucous membranes. Can cause corrosive burns if too concentrated. Stains skin brown.

Table 3. Wound cleansing agents (Note: all agents are **STERILE, AQUEOUS SOLUTIONS** *unless indicated otherwise and for* **EXTERNAL USE** Abbreviations: S + N = Smith + Nephew, S + P = Seton & Prebbles, T(B) = Travenol (Baxter Health Care).

Graduated compression hosiery for venous ulceration

An update on compression hosiery for the management of venous leg ulcers

Graduated compression hosiery is used for several clinical conditions related to venous insufficiency and lymphoedema. In the management of venous ulceration, graduated compression hosiery is regarded as an essential component of prevention of ulcer occurrence. Occasionally it is used for ulcer healing. Graduated compression hosiery is also used prophylactically in the prevention of deep vein thrombosis[1].

Research supporting its use is sparse. However, medical and nursing clinicians recognise its value in clinical practice.

Clinical effects
The primary underlying cause of venous ulceration is the development of pathological changes caused by prolonged venous hypertension. Damage to deep, superficial or perforating venous systems can precipitate this change and will be aggravated by paralysis or immobility in patients with poor calf muscle function.

During venous hypertension, abnormally high pressures are transmitted to the capillary system when valve failure allows reverse blood flow. Normal venous capillary pressure is in the region of 25mmHg and may rise in a patient with venous disease to over 90mmHg[2]. Over time the familiar skin changes associated with venous hypertension develop, such as oedema, eczema, pigmentation changes, atrophy blanche, induration and ulceration.

Graduated compression hosiery is used to apply external pressure to the skin and underlying tissues, to support the superficial veins and to help counteract the raised capillary pressure, thereby reducing oedema. Reduction of oedema has been shown to be a crucial factor in relation to ulcer healing[3], in maintaining skin integrity and preventing further pathological deterioration[2].

Studies have identified that, in a pro-

C. Moffatt, RGN, NDN, is director of education and clinical practice; L. O'Hare, BA, RGN, is a lecturer practitioner, Centre for Research and Implementation of Clinical Practice, London

Compression hosiery; Leg ulcers

portion of those patients who are ambulant, compression hosiery can lower venous pressures by improving the closure of the semi-lunar valves in the superficial veins and decreasing vein diameter[4]. Compression hosiery has also been shown to improve the velocity of blood flow within the deep system[5].

Compression hosiery is widely used as a prophylactic measure in the prevention of deep vein thrombosis. Its exact therapeutic effect remains unclear, although recent work has suggested that the use of anti-embolism stockings pre- and post-operatively prevents venous distension, which causes endothelial tears precipitating the formation of a thrombosis[6].

Compression therapy has also been used in combination with vein ligation and sclerotherapy. This area is still controversial and open to debate, although a five-year follow up study by Dinn and Henry[7] demonstrated a 26% recurrence rate at five years using a combination of treatments. Despite the absence of large randomised controlled trials, venous surgery should be considered, particularly in young patients who may be doomed to recurrent bouts of ulceration.

Ulcer recurrence
While research relating to recurrence of ulceration remains sparse, studies suggest that rates of recurrence may be high[8]. Compliance with wearing compression hosiery as part of a leg ulcer care programme has been shown to affect the incidence of re-ulceration[9]. In a randomised controlled trial undertaken in Riverside Health Authority, the recurrence rate in patients who wore and

complied with stockings was 28% at 18 months, compared to 57% in patients who did not wear stockings[9].

This same study provided insight into the clinical risk factors associated with ulcer recurrence. Independent risk factors were the previous size of the ulcer (>10cm), a history of deep vein thrombosis and unsuitability for stockings. These illustrate that the severity of the underlying disease is an important factor in the recurrence of ulceration.

Johnson[10] identified that patients reported difficulties in the use of compression hosiery and Travers[11] found that of 32 women, 17 did not wear their stockings at all, while 60% found the cosmetic appearance unacceptable. Other factors identified were the presence of friable skin, difficulty in application and removal of stockings[12] and skin irritation following application[9].

The subject of leg ulcer recurrence is complex, and a positive and preventive management strategy requires that clinicians adopt a holistic approach to patient assessment and re-assessment.

Patient assessment
A detailed patient history can identify whether the patient has a high risk of ulcer recurrence. In addition, the patient's level of compliance must be considered. Factors affecting compliance are the patient's attitude, level of motivation and ownership of the problem. An account of the patient's knowledge and understanding of the treatment, previous experiences and future expectations can aid clarification of these issues, and enables the clinician to plan individualised patient education programmes to facilitate a shared approach to care. Incorporating concepts such as the Health Belief Model[13] within a life context framework emphasises the multi-factorial aspects of changing behaviour and life style.

Potential hazards of compression hosiery

- Pressure necrosis because of concurrent arterial disease

- Friction or pressure damage owing to poor fitting hosiery

- Skin allergies or irritation

- Tourniquet effect in patients who cannot apply or remove stockings

Prior to the application of compression hosiery a detailed patient assessment should be undertaken to identify any factors which may undermine the therapeutic effect and wearability of the garment. The potential hazards of compression hosiery need to be acknowledged as this may influence the type of stocking chosen.

Areas at risk of pressure damage

- Tibial crest

- Constricting cuffs around arthritic knees

- Dorsum of foot

- Ankle deformity

- Crowded, deformed toes

- Bunion area

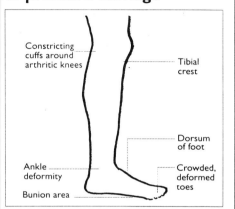

Aids to application of stockings

- Valet (Medi)
- Rubber gloves   ) assist patient
  Talcum powder) grip

- Chinese slipper) aid ease of
  Plastic bag   ) application of
  Nylon stocking) stocking over foot

Consider if the patient has any known allergies

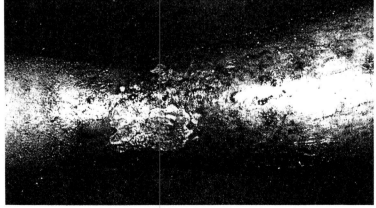

An acute reaction to compression hosiery: the patient is allergic to rubber

---

Useful prescribing information

- Garment required (brand name if necessary)

- Class of stocking

- Length of garment – below knee, thigh, tights

- Quantity required

- Size, with ankle calf measurements (thigh if necessary)

- Open or closed toe

- Colour

Availability in the community of stockings on Drug Tariff

Many of the earlier studies which focused on stocking performance were undertaken prior to a change in specifications on the NHS Drug Tariff. Cornwall et al.[15] identified a wide difference in the pressure ranges of different brands. Further research is now needed in the light of these recent developments.

Make	Class	Style	Foot	Size	Length
Credalast	Class 1	B/K or Thigh	Open toe	Sm/Med/Lg/ExLg	Std/Long
Credalast	Class 2	B/K or Thigh	Open toe	Sm/Med/Lg/ExLg	Std/Long
Credalast	Class 3	B/K or Thigh	Open toe	Sm/Med/Lg/ExLg	Std/Long
New Venosan	Class 1	B/K or Thigh	Full foot	Sm/Med/Lg	One length
New Venosan	Class 2	B/K or Thigh	Open toe	Sm/Med/Lg	Std/Long
New Venosan	Class 3	B/K or Thigh	Open toe	Sm/Med/Lg	Std/Long
Duomed	Class 1	B/K or Thigh	F/F or O/T	Sm/Med/Lg/ExLg	One length
Duomed	Class 2	B/K or Thigh	Open toe	Sm/Med/Lg/ExLg	One length
Duomed	Class 3	B/K or Thigh	Open toe	Sm/Med/Lg/ExLg	One length
Eesilite	Class 1	B/K or Thigh	F/F or O/T	Sm/Med/Lg/ExLg	One length
Eesilite	Class 2	B/K or Thigh	F/F or O/T	Sm/Med/Lg/ExLg	One length
Eesilite	Class 3	B/K or Thigh	F/F or O/T	Sm/Med/Lg/ExLg	One length
Scholl	Class 1	B/K or Thigh	Full foot	Sm/Med/Lg/ExLg	One length
Scholl	Class 2	B/K or Thigh	Open toe	Sm/Med/Lg/ExLg	One length
Scholl	Class 2	B/K or Thigh	Full foot	Sm/Med/Lg/ExLg	One length
Scholl	Class 2	Thigh	Full foot	Sm/Med/Lg/ExLg	One length
Scholl Soft grip	Class 2	B/K or Thigh	Open toe	Sm/Med/Lg/ExLg	One length
Scholl	Class 3	B/K or Thigh	Open toe	Sm/Med/Lg/ExLg	One length
Lastosheer	Class 1	B/K or Thigh	Full foot	Sm/Med/Lg/ExLg	One length
Lastosheer	Class 2	B/K or Thigh	Full foot	Sm/Med/Lg/ExLg	One length
Lastosheer	Class 3	B/K or Thigh	Full foot	Sm/Med/Lg/ExLg	One length

Key
B/K – Below knee
F/F – Full foot
O/T – Open toe

Patient assessment

- Ensure adequate arterial circulation (preferably with Doppler ultrasound)
- Check skin integrity
- Check for known allergies
- Examine for joint deformity
- Measure limb for hosiery
- Check manual dexterity
- Assess patient compliance

Measuring the normal limb for hosiery

- Use a tape measure
  A – measure the ankle circumference at narrowest point
  B – measure the calf at widest point
  C – for thigh length measure at widest point
- Check these measurements fall within the given range for stocking type (measurement outside range requires made-to-measure stocking)
- Measurements D & E are important in excessively tall or short patients

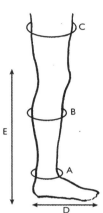

Compression hosiery

	Pressure applied	Recommended use
Class I	14-17mmHg	Varicose veins, mild oedema
Class II	18-24mmHg	Moderate/severe, varicose veins, prevention of ulcer, recurrence
Class III	25-35mmHg	Gross varices, post-phlebitic limb, recurrent ulceration, lymphoedema

A disproportionate limb requiring a made-to-measure stocking

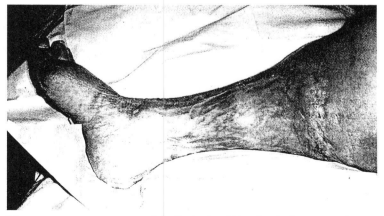

The accurate measurement of the limb should be clearly documented

Many of the problems that patients have to confront in relation to compliance with compression hosiery can be alleviated by knowledgeable and imaginative clinical management. Nurses are important resources for accurate patient information and are responsible for providing verbal and written advice on the application, removal and general care of the stockings.

Measuring the limb

The accurate measurement of the limb should be clearly documented on the patient's records. Where two limbs are involved, they should be measured separately. The optimum time to measure the affected limb is at the start of the day or as soon as the ulcer has healed. The cause of ill-fitting or uncomfortable hosiery is inaccurate measurement, the wrong prescription or an alteration in the patient's limb circumference owing to oedema. An assessment of areas at high risk of pressure damage and the correct measurement procedure for compression hosiery can positively promote patient compliance.

While the majority of patients' limbs will be accommodated by the standard size available on prescription, some patients with disproportionate limbs are unsuitable for standard size compression hosiery and may require a made-to-measure stocking.

It is generally accepted by clinicians that knee-length stockings are as effective as those that are thigh length[5]. The latter are advocated where oedema accumulates above the knee joint or arthritic changes to the knee increase discomfort.

The limb is ready for the application of stockings once the newly epithelialised area of the ulcer has regained a degree of its previous tensile strength.

Often the trauma of application and removal can damage friable skin and it is advisable to allow two to four weeks after the ulcer has healed before commencing the treatment.

It is recommended that stockings are removed at night and re-applied in the morning. For many patients, because of physical constraints, this will not be possible and stockings will be left on overnight and changed weekly. Attention to skin hygiene is then essential. Basic skin care should incorporate the topical application of a bland ointment or emollient to the limb to promote and maintain its integrity. Patients should be advised which cream or ointment to use and be warned to avoid highly perfumed products or those containing lanolin, which may lead to allergy.

The involvement of a chiropodist or orthotist is important where nail care and specialist foot wear are indicated. The patient or carer should be encouraged to report to a nurse at the earliest opportunity any area of discoloration or change in the skin texture.

Aids to application

There are several aids to assist in the application of compression hosiery. A Valet (Medi) is a useful applicator aid, particularly for otherwise independent patients who have only a limited degree of mobility and dexterity in their hands, hips and ankles. This aid is not available on prescription. In some areas nurses have liaised with occupational therapists and the Valet (Medi) is available through an equipment store.

Other less expensive devices include the use of a plastic bag placed on the foot or chinese slippers, wearing rubber gloves or using talcum powder. In circumstances where the patient is unable to use any aid, it is appropriate that an auxiliary nurse, home help, relative or other carer is co-opted to provide this essential care. A short training session or demonstration with written guidelines enables the nurse to share this responsibility while maintaining patient safety.

Classes of compression hosiery

Choice of class of compression stocking generally relates to the underlying pathology. A Class II stocking which exerts approximately 18-24mmHg of pressure at the ankle is generally recognised as sufficient to prevent ulcer recurrence, although little research is available to support this argument.

Patients with limited mobility in their hands may find it easier to use two Class I stockings, removing one layer at night. Patients with significant deep vein damage or those suffering recurrent bouts of ulceration, may benefit from a Class III stocking applying pressures of 25-35mmHg. However, these stockings may be difficult for elderly patients to apply. Essential information to be included within a prescription for hosiery can facilitate the provision of correctly fitting garments. It is suggested by manufacturers that compression hosiery is renewed six monthly. The affected limb should be re-measured on each occasion.

Compression hosiery should not be applied to patients with significant arterial disease. Careful assessment of the patient includes ensuring an adequate arterial circulation is present, preferably using Doppler ultrasound[14].

Stocking availability

Many of the earlier studies which focused on stocking performance were undertaken prior to 1988 when the British Standards performance was changed. Previously there had been only a limited choice of compression hosiery available on prescription. From 1988 a change in specifications for products on the NHS Drug Tariff meant the inclusion criteria were based on performance as well as the construction of the garment.

Conclusion

Several studies[9,12] have demonstrated that compression hosiery has a significant role as part of a preventive programme to reduce the incidence of leg ulcer recurrence. However, this continues to be a contentious issue, and further research in this area of care is needed.

REFERENCES
1. Cornwall, J.V., Dore, C.J., Lewis, J.D. Leg ulcers: epidemiology and aetiology. Br J Surg 1986; 73: 693-696.
2. Browse, N.L., Burnand, K.G., Lea Thomas, M. *Diseases of the Veins: Diagnosis, pathology and treatment.* London: Edward Arnold, 1988.
3. Myers, M.B., Rigtnor, M., Cherry, G.W. Relationship between oedema and the healing rate of stasis ulcers of the leg. Am J Surg 1972; 124: 666-668.
4. Somerville, J.J.F., Brow, G.O., Byrne, P.J. et al. The effects of elastic stockings on superficial venous pressures in patients with venous insufficiency. Br J Surg 1974; 61: 9979-9981.
5. Lawrence, D., Kakkar, V.V. Graduated static external compression of the lower limb: a physiological assessment. Br J Surg 1980; 67: 119-121.
6. Coleridge-Smith, P.D., Hasty, J.H., Scurr, J.H. Deep vein thrombosis: effect of graduated compression stockings on the deep veins of the calf. Br J Surg 1991; 78: 724-726.
7. Dinn, E., Henry, M. Treatment of venous ulceration by injection sclerotherapy and compression hosiery: a 5-year study. Phlebol 1992; 7: 23-26.
8. Callam, M.J., Ruckley, C.V., Harper, D.R., Dale, J.J. Chronic ulceration of the leg: clinical history. BMJ 1987; 294: 1855-1856.
9. Moffatt, C.J., Dorman, M.C. Recurrence of leg ulcers within a community ulcer service. JWC 1995; 4: 9, 57-61.
10. Johnson, G.V. Elastic stockings. BMJ 1988; 296: 720.
11. Travers, J.P., Harrison, J.D., Makin, D.S. Post-operative use of compression stockings in preventing recurrence of varicose veins. Paper presented to the Venous Forum of the Royal Society of Medicine. London, 1990.
12. Cherry, G.W. Leg ulcers: in support of stockings. Comm Outlook 1986; 8: 29-31.
13. Shillitoe, R.W. Christie, H.J. Determinants of self care: the Health Belief Model. Holistic Medicine 1989; 4: 1, 3-17.
14. Moffatt, C.J., O'Hare, L. Ankle pulses are not sufficient to detect impaired arterial circulation in patients with leg ulcers. JWC 1995; 4: 3, 134-137.
15. Cornwall, J.V., Dore, C.J., Lewis, J.D. Graduated compression and its relation to venous refilling time. BMJ 1987; 295: 1087-1090.

CURRENT CONCEPTS

ASSESSMENT AND MANAGEMENT OF FOOT DISEASE IN PATIENTS WITH DIABETES

Gregory M. Caputo, M.D.,
Peter R. Cavanagh, Ph.D.,
Jan S. Ulbrecht, M.D.,
Gary W. Gibbons, M.D.,
and Adolf W. Karchmer, M.D.

THE human and financial costs of lower-extremity amputation in patients with diabetes mellitus are well recognized.[1] However, the rates of major amputation in the United States remain high,[2] in part because present knowledge regarding the prevention and management of foot disease is not widely applied in clinical practice. The U.S. Department of Health has set a goal for the year 2000 of a 40 percent reduction in amputation rates among diabetic patients.[3] Methods to achieve this goal are available today. For example, in the majority of diabetic patients, the initial condition that eventually leads to amputation is a skin ulcer.[4] The simple technique of testing for sensory neuropathy with a monofilament can be used to identify patients at risk for ulceration and therefore most in need of preventive intervention. Computerized analysis of plantar pressure distribution can identify focal areas at high risk for ulceration that merit protection with preventive footwear. Up to 90 percent of ulcers will heal when treated with a comprehensive approach that includes techniques for relieving weight from the ulcerated area, treatment of infection, and restoration of arterial perfusion.[5,6] The total-contact cast allows continued ambulation while effectively relieving pressure at the site of the ulcer. Arterial reperfusion with the use of bypass grafts to pedal vessels represents an important advance in limb salvage.

THE NEUROPATHIC ULCER

The Role of Neuropathy

Sensory neuropathy, ischemia, and infection are the principal pathogenic factors in foot disease associated with diabetes. Peripheral neuropathy has a central role and is present in over 80 percent of diabetic patients with foot lesions.[4,7,8] In most cases, ulceration is a consequence of the loss of protective sensation —

that is, the loss of awareness of trauma that can cause the breakdown of the skin.[9-11]

A simple method can identify patients who have lost protective sensation.[10] A nylon monofilament (designated 5.07) is pressed against the skin to the point of buckling (Fig. 1). Patients who cannot feel the monofilament are at risk for ulceration and require special care.[10] A test with a monofilament is as effective as more time-consuming tests of vibration and thermal sensation in identifying patients prone to ulceration.[11] All patients with diabetes should be assessed annually with this inexpensive, rapidly performed test.

The Role of Mechanical Stress

Among patients who have lost protective sensation, injuries from small foreign bodies in footwear, pressure necrosis from poorly fitting footwear, and puncture wounds often go unnoticed. However, the most common mechanism of injury appears to be unperceived, excessive, and repetitive pressure on plantar bony prominences, such as the metatarsal heads.[12,13] Foot deformities, such as clawing of the toes, contribute to elevated focal pressure, making ulceration even more likely. The most devastating acute and chronic deformities, including bony dislocation and collapse of the arch, result from Charcot's neuroarthropathy.[14,15] Methods for clinically predicting areas of high pressure are summarized in Table 1. Measurement of plantar pressure distribution, which identifies areas of high focal pressure, is performed at specialized centers (Fig. 2A).[12,16-19]

Management of Neuropathic Ulcers

Initially, a neuropathic ulcer of the foot must be assessed for infection, débrided of devitalized tissue, and examined by radiography to detect foreign bodies, soft-tissue gas, or bony abnormalities. Effective treatment requires that weight bearing be eliminated.[20,21] Foot ulcers commonly fail to heal simply because patients continue to put weight on their feet. Because a prolonged period with no weight put on the affected foot (i.e., strict bed rest) is usually unrealistic, devices are required that reduce pressure at the site of the ulcer while allowing ambulation.[22-24] Small, shallow ulcers have been treated successfully with felted foam inserts. However, the total-contact cast is the optimal device for protecting neuropathic ulcers during ambulation (Fig. 3).[24,25] This device, advocated by Brand and colleagues for the management of neuropathic ulcers due to leprosy, differs from a typical orthopedic cast. The total-contact cast is minimally padded and carefully molded to the shape of the foot and leg, with a heel for walking. It is designed to distribute pressure over the entire surface of the foot and lower leg and thereby protect the site of the ulcer. The cast should be removed 24 to 48 hours after application to assess the adequacy of the fit. Another cast is then applied and changed every week thereafter. Healing generally occurs in 8 to 10 weeks (Fig. 2B and 2C). The Carville splint and Scotch cast boot are alternatives to the total-contact cast that are removable and therefore

From the Department of Medicine, Pennsylvania State University College of Medicine, Milton S. Hershey Medical Center, Hershey, Pa. (G.M.C., P.R.C., J.S.U.); and the Departments of Surgery (G.W.G.) and Medicine (A.W.K.), New England Deaconess Hospital, Harvard Medical School, Boston. Address reprint requests to Dr. Caputo at the Division of General Internal Medicine, Milton S. Hershey Medical Center, 500 University Dr., Hershey, PA 17033.

Supported in part by a grant (R01-DK 42912) to Drs. Cavanagh and Ulbrecht from the National Institute of Diabetes and Digestive and Kidney Diseases.

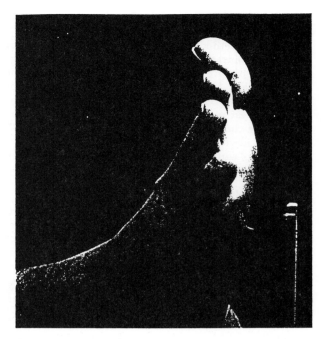

Figure 1. A Simple Office Test to Determine Whether a Patient Has Protective Sensation in the Feet.

A nylon monofilament (NC 12750 #14 [5.07]; North Coast Medical, San Jose, Calif.) is pressed against the skin of the foot. When buckling occurs (as shown), a known force has been applied to the skin. The inability of the patient to feel the force of the buckling monofilament correlates with an increased risk of neuropathic foot injury.

allow daily inspection of the ulcer.[23,24] A slow transition from a cast to a shoe is required, with the interim use of a sandal with a thick, pliant insole. The term "healing shoe" is a misnomer; patients with plantar ulcers who walk in shoes are not being adequately treated.

Wound care includes débridement of necrotic tissue and callus, application of sterile dressings, and frequent inspection. Dry dressings are used in casts; otherwise, saline-moistened sterile gauze is applied and changed two to three times a day. Occlusive dressings also appear to be satisfactory.[26,27] The efficacy of topically applied growth factors has not been conclusively proved.[28-30] Topical iodine preparations, astringents, and hydrogen peroxide interfere with the healing of the wound.[31,32]

Prevention of Neuropathic Ulcers

Patients who have healed ulcers or are at risk for ulceration because they have lost protective sensation require education in lifelong foot care, therapeutic footwear, and periodic callus and nail care.[20] Because calluses can increase local pressure by up to 30 percent,[33] periodic débridement of calluses is crucial. Blisters, macerated skin, or hemorrhagic calluses should be treated with débridement, as needed, and relief of pressure.

Patients must be educated to avoid the preventable causes of ulceration. They should refrain from walking barefoot; inspect their feet, including the interdigital spaces, daily (with the help of a partner if necessary); change their shoes at least twice daily; and avoid potential trauma (caused by hot water, heating pads, and so forth). Patients should be encouraged to contact their physicians promptly if they have any new abnormalities of the feet, even seemingly minor ones. General medical care should include strict glycemic control to decrease the frequency and severity of neuropathy.[34] To protect the arterial circulation, patients must refrain from using tobacco.

Shoes must accommodate any deformities and provide cushioning at the points of contact between the foot and the shoe.[18,35,36] Physicians should prescribe the appropriate footwear and direct the gradual introduction of new shoes into use, with frequent evaluations of fit. With certification by physicians, Medicare covers therapeutic footwear for diabetic patients. For patients with minimal foot deformities, athletic shoes with sufficient room for the toes and forefoot may suffice.[37,38] Cushioned socks aid in reducing pressure.[39] Added-depth shoes with resilient flat foam or custom-molded insoles or rigid rocker soles, which stabilize the foot, are necessary for more difficult cases. Custom-molded shoes are reserved for patients who have severely deformed feet or have undergone a partial foot amputation.[18,35] In-shoe pressure measurements should lead to a more quantitative approach to footwear prescription.[18,40] Patients in whom new ulcers develop despite prescribed footwear should be referred to a specialized center.

INFECTION

Not all neuropathic foot ulcers are infected. Infection is suggested by local inflammation, purulent drainage, sinus-tract formation, or crepitation. The severity of cellulitis may range from a mild, localized infection to a limb-threatening, necrotizing process with fasciitis. Foot ulcers can be divided into superficial lesions that do not threaten the limb and deeper, limb-threatening ulcers (Fig. 4).[41] Fever, chills, and leukocytosis are absent in two thirds of patients with limb-threatening infection, which may include deep

Table 1. Clinical Findings Predicting Areas of High Plantar Pressure.

History
Prior ulceration
Prior surgery involving the metatarsal bones
Physical finding
Callus*
Hemorrhagic callus*
Blister or macerated skin*
Limited hallux dorsiflexion (<30 degrees)
Prominent metatarsal heads inadequately
covered with soft tissue†
Other plantar bony prominences
Radiograph finding
Charcot's fracture

*Indicates that high pressure or shear is being generated that is capable of injuring soft tissue.

†Detected by gently stroking a finger across the plantar surface of the forefoot.

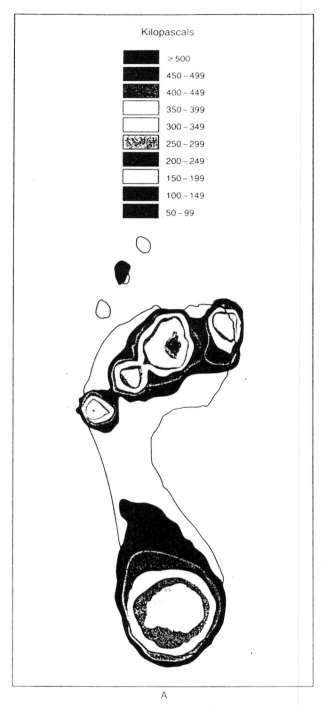

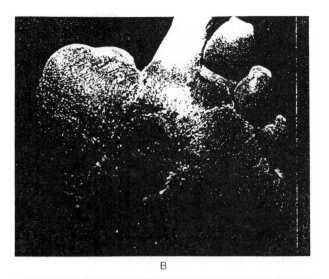

B

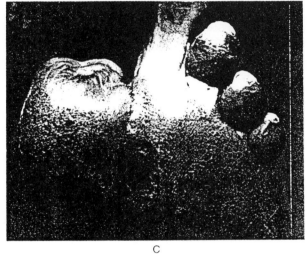

C

Figure 2. A Neuropathic Ulcer of the Left Foot of a Patient with an Amputated Hallux.

An isobaric contour plot shows the peak plantar pressure at each location on the foot during the phase of walking when the foot is flat on the ground (Panel A). The plot is viewed as if it were a footprint on a pressure-sensitive platform. The correspondence between the site of the ulcer and the region of high focal pressure indicates a mechanical cause of the lesion and represents the target area for reducing pressure with the use of therapeutic footwear. The lesion had been resistant to healing for six months, during which period the patient continued to walk and perform normal activities of daily life while wearing a cast sandal with a soft insole (Panel B). After four weeks of treatment, including ambulation in a total-contact cast, the ulcer was almost completely healed (Panel C).

abscesses, extensive soft-tissue infection, or metastatic infection of remote sites.[42] Hyperglycemia is a common sign of limb- or life-threatening infection. Erythema, swelling, and warmth in a nonulcerated foot may indicate acute Charcot's disease rather than infection. Conversely, some uninflamed ulcers are associated with underlying osteomyelitis.[43]

Most mild infections are caused by aerobic gram-positive cocci such as *Staphylococcus aureus* or streptococci.[44,45] Deeper, limb-threatening infections are usually polymicrobial and caused by aerobic gram-positive cocci, gram-negative bacilli (e.g., *Escherichia coli*, klebsiella species, and proteus species), and anaerobes (e.g., bacteroides species and peptostreptococcus).[46] The pathogenic role of coagulase-negative staphylococci, enterococci, and corynebacterium species is often difficult to discern, particularly when they are cultured along with typically virulent organisms.

Clinically uninfected ulcers should not be cultured. Superficial swabs from an infected ulcer are not ideal for culturing, since both colonizing and infecting organisms are recovered. Infecting organisms are more reliably detected in specimens obtained by curettage

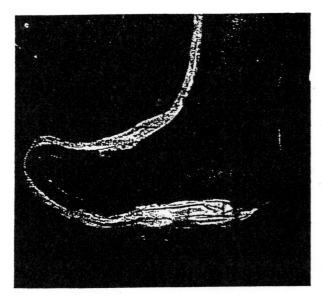

Figure 3. Cross-Section of a Total-Contact Cast Formed to a Patient's Foot.

The rubber heel, which is placed under the midfoot, permits ambulation. Soft black foam covers the anterior portion of the foot to prevent injury. The cast is changed 24 to 48 hours after application and then weekly.

of the base of the ulcer after débridement.[45,47] Needle aspiration is a reliable method of detection, but its sensitivity is low.[46,47] Culturing of bone specimens, obtained by percutaneous biopsy or surgical excision (through approaches that do not traverse the ulcer), is the best method for determining the cause of osteomyelitis.

The diagnosis of osteomyelitis is problematic, since plain radiographs are neither sensitive nor specific.[43,48] Differentiating between diabetic osteoarthropathy and osteomyelitis is difficult. Technetium bone scans are sensitive but expensive and lack adequate specificity.[48] Indium-111–labeled leukocyte scanning is considered to be the most accurate radionuclide study,[43,48] but it too is expensive and it may be difficult to interpret in the presence of local soft-tissue inflammation. The usefulness of computed tomography and magnetic resonance imaging requires further study.

The ability to reach bone by gently advancing a sterile surgical probe has a high specificity and positive predictive value in diagnosing osteomyelitis, but the sensitivity of this technique is low.[49] Combining plain radiography with a probe for bone is a reasonable initial approach to the diagnosis of osteomyelitis. If bone is detected on probing, treatment for osteomyelitis is recommended. If bone cannot be detected by probing and the plain radiograph does not suggest osteomyelitis, the recommended treatment is a course of antibiotics directed at soft-tissue infection. Because occult osteomyelitis may be present,[43] radiography should be repeated in two weeks. Further studies are warranted if osteomyelitis is suggested radiographically or if infection recurs shortly after treatment has been completed.

Antibiotics should be administered immediately after appropriate specimens have been obtained for culture. The choice of a regimen should be based on the suspected pathogens. Infections can be classified as non–limb-threatening, limb-threatening, or life-threatening for the purpose of empirical selection of an antibiotic regimen. There are many appropriate regimens for each classification (Table 2). Aminoglycosides should generally be avoided in favor of non-nephrotoxic antibiotics. Fluoroquinolones, which lack adequate activity against gram-positive and anaerobic pathogens, should not be used empirically as single agents. If the infection does not respond adequately to treatment, the antimicrobial agent should be changed according to the culture results. However, expansion of initial therapy to treat resistant isolates is not required if the infection is responding to treatment. An empirical regimen that is unnecessarily broad, given the culture results, can be simplified if the infection has responded to treatment.

The treatment of osteomyelitis has traditionally included aggressive surgical débridement or limited amputation of infected bone. In some cases, removal of infected bony prominences also eliminates the areas of high pressure responsible for the ulceration.[50] A 10- to 12-week course of antibiotics has been reported to cure pedal osteomyelitis without the need for surgical débridement.[51,52] However, these studies included patients in whom the diagnosis of osteomyelitis was based solely on plain radiographs and technetium bone scans; thus, the conclusion is open to question. Further study is needed to determine which subgroups of diabetic patients with pedal osteomyelitis may be cured by prolonged antimicrobial therapy without surgery.

The optimal duration of antimicrobial therapy after surgical débridement of infected pedal bone has not been established. Traditionally, a regimen of four to six weeks of parenteral antibiotic therapy has been recommended. If the entire portion of infected bone has been removed during digital or ray amputation, however, a two- to three-week course of antibiotics directed at residual soft-tissue infection is reasonable. In contrast, prolonged therapy is recommended for tarsal or calcaneal osteomyelitis, since the infected bone is débrided piecemeal.

At present, it is difficult to recommend a single approach to the diagnosis and treatment of pedal osteomyelitis in diabetic patients, and clinical judgment is required. Patients with limb- or life-threatening infection must undergo early aggressive drainage and débridement of all necrotic tissue, including bone. In some patients with less serious infection, a trial of prolonged antimicrobial therapy may be a reasonable approach.[51,52]

SURGICAL ASPECTS

The extent and severity of infection and the adequacy of arterial supply determine the role of surgery in the management of diabetic foot disease.[42] Because of neuropathy, evaluation of the wound, including probing for bone or sinus tracts and débridement, can usually be done at the bedside. To avoid any misunder-

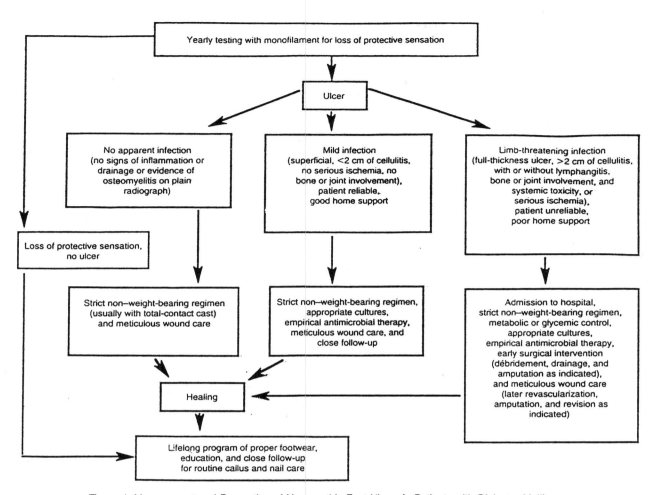

Figure 4. Management and Prevention of Neuropathic Foot Ulcers in Patients with Diabetes Mellitus.
Occult osteomyelitis should be considered in all cases of neuropathic ulceration. The total-contact cast is not used if infection is present.

standing and potential litigation, the importance of inspection and débridement must be communicated to the patient and family. They should understand what the newly débrided ulcer will look like.

Limb-threatening infections require immediate hospitalization and bed rest even if signs and symptoms of systemic infection are absent. Up to one third of patients must still undergo major limb amputation before any treatment is initiated — a fact that underscores the need for aggressive in-hospital treatment of limb-threatening infections.[53] Although medical stabilization, glycemic control, and antimicrobial therapy are important, débridement should not be delayed. Diabetic patients do not tolerate undrained suppuration. Failure to débride necrotic, infected tissue and drain purulent collections increases the risk of amputation. Drainage by needle aspiration or percutaneous drains is inadequate. All necrotic and devitalized tissue must be débrided, and dependent drainage established. The initial débridement must be performed independently of the status of the arterial circulation, with revascularization postponed until sepsis is controlled.[54] Adequate débridement may require multiple

procedures. If the infection has destroyed the architecture and function of the foot or acutely threatens the patient's life, guillotine amputation to control sepsis, followed by definitive closure, is recommended.[55]

Postoperative management includes meticulous local care, adequate nutrition, control of lower-extremity edema by elevation and diuretic therapy, and avoidance of weight bearing. Glycemic control is important to optimize host defenses against infection. Saline-moistened gauze sponges are placed on the wound and changed two to three times a day. Daily inspection of the wound, with débridement as necessary, is essential. Heat, soaks, and whirlpool therapy may damage the tissue and promote infection. In a double-blind randomized trial,[56] topical hyperbaric oxygen was not beneficial. When healing has occurred, weight bearing is gradually introduced and increased with the use of accommodative footwear to protect the wound.

The arterial circulation must be assessed in every diabetic patient with a foot infection. Arterial insufficiency is a pathogenic factor in up to 60 percent of diabetic patients with nonhealing ulcers and in 46 per-

Table 2. Selected Empirical Antimicrobial Regimens for Foot Infections in Patients with Diabetes Mellitus.*

Non–limb-threatening infection
Oral regimen
  Cephalexin
  Clindamycin
  Dicloxacillin
  Amoxicillin–clavulanate
Parenteral regimen
  Cefazolin
  Oxacillin or nafcillin
  Clindamycin

Limb-threatening infection
Oral regimen
  Fluoroquinolone and clindamycin
Parenteral regimen
  Ampicillin–sulbactam
  Ticarcillin–clavulanate
  Cefoxitin or cefotetan
  Fluoroquinolone and clindamycin

Life-threatening infection
Parenteral regimen
  Imipenem–cilastatin
  Vancomycin, metronidazole, and aztreonam
  Ampicillin–sulbactam and an aminoglycoside

*These regimens may require adjustment if the patient has a history of allergies or if there are clinical or epidemiologic factors suggesting unusual pathogens. Doses should be commensurate with the severity of infection, with adjustment for renal dysfunction when indicated.

cent of those undergoing major amputation.[5] Atherosclerotic occlusion in diabetic patients characteristically involves the distal tibial and peroneal arteries but spares the foot vessels, especially the dorsalis pedis artery. Occlusive microvascular lesions that affect the foot and preclude successful revascularization are not prevalent in diabetic patients.[57]

Noninvasive vascular laboratory tests frequently underestimate the extent and severity of arterial insufficiency in diabetic patients. Noninvasive studies, including transcutaneous oximetry, should be used only as a complement to careful bedside evaluation and sound clinical judgment. If serious ischemia is suspected, arteriography of the lower extremity, including the foot vessels, should be performed. A diabetic patient should never undergo foot amputation solely on the basis of the results of noninvasive tests.

The decision to perform vascular surgery depends on the severity of the vascular impairment, the risk associated with surgery, and the potential for rehabilitation. Advanced age does not preclude surgery. Modern revascularization procedures are tailored to individual requirements on the basis of preoperative assessment. With aggressive perioperative cardiovascular monitoring, revascularization can be as safe as a major amputation and less costly.[58,59]

Endovascular techniques (balloon angioplasty and atherectomy) may restore the patency of proximal arteries with limited occlusive disease but are generally contraindicated for limb-threatening occlusion of infrainguinal arteries. At three years, 87 percent of patients with autogenous vein bypass grafts to the foot vessels continue to have patent arteries, and 92 percent are spared amputation.[60] In patients with extensive tissue loss or gangrene of the foot, restoration of

pulsatile blood flow to the foot is required for healing.[5] Aggressive arterial reconstruction, including bypass grafts to foot vessels, allows effective débridement of soft tissue and resection of osteomyelitic bone without amputation.

An aggressive multidisciplinary approach to foot disease associated with diabetes appears to save the lower extremity and to be cost effective. Two recent studies reported that for every category of amputation, the rates were reduced between 1984 and 1990, and the average length of hospitalization decreased by 33 percent.[58,61] Early, aggressive control of infection and appropriate distal arterial revascularization allow orthopedic, podiatric, or reconstructive surgeons to perform foot-sparing surgery in selected patients with severe deformities that cannot be accommodated by custom footwear. These procedures can preserve the weight-bearing function of the foot in cases in which amputation would previously have been considered necessary.

SUMMARY

Limb- or life-threatening complications in patients with diabetes can be prevented with an integrated, multidisciplinary approach. Most patients seen in clinical practice are in the early stages of the disease process. Glycemic control retards the progression of neuropathy, which is the most important risk factor for ulceration. Early detection of the loss of protective sensation and implementation of strategies to prevent ulceration will reduce the rates of limb-threatening complications. Clinicians should routinely examine the feet of diabetic patients. Education in foot care, proper footwear, and close follow-up are required to prevent or promptly detect neuropathic injury. If ulceration occurs, removal of pressure from the site of the ulcer and careful management of the wound will allow healing in most cases. The failure to heal despite these measures should prompt a search for associated arterial insufficiency. If infection is present, appropriate antimicrobial therapy combined with immediate surgical intervention, including revascularization when necessary, will increase the chances of saving the limb. With this comprehensive approach, it is possible to achieve the goal of a 40 percent decrease in amputation rates among diabetic patients by the year 2000.

We are indebted to Ms. Donna Harris for assistance in the preparation of the manuscript.

REFERENCES

1. Reiber GE. Diabetic foot care: financial implications and practice guidelines. Diabetes Care 1992;15:Suppl 1:29-31.
2. Fylling CP. Wound healing: an update. Comprehensive wound management for prevention of amputation. Diabetes Spectrum 1992;5:358-9.
3. Department of Health and Human Services. Healthy People 2000: national health promotion and disease prevention objectives. Washington, D.C.: Government Printing Office, 1991:73-117. (DHHS publication no. 91-50213.)
4. Pecoraro RE, Reiber GE, Burgess EM. Pathways to diabetic limb amputation: basis for prevention. Diabetes Care 1990;13:513-21.
5. Pomposelli FB Jr, Jepsen SJ, Gibbons GW, et al. Efficacy of the dorsal pedal bypass for limb salvage in diabetic patients: short-term observations. J Vasc Surg 1990;11:745-52.

6. Myerson MS, Papa J, Eaton K, Wilson K. The total-contact cast for management of neuropathic plantar ulceration of the foot. J Bone Joint Surg Am 1992;74:261-9.

7. Edmonds ME. Experience in a multidisciplinary diabetic foot clinic. In: Connor H, Boulton AJM, Ward JD, eds. The foot in diabetes: proceedings of the First National Conference on the Diabetic Foot, Malvern, England, May 1986. Chichester, England: John Wiley, 1987:121-34.

8. Boulton AJM. The diabetic foot: neuropathic in aetiology? Diabet Med 1990;7:852-8.

9. Boulton AJ, Kubrusly DB, Bowker JH, et al. Impaired vibratory perception and diabetic foot ulceration. Diabet Med 1986;3:335-7.

10. Birke JA, Sims DS. Plantar sensory threshold in the ulcerative foot. Lepr Rev 1986;57:261-7.

11. Sosenko JM, Kato M, Soto R, Bild DE. Comparison of quantitative sensory-threshold measures for their association with foot ulceration in diabetic patients. Diabetes Care 1990;13:1057-61.

12. Ctercteko GC, Dhanendran M, Hutton WC, Le Quesne LP. Vertical forces acting on the feet of diabetic patients with neuropathic ulceration. Br J Surg 1981;68:608-14.

13. Brand PW. Repetitive stress in the development of diabetic foot ulcers. In: Levin ME, O'Neal LW, eds. The diabetic foot. 4th ed. St. Louis: C.V. Mosby, 1988:83-90.

14. Sammarco GJ. Diabetic arthropathy. In: Sammarco GJ, ed. The foot in diabetes. Philadelphia: Lea & Febiger, 1991:153-72.

15. Cavanagh PR, Young MJ, Adams JE, Vickers KL, Boulton AJM. Radiographic abnormalities in the feet of patients with diabetic neuropathy. Diabetes Care 1994;17:201-9.

16. Cavanagh PR, Ulbrecht JS. Biomechanics of the diabetic foot: a quantitative approach to the assessment of neuropathy, deformity, and plantar pressure. In: Jahss MH, ed. Disorders of the foot and ankle: medical and surgical management. 2nd ed. Vol. 2. Philadelphia: W.B. Saunders, 1991:1864-907.

17. Boulton AJM, Hardisty CA, Betts RP, et al. Dynamic foot pressure and other studies as diagnostic and management aids in diabetic neuropathy. Diabetes Care 1983;6:26-33.

18. Cavanagh PR, Ulbrecht JS. Biomechanics of the foot in diabetes mellitus. In: Levin ME, O'Neal LW, Bowker JH, eds. The diabetic foot. 5th ed. St. Louis: Mosby–Year Book, 1993:199-232.

19. Ulbrecht JS, Norkitis A, Cavanagh PR. Plantar pressure and plantar ulceration in the neuropathic diabetic foot. In: Kominsky SJ, ed. The diabetic foot. Vol. 1. Chicago: Mosby–Year Book, 1994:29-45.

20. Davidson JK, Alogna M, Goldsmith M, Borden J. Assessment of program effectiveness at Grady Memorial Hospital — Atlanta. In: Steiner G, Lawrence PA, eds. Educating diabetic patients. New York: Springer, 1981:329-48.

21. Coleman WC, Brand PW, Birke JA. The total contact cast: a therapy for plantar ulceration on insensitive feet. J Am Podiatry Assoc 1984;74:548-52.

22. Frykberg RG. Podiatric problems in diabetes. In: Kozak GP, Hoar CS Jr, Rowbotham JL, Wheelock FC Jr, Gibbons GW, Campbell D, eds. Management of diabetic foot problems: Joslin Clinic and New England Deaconess Hospital. Philadelphia: W.B. Saunders, 1984:45-67.

23. Burden AC, Jones GR, Jones R, Blandford RL. Use of the "Scotchcast boot" in treating diabetic foot ulcers. BMJ 1983;286:1555-7.

24. Novick A, Birke JA, Graham SL, Koziatek E. Effect of a walking splint and total contact casts on plantar forces. J Prosthet Orthot 1991;3:168-78.

25. Mueller MJ, Diamond JE, Sinacore DR, et al. Total contact casting in treatment of diabetic plantar ulcers: controlled clinical trial. Diabetes Care 1989;12:384-8.

26. Hutchinson JJ, McGuckin M. Occlusive dressings: a microbiologic and clinical review. Am J Infect Control 1990;18:257-68.

27. Witkowski JA, Parish LC. Rational approach to wound care. Int J Dermatol 1992;31:27-8.

28. Steed D, Goslen JB, Holloway GA, Malone JM, Bunt TJ, Webster MW. Randomized prospective double-blind trial in healing chronic diabetic foot ulcers: CT-102 activated platelet supernatant, topical versus placebo. Diabetes Care 1992;15:1598-604.

29. McGrath MH. Peptide growth factors and wound healing. Clin Plast Surg 1990;17:421-32.

30. Knighton DR, Fiegel VD. Growth factors and repair of diabetic wounds. In: Levin ME, O'Neal LW, Bowker JH, eds. The diabetic foot. 5th ed. St. Louis: Mosby–Year Book, 1993:247-57.

31. Kucan JO, Robson MC, Heggers JP, Ko F. Comparison of silver sulfadiazine, povidone-iodine and physiologic saline in the treatment of chronic pressure ulcers. J Am Geriatr Soc 1981;29:232-5.

32. Lineaweaver W, Howard R, Soucy D, et al. Topical antimicrobial toxicity. Arch Surg 1985;120:267-70.

33. Young MJ, Cavanagh PR, Thomas G, Johnson MM, Murray H, Boulton AJM. The effect of callus removal on dynamic plantar foot pressures in diabetic patients. Diabet Med 1992;9:55-7.

34. The Diabetes Control and Complications Trial Research Group. The effect of intensive treatment of diabetes on the development and progression of long-term complications in insulin-dependent diabetes mellitus. N Engl J Med 1993;329:977-86.

35. Ulbrecht JS, Perry JE, Hewitt FG Jr, Cavanagh PR. Controversies in footwear for the diabetic foot at risk. In: Kominsky SJ, ed. The diabetic foot. Vol. 1. Chicago: Mosby–Year Book, 1994:441-53.

36. Coleman WC. Footwear in a management program for injury prevention. In: Levin ME, O'Neal LW, Bowker JH, eds. The diabetic foot. 5th ed. St. Louis: Mosby–Year Book, 1993:531-47.

37. Perry JE, Ulbrecht JS, Cavanagh PR. Non-therapeutic footwear can play a role in reducing plantar pressure in the diabetic foot. J Bone Joint Surg Am (in press).

38. Soulier SM. The use of running shoes in the prevention of plantar diabetic ulcers. J Am Podiatr Med Assoc 1986;76:395-400.

39. Veves A, Masson EA, Fernando DJS, Boulton AJM. Use of experimental padded hosiery to reduce abnormal foot pressures in diabetic neuropathy. Diabetes Care 1989;12:653-5.

40. Cavanagh PR, Hewitt FG Jr, Perry JE. In-shoe plantar pressure measurement: a review. Foot 1992;294:185-94.

41. Gibbons GW. Diabetic foot sepsis. Semin Vasc Surg 1992;5:244-8.

42. Gibbons GW, Eliopoulos GM. Infection of the diabetic foot. In: Kozak GP, Hoar CS Jr, Rowbotham JL, Wheelock FC Jr, Gibbons GW, Campbell D, eds. Management of diabetic foot problems: Joslin Clinic and New England Deaconess Hospital. Philadelphia: W.B. Saunders, 1984:97-102.

43. Newman LG, Waller J, Palestro CJ, et al. Unsuspected osteomyelitis in diabetic foot ulcers: diagnosis and monitoring by leukocyte scanning with indium in 111 oxyquinoline. JAMA 1991;266:1246-51.

44. Jones EW, Edwards R, Finch R, et al. A microbiologic study of diabetic foot lesions. Diabet Med 1984;2:213-5.

45. Lipsky BA, Pecoraro RE, Wheat LJ. The diabetic foot: soft tissue and bone infection. Infect Dis Clin North Am 1990;4:409-32.

46. Wheat LJ, Allen SD, Henry M, et al. Diabetic foot infections: bacteriologic analysis. Arch Intern Med 1986;146:1935-40.

47. Sapico FL, Witte JL, Canawati HN, Montgomerie JZ, Bessman AN. The infected foot of the diabetic patient: quantitative microbiology and analysis of clinical features. Rev Infect Dis 1984;6:Suppl 1:S171-S176.

48. Keenan AM, Tindel NL, Alavi A. Diagnosis of pedal osteomyelitis in diabetic patients using current scintigraphic techniques. Arch Intern Med 1989;149:2262-6.

49. Grayson ML, Balogh K, Levin E, Karchmer AW. "Probing to bone" — a useful clinical sign of osteomyelitis in diabetic fetid feet. In: Program and abstracts of the 30th Interscience Conference on Antimicrobial Agents and Chemotherapy, Atlanta, October 21–24, 1990. Washington, D.C.: American Society for Microbiology, 1990:127. abstract.

50. Tillo TH, Giurini JM, Habershaw GM, Chrzan JS, Rowbotham JL. Review of metatarsal osteotomies for the treatment of neuropathic ulcerations. J Am Podiatr Med Assoc 1990;80:211-7.

51. Peterson LR, Lissack LM, Canter K, et al. Therapy of lower extremity infections with ciprofloxacin in patients with diabetes mellitus, peripheral vascular disease, or both. Am J Med 1989;86:801-8.

52. Bamberger DM, Daus GP, Gerding DN. Osteomyelitis in the feet of diabetic patients: long-term results, prognostic factors, and the role of antimicrobial and surgical therapy. Am J Med 1987;83:653-60.

53. Gibbons GW. The diabetic foot: amputations and drainage of infection. J Vasc Surg 1987;5:791-3.

54. *Idem.* Toe and foot amputations. In: Ernst SB, Stanley JC, eds. Current therapy in vascular surgery. 2nd ed. Philadelphia: B.C. Decker, 1991:694-6.

55. McIntyre KE Jr, Bailey SA, Malone JM, Goldstone J. Guillotine amputation in the treatment of nonsalvageable lower-extremity infections. Arch Surg 1984;119:450-3.

56. Leslie CA, Sapico FL, Ginunas VJ, Adkins RH. Randomized controlled trial of topical hyperbaric oxygen for treatment of diabetic foot ulcers. Diabetes Care 1988;11:111-5.

57. LoGerfo FW, Coffman JD. Vascular and microvascular disease of the foot in diabetes: implications for foot care. N Engl J Med 1984;311:1615-9.

58. Gibbons GW, Marcaccio EJ Jr, Burgess AM, et al. Improved quality of diabetic foot care, 1984 vs 1990: reduced length of stay and costs, insufficient reimbursement. Arch Surg 1993;128:576-81.

59. Gupta SK, Veith FJ. Inadequacy of diagnosis related group (DRG) reimbursements for limb salvage lower extremity arterial reconstructions. J Vasc Surg 1990;11:348-57.

60. Pomposelli FB Jr, Jepsen SJ, Gibbons GW, et al. A flexible approach to infrapopliteal vein grafts in patients with diabetes mellitus. Arch Surg 1991;126:724-9.

61. LoGerfo FW, Gibbons GW, Pomposelli FB Jr, et al. Trends in the care of the diabetic foot: expanded role of arterial reconstruction. Arch Surg 1992;127:617-21.

The Importance of Contact Dermatitis in the Management of Leg Ulcers

Janice Cameron
Senior Nurse, Dermatology, Churchill Hospital, Oxford

INTRODUCTION

There is a continuing high incidence of contact sensitivity (allergy) in patients with venous (stasis) ulcers. Studies have suggested that the prevalence of contact sensitivity is considerably higher in leg ulcer patients than in other dermatology out patients[1,2]. A review of the literature over the last 15 years shows that between 50% - 69% of leg ulcer patients show either a single sensitivity or multiple sensitivities to allergens that may be of relevance in their current or future management. Lanolin and the topical antibiotics neomycin and framycetin remain the most common sensitisers in leg ulcer patients. (Table 1)

ECZEMA

Eczema and dermatitis are terms used to describe the same condition. It is characterised by erythema, weeping, crusting and irritation of the skin. Eczema (dermatitis) is a common complication in the management of venous leg ulcers. It may be due to an irritant or allergic contact dermatitis or stasis eczema or of mixed aetiology.

VENOUS STASIS ECZEMA

This is an endogenous eczema, related to constitutional (internal) factors. It appears in the gaiter area of the lower leg and is associated with venous disease.

CONTACT DERMATITIS

Contact dermatitis is an exogenous eczema, caused by external factors that have either irritated the skin or caused an allergic reaction. The eczema normally occurs in areas of direct contact, but if sufficiently severe the eczema may become generalised. Researchers have observed that patients with eczema around their leg ulcer have more allergies than those without[3,4].

ALLERGIC CONTACT DERMATITIS

This occurs following sensitisation to an allergen. Further exposure will result in an eczematous reaction. This process occurs as a result of cell mediated immunity and is a type 4 hypersensitivity. It has been suggested that the occlusive nature of many leg ulcer applications, on broken or eczematous skin,

Table 1 - Frequency of Contact Sensitivity

reference	no. of patients	frequency of contact sensitivity	commonest sensitisers
Fraki et al 1979[13]	192	69%	neomycin, framycetin, wool alcohols, balsam of Peru
Dooms-Goosens et al 1979[1]	163	63%	wool alcohols, balsam of Peru parabens, benzocaine, neomycin
Malten and Kuiper 1985[14]	100	69%	wool alcohols, fragrance, neomycin, balsam of Peru
Kulozic et al 1988[3]	59	51%	wool alcohols, neomycin, framycetin
Cameron 1990[10]	52	58%	wool alcohols, neomycin, framycetin, parabens, cetylstearyl alcohol
Wilson et al 1991[11]	81	67%	wool alcohols, neomycin, framycetin, gentamicin cetylstearyl alcohol

creates the perfect environment for sensitisation to develop[5]. Patients with chronic venous insufficiency have been found to have excessive folding of the epidermis. This is thought to increase the concentration of frequently applied topical substances, and increase the contact time of the medicament with antigen presenting cells[6]. Patients may become allergic to any part of their topical therapy including dressings, emollients, creams, bandages and bath additives. Sensitisation requires at least 10 - 14 days of exposure to the allergen. It is possible however for a substance to be used for several years before resulting in an allergic reaction. To investigate a possible allergic contact dermatitis the patient should be referred to a dermatologist for patch testing. Identification of the allergen is important for future management. Simply changing the treatment may expose the patient to the same allergen as it may be present in several different topical applications.

PATCH TESTING

This is a scientific method of investigation, with defined guidelines recommended by the International Contact Dermatitis Research Group (ICDRG)[7]. The patch test substances are commercially prepared. Patch testing can lead to false positive and false negative results if the correct concentrations are not used. Patients attending the leg ulcer outpatient clinic at the Dermatology Department in Oxford are patch tested as part of their initial assessment. Allergens grouped together are referred to as a 'battery'. All patients are patch tested with the European Standard Battery which contains 24 of the most commonly encountered environmental allergens, many of which are of relevance to leg ulcer management. Further batteries are applied according to the patient's specific treatment.

The test procedure is carried out over a period of 5 days.
Day 1 - Small amounts of the patch test substances are applied, under occlusion, in hypoallergenic aluminium discs, to clean, clear skin on the upper part of the patients back.
Day 3 - The patch test strips are removed and discarded. A minimum period of 30 minutes is left between removal and examination of the area to allow for any redness caused by removal of the test strips to resolve. The back is then examined for erythema and eczema at the test sites. The patient is advised to keep the test area dry until after the final reading.
Day 5 - The test area is re-examined.
The IDRG define the guidelines for reading the results. They are graded as follows:

-	no reaction
?+	doubtful reaction
+	weak (non vesicular) reaction
++	strong (oedematous or vesicular) reaction
+++	extreme reaction

Different studies can only be compared if they have followed these guidelines.

ANGRY BACK

A strong positive reaction to a patch test can sometimes cause false positive reactions in other test patches in the immediate vicinity. This phenomenon is known as the angry back syndrome[8].

PATCH TEST RESULTS

Allergy to topical application is common in patients with stasis leg ulcers. A review of the incidence of sensitivity in this group of patients from 8 centres between 1972 - 1977 showed an average incidence of 62.5% per year from a total of 1095 patients[9]. The most common sensitisers were found to be wool alcohols (lanolin), the topical antibiotics neomycin and framycetin, and balsam of Peru - (an indicator of perfume sensitivity[9]). Further studies between 1979 and 1991 confirm that lanolin, neomycin and framycetin remain the most common sensitisers in leg ulcer patients (table 1). The fact that there has been no reduction in incidence of sensitivity to lanolin and topical antibiotics in the last 20 years suggests that health care professionals are not aware of its sensitising potential. This is perhaps because most sensitivity studies of patients with leg ulcers have been published in dermotological rather than general medical and nursing journals. Products containing lanolin are still widely used in the community and new cases of sensitivity are constantly appearing. It is essential that results are made known to Primary Health Care Teams if they are to keep abreast of changing recommendations and practices.

ALLERGENS OF RELEVANCE IN LEG ULCER MANAGEMENT

Lanolin (wool alcohols) is present in some creams, emollients, bath additives, barriers and baby products. It is now considered inadvisable to use any product containing lanolin on a patient with a leg ulcer.
Neomycin and framycetin are aminoglycoside antibiotics, Patients allergic to one should also avoid the other. They are common in medicated tulle dressings and powders and are added to some creams and antifungal preparations.
Parabens (hydroxybenzoates) have been found to be common sensitisers. They are preservatives used in some creams and paste bandages.
Cetylstearyl alcohols have recently been shown to have become important sensitisers. They are difficult to avoid as they form the base of many creams, and some paste bandages and emulsifying ointments[10,11].
Colophony, or a derivative, is the adhesive on plasters, tapes, adhesive bandages and some dressings[12].
Rubber is present in tubular, elastic and cohesive bandages although it is usually covered in cotton to help prevent contact with the skin.

OVER THE COUNTER PRODUCTS

Some 'over the counter' products contain allergens that may also be of relevance, eg Benzocaine, Chloroxylenol and frangrance mix. *Benzocaine* is present in creams and ointments to reduce irritation. *Chloroxylenol* is an antiseptic also used as a preservative. *Fragrance mix* is a marker for perfume sensitivity, found in many moisturisers and baby products.

MANAGEMENT OF ALLERGIC CONTACT DERMATITIS

If contact dermatitis is suspected, the patient should be referred for patch testing to identify the allergen responsible. The affected limb should be rested and acute eczema treated with a topical corticosteroid preparation. Corticosteriod ointments in a white soft paraffin base should be used in preference to creams which contain more sensitisers. The potency of the steroid should be determined by the degree of eczema. For an acute eczema Propaderm™ (Glaxo) or Betnovate™ (Glaxo) ointment could be used. For a more chronic eczema, Betnovate RD™ (Glaxo) or Eumovate are suitable. The ointment may need to be applied daily for a few days. The concentration can then be reduced slowly over a period of several days by gradually replacing the steroid ointment with a simple emollient such as 50% white soft paraffin /50% liquid paraffin (50/50). If the steroid ointment is stopped without first reducing the dose, the eczema may have a rebound effect. If there is a poor response to treatment the patient should be further investigated including the possibility of sensitivity to their current steroid therapy.

SECONDARY INFECTION
Irritation of the affected area causes scratching. This results in further tissue breakdown and secondary infection, a common complication of eczema. Topical antibiotics should never be used. Significant infection should be treated with a systemic antibiotic.

IRRITANT CONTACT DERMATITIS
Antiseptics, wound exudate, elastic and cohesive bandages and elastic tubular support bandages may all act as irritants. To avoid these substances coming into contact with the skin, the patient should be treated as follows:
- antiseptics should be avoided.
- the skin around the leg ulcer should be protected from contact with wound exudate, using a barrier preparation such as zinc oxide paste.
- to prevent bandages coming into direct contact with the skin a layer of cotton stockinette should be applied to the limb first.
- only simple emollient, such as a 50% liquid paraffin/50 % white soft paraffin mixture should be used.

ALLERGEN IDENTIFICATION IN CLINICAL PRACTICE
All products containing identified sensitisers must be avoided. This is not easy due to poor ingredient labelling in this country. Table 2 gives a list of current allergens that are significant in leg ulcer management and where they may be found. Lanolin is often listed in ingredient labelling as 'wool alcohols' and parabens as 'hydroxybenzoates'. When neomycin has been added to a medicament the letter N usually appears after the name of the product eg Dermovate NN™ (Glaxo) and Synalar N™ (Zeneca). Antibiotics and corticosteroids are usually listed on the packaging but preservatives are not always listed. The British National Formulary is useful in identifying product ingredients, although even this is not always comprehensive. Cetylstearyl alcohols are present in most creams and in anything containing emulsifying wax. If a patient has an allergy to colophony or its derivatives it would be advisable to avoid any adhesive dressings and bandages. There are several products that claim to be hypoallergenic, however the manufacturers should be asked about the suitability of their product for a patient with a known sensitivity. Any information given to the Primary Health Care Team regarding allergic reactions to treatment should be well documented in the patient's notes or care plans, and be easily accessible. Before any change in treatment, or a new medicament is introduced, the documented information should be checked. Changes could then be made on a rational basis. Identification and subsequent avoidance of an allergen will reduce the complications of an allergic contact sensitivity and may result in healing of the ulcer.

PATIENT EDUCATION
A list of known sensitisers and their sources should be given to the patient and their carers. Patients should be discouraged from self-medication with over the counter products which may contain sensitisers. Advice should be given on the use of emollients. A simple inexpensive emollient that is unlikely to sensitise is white soft paraffin/ liquid paraffin mixture made up 50%/50% as previously mentioned

CONCLUSION
Where patients have ulcers which are failing to heal, or there is a poor response to treatment, a reaction to their topical therapy should be considered. A greater awareness is needed by Primary Health Care Teams of the problems of contact sensitivity in leg ulcer management and the benefits of patch testing. Patients and carers also need to know what the main sensitisers are and how to avoid them.

Table 2: Common Leg Ulcer Allergens

Leg ulcer allergens	Where they may be found
lanolin/ wool alcohols	creams, ointments, bath additives, barrier preparations, baby products
topical neomycin and framycetin	medicaments, medicated tulle , medicated powders
parabens	preservative in medicaments and some paste bandages
cetylstearyl alcohols	most creams, emulsifying ointments and paste bandages containing emulsifying wax
colophony/ ester of rosin	adhesive used in tapes, bandages and dressings
rubber	elastic, tubular and cohesive bandages
perfume	many 'over the counter preparations' including creams and baby products

Address for Correspondence
Ms Janice Cameron, Senior Nurse Dermatology Unit, Churchill Hospital, Oxford OX3 7LJ

References

1 Dooms -Goosens A, Degreef H, Parijs M, Kerkhofs L. A retrospective study of patch test results from 163 patients with stasis dermatitis or leg ulcers. *Dermatologica* 1979; **159**(2): 93-100.

2 Blondeel A, Oleffe J, Achten G. Contact allergy in 330 dermatological patients. *Contact Dermatitis* 1978; **4**: 270-276.

3 Kulozic M, Powell SM, Cherry G, Ryan TJ. Contact sensitivity in community based leg ulcer patients. *Clinical and Experimental Dermatology* 1987; **13**: 82-84.

4 Paramsothy Y, Collins M, Smith A G. Contact dermatitis in patients with leg ulcers. *Contact Dermatitis* 1988; *18*: 30-36.

5 Stolze R. Dermatitis medicamentosa in eczema of the leg. *Acta Dermato-venereologica* 1966; **46**: 54-61.

6 Bahmer F A. Local factors that might promote the development of contact allergies in patients with chronic venous insufficiency. In: Davy A, Stenner R, editors. *Phlebologie*. London: Libbey, Eurotext Ltd 1989: 110-112.

7 Wilkinson D S, Fregert S, Magnusson B, Bandmann H J. Calnan C D, Cronin E, Hjorth N, Maibach H J., Malten K E, Meneghini C L, Pirila V. Terminology of contact dermatitis. *Acta Dermato-venereologica* 1970; **50**: 287-292.

8 Mitchell J C. The angry back syndrome: eczema creates eczema. *Contact Dermatitis* 1975; **1**: 193.

9 Breit R. Allergen change in stasis dermatitis. *Contact Dermatitis* 1977; **3**: 309-311.

10 Cameron J. Patch testing for leg ulcer patients. *Nursing Times* 1990; **86**: 25, 63-64.

11 Wilson C L, Cameron J, Powell S M. Cherry G, Ryan T J. High incidence of contact dermatitis in leg ulcer patients - implications for management. *Clinical and Experimental Dermatology* 1991; **16**: 250-253.

12 Mallon E, Powell S. Allergic contact dermatitis from Granuflex hydrocolloid dressing. *Contact Dermatitis* 1994; **30**: 110-111.

13 Fraki J E, Peltonen L, Hopsu-Havu V K. Allergy to various components of topical preparations in stasis dermatitis and leg ulcer. *Contact Dermatitis* 1979; **5**: 97-100.

14 Malten K E, Kuiper J P, Van der Staak W B J M. Contact allergic investigations in 100 patients with ulcus cruis. *Dermatologica* 1973; **147**: 241-254.

Assessments

Level 2 assessment

This assessment is in the form of a 3000–3500 word essay (excluding references, diagrams and appendices). The essay is in two parts.

PART A

1. Begin your essay by selecting one patient in your care who is receiving treatment for leg ulcers. Briefly describe the origins of the leg ulcer.
2. Next, examine how relevant anatomy and physiology contributed to the formation of the leg ulcer or the healing of that ulcer.

This part of your essay should be no more than 1200 words in total.

PART B

In Part B you will use the same patient as in Part A. This part of the essay will require you to undertake a critical analysis of the assessment and professional interventions selected for this patient and his/her leg ulcer.

1. Begin Part B by using the seven stages of leg ulcer assessment (see Sect. 4 of the package) to undertake an assessment of your patient's leg ulcer.
2. Continue by presenting your interpretation of the assessment data and drawing conclusions about the appropriate professional interventions for the leg ulcer which might be required by your patient.
3. Conclude your essay by offering a summary of at least two pieces of research which you think should influence the professional intervention for this patient's leg ulcer.

Part B of your essay should be no longer than 2200 words.

LEVEL 2 ASSESSMENT—MARKING GRID

	Max.	Your marks	Min.	
Appropriate patient is selected for this essay and the origins of the leg ulcer are clearly and accurately presented	15		0	Inappropriate patient selected and/or origins of the leg ulcer are unclearly or inaccurately presented
Comprehensive examination of how relevant anatomy and physiology contributed to the formation of the leg ulcer OR to its healing	20		0	Superficial examination of how the relevant anatomy and physiology contributed to the leg ulcer OR to its healing
Demonstrates a comprehensive understanding of the seven stages of leg ulcer assessment and comprehensively uses the stages to assess the patient's leg ulcer	20		0	Superficial understanding of the seven stages of leg ulcer assessment; superficial assessment of the patient's leg ulcer
Demonstrates accurate interpretation of the assessment data and draws appropriate conclusions about interventions from the assessment data	20		0	Inaccurate or incomplete interpretation of the assessment data and/or inappropriate conclusions about interventions drawn from the data
Accurate and appropriate summary of two pieces of research related to the professional interventions for this patient	15		0	Summary of two pieces of research is absent or is inaccurately or inappropriately presented
Essay is logically developed within word limit (± 10%) and correctly referenced using a recognised referencing system	10		0	Essay is illogical, not within word limit and/or incorrectly referenced/does not use a recognised referencing system

Level 3 assessment

Nurses who wish to be assessed at Level 3 should submit the following assessment which should be 3500–4000 words in length (excluding references, diagrams and appendices).

The Level 3 essay is in two parts.

PART A

1. Begin Part A of this assessment by selecting **one** aspect of leg ulcer management from the following list:

   • effective wound cleansing
   • skin care regimen for patients with leg ulcers
   • dressings and their application
   • interventions related to venous ulceration
   • leg ulcers related to patients with specific medical conditions.

2. Describe current practices in your place of work with regard to the aspect of leg ulcer management selected from the above list.

3. Critically evaluate these current practices in your place of work against national or local guidelines for leg ulcer management, technological advances and research evidence. Your critical evaluation must draw conclusions about the extent to which current practice in your place of work reflects any local or national guidelines, technological advances and research evidence. Any conclusions you draw must be justified or defended.

This part of your essay should be approximately 2000 words in length.

PART B

In this part of the essay you will be using the same aspect of leg ulcer management as you used in Part A. In this part, however, you will be exploring the role of the leg ulcer specialist nursing within the multidisciplinary team with regard to the contribution which a leg ulcer specialist nurse can make to quality leg ulcer care.

1. Begin Part B by exploring in depth, with reference to your own experience and the case studies presented in this leg ulcer learning package, how a multidisciplinary approach to leg ulcer management enhances the quality of leg ulcer care with reference to the aspect of leg ulcer management you examined in Part A of this essay.

2. Continue Part B by selecting **three** aspects of the specialist leg ulcer nurse's role from the list below:

   • discharge planning (hospital or the community)
   • quality of life
   • leg ulcer assessment
   • health promotion
   • selecting appropriate dressings and bandages
   • referral to other professionals/agencies
   • evaluation of leg ulcer treatment.

3. How can a specialist leg ulcer nurse enhance the quality of leg ulcer care within the three aspects of role you selected in (2) above?

This part of your essay should be no more than 2200 words in length.

LEVEL 3 ASSESSMENT—MARKING GRID

	Max.	Your marks	Min.	
An appropriate aspect of leg ulcer management has been selected	5		0	Aspect of leg ulcer management practice has not been identified or is not appropriate
Comprehensive description of current practices is presented with regard to the selected aspect of leg ulcer management	15		0	Superficial description of current practices; description is not related to the selected aspect of leg ulcer management
Part A demonstrates a comprehensive critical evaluation of current practices against local and national guidelines, technological advances and research evidence	20		0	Part A critical evaluation is superficial or uncritical with inadequate or no comparison of actual practices with local/national guidelines, technological advances and/or research evidence
Critical evaluation in Part A includes conclusions drawn and a justification for these conclusions	15		0	Part A critical evaluation does not include any conclusions, or conclusions are offered but not justified or defended
In-depth exploration of how a multidisciplinary approach to leg ulcer management enhances the quality of leg ulcer care with regard to the aspect of care selected	20		0	Superficial exploration of multidisciplinary leg ulcer management and how it enhances the quality of leg ulcer care with regard to the aspect of leg ulcer care selected in this essay
Three components of the role of the leg ulcer specialist nurse are selected	5		0	Fewer than three components of the role of the leg ulcer specialist nurse are selected
Comprehensive exploration of how the three selected components of the specialist leg ulcer nurse's role can enhance the quality of leg ulcer care	10		0	Superficial exploration of how the three role components selected can enhance the quality of leg ulcer care
Essay is logically developed within word limit (± 10%) and correctly referenced using a recognised referencing system	10		0	Essay is illogical, not within word limit, incorrectly referenced or no recognised referencing system used

Index